"Remarkable"

"Diane Stoler has written a remarkable book. Her description of the neurologic, emotional, and psychological consequences of traumatic brain injury is encyclopedic, and will be instructive not only to survivors and their families, but also to every professional who works in this field. At the same time, something else emerges in this text, and that is the indomitable strength of the human spirit."

JOSEPH RATNER, M.D.,
Chief of Psychiatry, HealthSouth/New England Rehabilitation Hospital

"Thorough and Practical"

"*Coping with Mild Traumatic Brain Injury* is a thorough, practical guide through unfamiliar and often frightening territory, offering wisdom and hope."

SALLY JESSY RAPHAEL,
Talk show host and mother of a person who sustained an mTBI

"A Must"

"This book is a must-read for anyone who has experienced a mild brain injury, as well as for family members, friends, and professionals working in this area of treatment. In addition to providing valuable knowledge, it provides hope and inspiration for the future, from someone who has been there. It is the first book available for the many people who struggle with the 'unseen injury,' providing for them a reference guide to follow during their treatment and recovery."

PAT LAZAREK,
Resource Coordinator, Massachusetts Brain Injury Association

COPING WITH CONCUSSION AND MILD TRAUMATIC BRAIN INJURY

A Guide to Living with the Challenges Associated with Post Concussion Syndrome and Brain Trauma

Diane Roberts Stoler, Ed.D.,
and Barbara Albers Hill

AVERY
a member of Penguin Group (USA)
New York

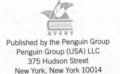

Published by the Penguin Group
Penguin Group (USA) LLC
375 Hudson Street
New York, New York 10014

USA · Canada · UK · Ireland · Australia
New Zealand · India · South Africa · China

penguin.com
A Penguin Random House Company

The excerpt on pages 321–22 is from "From Inside Out" by Beverley Bryant, which appeared in *Through This Window: Views on Traumatic Brain Injury*, edited by Patricia Felton, published by EBTS, Inc., 1992. Reprinted by permission.

"The Caregivers" by Rita Smithuysen is reprinted on page 327 with permission from W. Barry Smithuysen.

Most Avery books are available at special quantity discounts for bulk purchase for sales promotions, premiums, fund-raising, and educational needs. Special books or book excerpts also can be created to fit specific needs. For details, write Penguin Group (USA) LLC, Special Markets, 375 Hudson Street, New York, NY 10014.

Library of Congress Cataloging-in-Publication Data

Stoler, Diane Roberts.
[Coping with mild traumatic brain injury]
Coping with concussion and mild traumatic brain injury : a guide to living with the challenges associated with post concussion syndrome and brain trauma / Diane Roberts Stoler, Ed.D., and Barbara Albers Hill.
p.   cm.
Includes index.
ISBN 978-1-58333-476-8
1. Brain damage.   2. Brain—Wounds and injuries—Complications.   3. Brain damage—Patients—Rehabilitation.
4. Brain damage—Psychological aspects.   I. Hill, Barbara Albers.   II. Title.
RC387.5.S75   2013   2013016860
617.4'81044—dc23

Printed in the United States of America
3   5   7   9   10   8   6   4   2

BOOK DESIGN BY TANYA MAIBORODA

Some names and identifying characteristics have been changed to protect the privacy of the individuals involved.

Neither the publisher nor the authors are engaged in rendering professional advice or services to the individual reader. The ideas, procedures, and suggestions contained in this book are not intended as a substitute for consulting with your physician. All matters regarding your health require medical supervision. Neither the authors nor the publisher shall be liable or responsible for any loss or damage allegedly arising from any information or suggestion in this book.

While the authors have made every effort to provide accurate telephone numbers, Internet addresses, and other contact information at the time of publication, neither the publisher nor the authors assume any responsibility for errors, or for changes that occur after publication. Further, the publisher does not have any control over and does not assume any responsibility for author or third-party websites or their content.

To all people who have experienced a brain injury:
The human spirit is stronger than anything that can happen to it.
If there is a will, there is a way.

ACKNOWLEDGMENTS

■

BOTH *COPING WITH MILD TRAUMATIC BRAIN INJURY* AND THIS, OUR SECOND book, are the result of countless hours of research, along with input from professionals who freely gave their time and commitment to the books' success. Each chapter was reviewed several times by experts in the specific field for accuracy of information. With deep gratitude, I want to thank the following experts for their contributions in specific subject areas:

For neurology, very special thanks and deep appreciation to two neurologists who read and approved every chapter in this edition, Jorge A. Gonzalez, M.D., ABPN; and Carol Moheban, M.D., ABPN. Deep respect to the late Edward Bromfield, M.D., ABPN. Many thanks to Linda Cowell, M.D., FABPN; April Mott, M.D., ABIN; and Bernard S. Chang, M.D., MMSc, ABPN.

For sports medicine, William Paul Meehan III, M.D., ABSM.

For neuropsychology, Barbara Bruno-Golden, Ed.D., and Neil McGrath, Ph.D.

For biofeedback and neurofeedback, Robert Thatcher, Ph.D.; Mike Beasley, Ph.D.; Tom Collura, Ph.D., P.E.; and D. Corydon Hammond, Ph.D.

For energy psychology, Fred Gallo, Ph.D.

For ophthalmology, Dennis F. Stoler, M.D., FACO.

For otolaryngology, Terry J. Garfinkle, M.D., FACS; and James L. Demetroulakos, M.D., FACS.

For orthopedics, Kenneth Glazier, M.D.

For sleep and memory, Rajinder Hullon, M.D., and Stephen J. Kiraly, M.D., FRCPC.

For speech, language, and cognitive rehabilitation, Amy Karas, M.S., CCC-SLP.

For seizures and epilepsy, neurologist Bernard S. Chang, M.D., MMSc, ABPN.

For chronic pain, psychiatrist Arnold Sadwin, M.D., ABPN.

For alcohol and drug abuse, Victor A. McGregor, Ph.D., ANP, NPP.

For post traumatic stress disorder, Duane T. Bowers, LPC, CCHt.

For psychiatry, Stephen J. Kiraly, M.D., FRCPC; Paul Corcorian, M.D.; and Arnold Sadwin, M.D., ABPN.

For psychopharmacology, Sharon Barrett, M.D., ABPN; Jeffrey Hoffman, M.D., ABPN; and Albert Koegler, M.D., ABPN.

For psychology, Jack Jordon, Ph.D., and Alma Dell Smith, Ph.D., ABPP.

For psychiatric nursing, Ann Kennedy, MSN, R.N.

For internal medicine, Susan Beluk, M.D., FAB.

For nutrition, Martha Lindsay, M.S., CNE; and Tina Sullivan, AAPD.

For rehabilitation, Karen Lucas, Ph.D., CCC-SLP; Elise Paquette, R.N., CRR; and Judy Romano, OT-R.

For neurological and medical research, international librarian Alexi Berd, Ph.D. For extensive research in the developmental stage, my research intern, Amanda Pirrotta.

For legal issues, Kenneth Kolpan, Esq., and Charles N. Simkins, Esq. For insurance issues, Nancy Burns and Janet Papineau at William J. Cleary Insurance, Boston.

For treatment approaches, Igor Burdenko, Ph.D. (the Burdenko method); Nancy Risley, RPP, and Kris Stecker, RPP (polarity therapy); Juliet McCoy-Needham (the Feldenkrais method); David Sollars, L.Ac. (homeopathics, herbs, and acupuncture); William Mogan, L.Ac. (acupuncture); psychophysiologist Paul Swingle, Ph.D. (EEG biofeedback); Judy Smith, OT-R (EMG biofeedback); Ken Spracklin, P.T. (physical therapy); and Mark Delorenzo, D.C. (chiropractic), Paul M. Schoonman, D.C., and Melissa Wood, N.D. (naturopath and Bach Flower practitioner).

For information about specific symptom topics, Steve Labov, Member, Board of Governors, American Council for Headache Education; and Joan Clover, co-facilitator for previous ACHE/Prodigy, Headache Support (headaches); Darlene Herrick (sensory problems); speech/language pathologist Ruth Ruderman (academic skills deficits); Karen Estrada, M.S. (blast injury resources); and Christopher Nowinski (CTE) resources.

For background and general information about traumatic brain injury, Mary Reitter, Program Director at the national headquarters of the Brain Injury Association, Washington, D.C.; Elizabeth Jenkins, Executive Director, and Beth Lundgren (Watusi), at the Brain Injury Association of Kansas and Greater

Kansas City; Elaine M. Boucher, Executive Assistant, New Hampshire Brain Injury Association; and Pat Lazarek, Resource Coordinator, Mary Forde, Administrative Assistant and Events Coordinator, Rosalie Berquist, Prevention Coordinator, and Anne Marie Flavin, Administrative Assistant of the Prevention Program, with the Massachusetts Brain Injury Association.

In addition to all of the professionals named above, special thanks and appreciation go to the following people with concussion/mild traumatic brain injury, all of whom volunteered their time to proofread our first book to ensure that its contents related to the needs of brain-injured people: Gracia Berry, Elaine Boucher, Barbara Sweeny, and Pat Davis. Pat also helped to proofread the final copy. Her love and friendship throughout the project kept me focused and my spirits high. Thanks also go to Lisa Anastos, who had no previous knowledge of the topic and was willing to listen for clarity of information.

Deep appreciation goes to Fran Rand for her support, encouragement, and the many hours that she spent proofing the first several drafts of *Coping with Mild Traumatic Brain Injury*, along with this new book.

My deepest gratitude goes to the following people, who have allowed me to share their stories with you. Some have asked that their names be changed in the text, while others agreed to have their actual identity be disclosed: Shari Aznoian-Wilson, Jack Bateman, Gracia Berry, Elaine Boucher, Beverley Bryant, John Carter, Sharron Carter, Mike Deloge, Patricia Felton, Mary Beth Farr, Lianne Hansen, Darlene Herrick, Diane Holmes, Robert Holmes, Kevin Hurley, Missy Kelly, Randi Kleinstein, the late Helen Roberts Kronenfeld and the late Morris Kronenfeld, Terrie McKenna, Deborah McLean, Laurel Perkins, Barbara Perry, the late Rita Smithuysen, Dena Taylor, Gail Willeke, Dawn Langelle, Chad Polito, and others whose names do not appear because of ongoing litigation or by their request.

For *Coping with Mild Traumatic Brain Injury*, upon which this book is based, I am grateful to the supportive staff of Avery Publishing Group. Special thanks go to the late Roger Nye and to Rudy Shur, Joanne Abrams, Karen Hay, and my editor, Amy Tecklenburg, whose questions and calmness helped me to define the focus of our work.

For this new book, I express profound gratitude and deep appreciation for the endless hours that Anastasia Gallardo and Cindy Reynolds, my two research interns, have given. Without their help, organizational skills, and devotion to excellence, it would have taken three times longer to produce the finished product. Special thanks to my intern Jaclyn Caruso, who did all the illustrations in this book. We were limited to black-and-white drawings, and her gift for being able to produce the needed figures and illustrations is outstanding. In addition, I'm grateful to my intern John Tripoli, who proofed this manuscript to help clarify the subject matter. Thank you.

I'm deeply grateful for the supportive staff at Penguin Group. Special thanks to my publisher, Megan Newman, and my editor, Marisa Vigilante, and Sophia Muthuraj, assistant editor, whose support, insight, and belief in the importance of this project enabled it to be published. I can't praise highly enough their pursuit of excellence in this book's detail and quality. Nothing, but nothing, missed their eyes. Thank you.

Very special thanks and profound appreciation to my coauthor, Barbara Albers Hill, whose help, guidance, and support were and have been invaluable. And thanks to her husband, Kevin, and their three children for sharing Barbara with me during this project.

Thanks also to the many professionals who helped me with my recovery, for without their help I truly doubt I could have written this book: Dr. Michael Scott, Dr. James Whitlock, the late Dr. Ed Bromfield, the late Lucille Leonard, Dr. Charlie Hersch, Erika Kaplan, Dr. Douglas Katz, Dr. Carol Moheban, Dr. Igor Burdenko, Dr. Paul Swingle, Dr. Martha Lindsay, Joan Flynn, Judy Smith, Ken Spracklin, Susan Jane Brewster, Lynn Mascato, Michelle Skane, Lisa Orcutt-Murphy, Lisa Grey, Beth Quintal Levitt, Nicole Russo, Margaret Wade, Wendy Keiver-Hewett, Jennifer Stanley, Dr. Mark Delorenzo, Dr. Paul Schoonman, Jean Crannell, David Sollars, William Mogan, Dr. Jane Thompson, Dr. Jana Oettinger, Sarah Eames, Maratha Rossman, Dominic Secondiani, Juliet McCoy-Needham, Betty Woodsum, and attorneys William Troupe, Carmine DiAdamo, and Ted Fairburn.

Special words of appreciation and love to the various people whose love, support, and understanding have helped my recovery. To my mentor and dear friend Eugene Isotti, Ph.D., thank you for your wisdom and for believing in me even when I did not. Thank you to Nancy Isotti, Jacqui Pilgrim, Fran Rand, David Rand, Kathy and Rick Murdock, Beatrice Liberace, Jillian Schleicher, Karen Campbell, Ann Kennedy, Betty Chestnut, Sandy Perchik, Suzy and Frank Feirman, Francine Kaplan, Judy Onanian, Joyce and Normal Spector, Gale Dewsnapp, Jimer Wood, Ellie Routt, Lynne Wilkoff, Barbara Bruno-Golden, Sharyn Russell, Sandra and Jack Hawxwell, the late Amy Silberman, the late Kathi

Savage, Julie Joseph, Karen Callahan, Michael Callahan, Kimberly Cronin, Fran Iseman, Rose Ann Negele, Arline Descheneau, Susan Glazier, Fay Grajower, Lynn Koplowitz, Ellie DiCataldo, and Gail Willeke for their friendship. And to my ex-husband, Denny, thank you for your support, love, and devotion during the initial phase of recovery and your encouragement to write *Coping with Mild Traumatic Brain Injury*.

Thank you to my many Prodigy TBI friends, such as the late Rita Smithuysen, Shirl Rappaport, Sunny Sheila Underwood, Jeri Dopp, Samantha Jane Scolamiero, Carollee Crabtree, and many I have never met, for their prayers and support. To my Facebook, LinkedIn, and Twitter friends with traumatic brain injury, your individual and group input and support have been invaluable. To my extended family members, the late Helen Roberts, the late Joe Stoler, Elaine Rembrandt and Rabbi Daniel Roberts, Evette Mittin, the late Pegi Stoler, Phyllis Goodman, the late Irv and Roz Pocrass, Tippy Awerbuch, Roberta and Steve Keenholtz, Alan and Detty Pocrass, Jim and Ellen Pocrass, Renée and Fred Levy, Julie Levy, the late Ken Pocrass, Barbara Pocrass, Michelle and Steve Garfinkel, and Brendan, Lindsay, Matthew, and Justin Garfinkel, my deepest thanks. Also, special hugs and appreciation go to new family members Cindy Stoler, my granddaughter Debbie Stoler, Melissa Arsenault, my grandson, (CJ) Craig Joseph Stoler, and my granddaughter Kayleigh Ann Stoler.

Lastly, my love and very special appreciation go to my three children, Craig, Brad, and Alan. They never lost faith in me and believed that I would recover. It was their continual love, support, and encouragement that kept my hopes alive. Thank you for being there for me. It must be evident that I have received valuable help and support from many directions. If I have neglected to mention your name, please know that you, yourself, are not forgotten. I thank you.

CONTENTS

◼

FOREWORD

■

THE MORPHING OF MILD TRAUMATIC BRAIN INJURY TO INCLUDE CEREBRAL concussions is a reflection of our culture's current trends in sports and the overall improved understanding of brain injury. Much knowledge has been acquired since *Coping with Mild Traumatic Brain Injury* was first published.

As a treating neurologist and sub-specialist in this field, I find this book a great tool for the layperson who, for the first time, is being confronted with a concussion and its many nuances and ramifications. The scenarios that Stoler portrays are based on her real-life experience as a treating neuropsychologist and her own personal reality as a brain-injured patient. It is the perfect combination of clinical experience, up-to-date information, practical thinking, and effort in simplifying complex concepts and terms so that the average unfamiliarized person can get a quick sense of the essential meaning of cerebral concussion and traumatic brain injury.

This book is a time-saver for both physician and patient, making the office visit more meaningful and productive for all families concerned about their loved ones and their recovery. This book is an equally good read for those who have suffered brain injury themselves.

It was a pleasure to work with Stoler in the preparation of several chapters, and I hope this book will serve you as well as it already has many of my patients.

JORGE A. GONZALEZ, M.D.
Neurology and Neurorehabilitation

PREFACE

■

I N ONE SECOND, MY WHOLE LIFE CHANGED. ONE MOMENT I WAS AWAKE AND ALERT; the next, I had been involved in a head-on auto accident. Days later, my doctors diagnosed me as having suffered a mild head injury, now called a concussion, or *mild traumatic brain injury* (mTBI). At the time, this meant nothing to me, since I looked and felt fine save for minor cuts, bruises, and back pain. All I wanted to know was when I could return to work.

In the months that followed, many of the signs of concussion and *post concussion syndrome* (PCS) appeared. It took me years to understand the consequences of my concussion, and my recovery was slow. None of my doctors fully explained my problems, told me what to expect, or explained how to cope with my many symptoms.

During this time of my life, I cowrote *Coping with Mild Traumatic Brain Injury* with Barbara Albers Hill. Since then, a lot has happened in the world of brain injury and in my world as well. Once, the brain was thought to be a stagnate circuit, irreparable once damaged. Some doctors still hold this belief, as in the case of one of my consults, whose neurologist likened her injured brain to a smashed tomato and stated that nothing could correct the injury. With today's knowledge of neuroplasticity, or the brain's ability to rebuild itself, we recognize that this is far from the truth.

Along with revolutionary knowledge of the brain and how it works has come technological advancement in brain injury diagnosis and treatment. In addition, there is awareness of the consequences of repeated blows to the brain as seen in many sports injuries, the effects of blast injury, and the effect of proper nutrition on the brain. This new information is discussed in detail in this new book.

I have acquired much new knowledge from research but have learned other information firsthand after incurring two subsequent brain injuries since the publication of our first book. In one, an out-of-control snowplow smashed the front of my car; in the other, the hinges of a zero-gravity lounge chair snapped, flinging me backward and knocking me out. In conjunction, I've experienced both Lyme disease and menopause, conditions that can play havoc with post concussion symptoms.

I have also learned the harsh reality of caregiver denial and fatigue. This is the disbelief by someone you count on that such an injury has actually occurred, and the reaction that can follow the overwhelming responsibility of your post-injury care. Statistics show that there is a higher divorce rate for, and increased emotional abandonment of, people who incur disabilities, and I've found that the loss of people you depended on to care for you is a major loss. I'm now divorced after thirty-five years of marriage, and my usually caring adult children some-times minimize or dismiss my daily struggle to live with my brain injuries. I'm often left to find services and resources for myself—a dilemma that is one of the silent consequences of concussion. After all, if you aren't thinking correctly or can't remember information, how do you find the appropriate doctors or advo-cate for needed services?

Brain injury is a life-changing event, and each such injury and consequences are as unique as the person affected. It is hard to accept the truth—that you will never again be the person you were prior to your injury. A broken bone will heal, but not exactly as it was before, and the same is true of a brain injury. Grieving the loss of your former self may be the hardest aspect of total recovery, yet it is important to keep in mind that you *will* recover. There is hope, support, and treatment for every symptom you may experience.

Since *Coping with Mild Traumatic Brain Injury* was published in 1997, the availability of online support has gone from a few websites and TBI chat rooms to a proliferation of social networks and sites that offer information, advice, and encouragement from others with brain injuries. In recent years, I've connected with hundreds of supportive people no matter what the hour of the day. In addi-tion, there has been tremendous growth in the numbers of in-person support groups, professional advocates for the brain injured, and independent-living centers.

Despite this explosion of available help, it is clear that survivors, family, and friends still need a concise form of knowledge about coping with concussion and PCS. This new book is designed as a practical guide that allows you to focus on the specific issues that affect you personally. In fact, much of the information provided in these pages may also be useful to those with developmental or acquired brain injury due to stroke, brain tumor, Parkinson's disease, or multiple sclerosis, since any type of injury to the brain can have consequences similar to those that accompany PCS.

In addition to objective knowledge, this book contains information from my own experience as well as those of others who have sustained a concussion. Although only first names are used, all the stories you will read are about real people. In addition, every chapter of this book has been reviewed by field experts to ensure accuracy. Their names and credentials appear in the acknowledgments.

Like many others, I am living proof that where there is a will, there is a way to move beyond the effects of brain injury. I'm not the person I was before my brain injuries; instead, I am a composite of the old and new. I have learned over time that the best route to positive change lies in understanding your symptoms and problems and learning how to deal with them. It is my hope that this book will help you toward the same realization by answering your questions, helping to solve your problems, and giving you hope for a productive life following your concussion.

DIANE ROBERTS STOLER, ED.D.
Neuropsychologist
Board-Certified Health Psychologist
Board-Certified Sports Psychologist
Georgetown, Massachusetts

A WORD ABOUT BRAIN INJURY LABELS

■

UNTIL 1994, ANY TRAUMATIC DAMAGE TO ANY PART OF THE HEAD OR BRAIN was called a head injury. Yet a head injury doesn't necessarily mean injury to the brain, nor does a brain injury always follow a head injury. You can strike your head hard enough to cause trauma to the skull but not the brain, because the hair, scalp, bony skull, and underlying membranes can protect the brain during certain impacts. However, this protection fades as the speed of impact is increased. Brain injury is injury to the brain that causes neurological dysregulation, meaning that the brain is not functioning properly. This can result in ongoing physical, emotional, and thinking problems. With this knowledge, in 1994 the World Health Organization adopted terms more descriptive of actual injuries to the brain. *Acquired brain injury* (ABI) is used to describe any damage to the brain not present at birth. A type of ABI called *traumatic brain injury* (TBI) includes any damage to the brain caused by an external force.

TBI can occur with or without injury to the skull. Even when there is no visible damage to the head, such as after a sports collision, blast injury, or car accident involving whiplash, the brain may still have been rotated or jostled inside the skull with a force strong enough to cause shearing and tearing of the nerves. At one time, the terms *open head injury* and *closed head injury* were used to distinguish whether external damage was present or not. Today, however, these terms are infrequently used.

Now we more commonly use the labels *mild, moderate,* and *severe* to preface the acronym TBI, but these descriptors are easily misunderstood. In everyday life, these terms are used to describe the level or quality or amount of something; thus, *mild* suggests "not so bad." Learning that you have a *mild traumatic brain injury* (mTBI), more commonly called a concussion, might not lead you to expect major consequences. However, when related to brain injury, these adjectives have nothing to do with the severity of injury. Rather, they refer to the length of time a person lacks awareness of his or her environment following impact. In a concussion, this lack of awareness can range from zero to sixty minutes or longer and still be considered mild, while moderate brain injury refers to loss of consciousness for up to twenty-four hours. Beyond that length of time, a brain injury is called a coma.

A person's condition immediately following brain injury doesn't always indicate the seriousness of the injury. Although most people who experience a concussion appear quite normal within hours of the event, new or lingering symptoms often force them to seek medical assistance later. The ongoing long-term consequences, or *sequelae*, of brain injury are labeled *post concussion syndrome* (PCS) or, in some areas of the world, *post concussion disorder* (PCD).

ABOUT THIS BOOK

∎

ITHIN THE NEXT FEW SECONDS, SOMEONE IN THE WORLD WILL INCUR A traumatic brain injury from an automobile accident, assault, fall, sports accident, blast injury, or incident of physical abuse. Depending on his or her immediate symptoms, such as loss of consciousness, dizziness, or physical complaints such as headache, this person may or may not receive medical treatment. If he or she is unconscious for anywhere from several seconds to sixty minutes and appears outwardly fine, even though amnesia may be present, the diagnosis will likely be concussion, also called *mild traumatic brain injury* (mTBI), and the individual will probably be told to rest for a few days or weeks. If the diagnostician is a proponent of nutritional effects, a few dietary changes and the intake of extra water may also be advised for good hydration, an increase in protein, and avoidance of sugar and processed foods.

This prescription of rest, time, and nutritional advice is indeed appropriate for many people with a concussion. However, many others encounter ongoing symptoms that continue to adversely affect their daily lives. These symptoms usually become apparent when people attempt to resume their responsibilities at home, work, or school.

This book is designed to help you understand and cope with the symptoms that follow a concussion, called *post concussion syndrome* (PCS). It is set up in six parts and contains a detailed glossary.

Part 1 contains information about the structure and workings of the brain and its neuroplasticity, as well as how these impact your recovery. Also included are the specifics of concussion and information on the effects of diet, age, gender, and left- or right-handedness. The types, leading causes, and symptoms of concussion are discussed, along with the effects of repeated injury to the brain. In addition, this section discusses methods of diagnosing and assessing TBI, from the Glasgow Coma scale to imaging tests to neuropsychological testing and impact assessments.

Part 2 details the various physical symptoms that can follow this type of injury. Problems with thinking and academic skills are covered in Part 3, and the emotional repercussions of concussion are explored in Part 4. Part 5 addresses such related topics as financial, insurance, and family issues; rehabilitation; and eventual outcomes. In Parts 2 through 5, each individual chapter deals with one particular aftereffect of concussion and provides a real-life story, an explanation of why the symptom or problem occurs, information on treatment, and practical suggestions for coping with the problem. Lastly, Part 6 explores future directions in the diagnosis and treatment of concussion and PCS.

If you are reading this book, you probably already know that the effects of a concussion can be far-reaching as well as long-lasting. It is my hope that your recovery, or that of your loved one, will be made easier by the information, advice, and support included in the pages that follow.

PART 1

CONCUSSION/MILD TRAUMATIC
BRAIN INJURY: AN OVERVIEW

INTRODUCTION

■

LYNN, A 26-YEAR-OLD DENTAL HYGIENIST, WAS DRIVING TO WORK ONE MORNING when her car was rear-ended at a red light. The fifteen-mile-per-hour impact caused no damage to either vehicle, and the seat belt kept Lynn's body in place. Only her head moved, quickly snapping forward and back. Lynn felt momentarily disoriented, but the feeling passed, and she went on her way without giving the matter much thought.

By lunchtime, Lynn had a severe headache. By evening, she also felt nauseated and extremely tired. At first, Lynn suspected a virus. But as the days passed, her headaches escalated and her fatigue increased. She also began to have problems sleeping, concentrating, expressing herself, and making decisions. To others, Lynn seemed uncharacteristically short-tempered and forgetful, and this led the puzzled young woman to see her physician. The eventual diagnosis? A concussion, also referred to as a *mild traumatic brain injury* (mTBI), a result of the now months-ago incident at the traffic light.

LYNN'S STORY is not at all unusual. In fact, each year millions of people worldwide are seen in hospitals, suffering from concussions. Many more visit doctors' offices and walk-in clinics, or may not even report the event, which is why concussion has come to be called "the Silent Epidemic." The principal causes of TBI are falls, motor vehicle accidents, blows, assaults, sports injuries, blast injuries, and violent movements such as whiplash. Like Lynn, a significant number of those who incur a concussion suffer debilitating aftereffects—*post concussion syndrome* (PCS)—for months or years afterward despite what is usually a perfectly normal outward appearance. Part 1 of this book will help you better understand this phenomenon by providing a detailed look at the brain and brain function as well as the causes, significance, and evaluation of concussion.

CHAPTER 1

WHAT IS A CONCUSSION/MILD TRAUMATIC BRAIN INJURY?

■

IN THE COURSE OF EVERYDAY LIFE, YOU HAVE LITTLE REASON TO THINK ABOUT the workings of your brain, even with television ads and magazine articles presenting the relationships between eating, sleeping, and brain health. However, if you have suffered a concussion, also called *mild traumatic brain injury* (mTBI), or know someone who has, the subject takes on sudden importance. As with almost any injury, knowledge about the affected organ—the brain, in this case—will help you and your family to better understand your symptoms and maintain a sense of control over the recovery process.

It is likely that you've attempted an Internet search for answers to your questions about your injury, symptoms, and treatment, only to feel overwhelmed by the quantity of information available. If so, you have probably wondered where you can find information that is accurate and leads to the answers you need. This book is intended to provide just that: the most recent research, verified by experts and presented in a concise, easy-to-use format.

A LOOK AT THE BRAIN

The human brain weighs about three pounds and is the most complex of organs—an intricate network of some 200 billion nerve cells and a trillion supporting cells. It is nourished by a vast network of blood vessels that supply the oxygen and glucose needed to fuel the brain. Your diet, quality of sleep, degree of stress, hormonal factors, and general quality of life directly affect your brain function, impacting all bodily activity from heart rate and movement to emotion and learning. The brain's complex components include veins, arteries, capillaries, threadlike nerve fibers, connective networks, neurotransmitters, neuromodulators, and hormones, which are involuntarily reactive to both internal and external events. Only a small portion of the brain operates in a voluntary, responsive

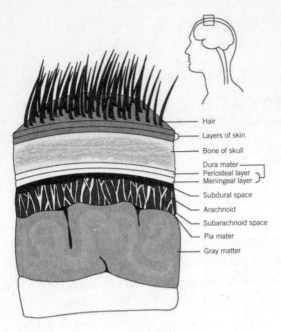

Hair
Layers of skin
Bone of skull
Dura mater
Periosteal layer
Meningeal layer
Subdural space
Arachnoid
Subarachnoid space
Pia mater
Gray matter

Figure 1.1. *A cross-section of the brain.*

manner; thus, brain function determines a person's abilities, personality, and state of health, all the while creating a capacity for thinking, feeling, imagining, and planning.

While the human skull is hard and bony, the brain within has been likened to custard in a bowl—soft, pliable, and slippery (Figure 1.1). Directly beneath the skull are three thin membranes called *meninges* that hold pockets of air and about a coffee-cupful of *cerebrospinal fluid* (CSF), which cushion the brain and its circulatory network.

This network, composed of arteries and veins (Figure 1.2), nourishes the brain, with each heartbeat providing oxygen and important nutrients as fuel. The countless small branches off the arteries and veins are called capillaries (Figure 1.3).

Directly beneath the meninges is the brain's wrinkled gray and white matter, made up of four distinct areas of brain functioning. These include the *brain stem*,

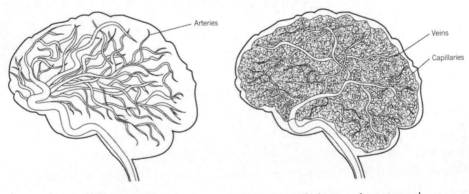

Arteries

Veins

Capillaries

Figure 1.2. *The brain and its arteries.*

Figure 1.3. *The brain and its veins and capillaries.*

midbrain, limbic system, and *cerebral cortex.* Of the four areas, the frontal area of the cerebral cortex is the most voluntary (responsive) to internal and external events.

The cerebral cortex, sometimes called the *cerebrum,* is the top layer of the brain and is its largest and most advanced part. It controls problem-solving, planning, and judgment, as well as movement and sensory activity. This area is divided into two halves, or hemispheres—the left and the right. One curious fact about brain function is that the right hemisphere, or the right side of the brain, controls the left side of the body, while the left hemisphere controls the right side of the body. In addition, the right hemisphere governs aspects of creativity, intuition, and nonverbal communication—gestures, facial expressions, and the like—and is referred to as the nonlinear mind. The left hemisphere, called the linear mind, is responsible for logical thinking, mathematics, and verbal and written expression.

Both of the hemispheres are subdivided into parts called lobes, each of which controls specific body functions (Figure 1.4). The *frontal lobe,* located closest to the forehead, controls emotions and behaviors, social and motor skills, abstract thinking, reasoning, planning, judgment, and memory. *Broca's area,* situated at the base of the frontal lobe, helps to govern speech. This area of the brain, especially the prefrontal area, is the area that governs voluntary responsiveness. It is similar to a symphony conductor, instructing areas of the brain that are voluntary and reactive.

The *parietal lobe* is located halfway between the front and back of the skull.

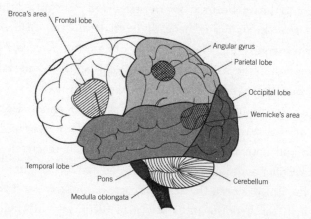

Figure 1.4. A look at the cerebrum.

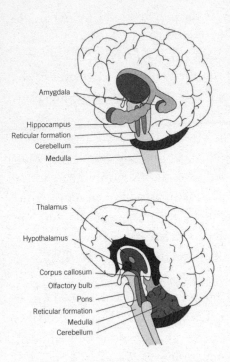

Amygdala

Hippocampus
Reticular formation
Cerebellum
Medulla

Thalamus

Hypothalamus

Corpus callosum
Olfactory bulb
Pons
Reticular formation
Medulla
Cerebellum

Figure 1.5. *The inner structures of the brain.*

This area is responsible for sensory and spatial awareness, giving feedback from and understanding of eye, hand, and arm movements during complex operations such as reading, writing, and numerical calculations. At the center of the parietal lobe is the *angular gyrus*, a fold in the surface of the brain where visual messages, such as words that are read, are matched with the sounds of spoken words. At the back of the head, behind the parietal lobe, is the *occipital lobe*, which controls vision and recognition.

The *temporal lobe* is located beneath the frontal and parietal lobes and has an influence on emotions. The temporal lobe plays a part in smelling, tasting, remembering information, noticing things, comprehending music, and categorizing objects. It also plays a role in aggressiveness and sexual behavior. At the back of the left temporal lobe is *Wernicke's area*, which is responsible for hearing and interpreting language.

Beneath the cerebrum are a number of internal brain structures (Figure 1.5). The *thalamus* acts as a nerve-impulse relay station for information coming into the brain, passing it to the cerebrum to be prioritized and transmitted throughout the body. The *hypothalamus* is located beneath the thalamus and influences sex drive, sleep, long-term memory, and the expression of emotion perceived by the brain, passing information to the *pituitary gland* that helps regulate and stabilize various hormones in your body—part of your *neuroendocrine system*.

The limbic system and components such as the *amygdala* are the source of involuntary survival reactions to perceived danger. Other components include the endocrine and autonomic nervous systems, which reactively control your breathing, heart rate, and digestive and intestinal systems (Figure 1.6). The limbic system is the link between the cerebral cortex, midbrain, and brain stem. Its components help the hypothalamus prioritize incoming information and also play a vital part in controlling memory, pain, and emotions.

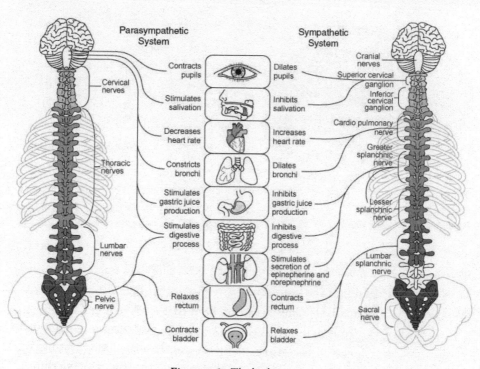

Figure 1.6. *The limbic system.*

At the central rear of the brain is the brain stem, which contains the midbrain, the *pons*, and the *medulla oblongata*. These structures control breathing and heartbeat and serve as a relay station for all motion and sensation. The cerebellum, a part of the brain situated in a cupped position slightly above the brain stem, oversees movement and balance, while the *hippocampus*, centrally located next to the temporal lobe near the base of the brain, is a key area in the creation of new memories and the transition of short-term memory to long-term.

Each part of the brain is highly specialized and is able to do its job only because of a vast network of nerve connections through the white matter (Figure 1.7), which includes specific neurotransmitters, neuromodulators (chemical messengers), and neuroconnective hubs (electrical connectors) for clearly defined tasks, functions, and processing.

It is the electrical system of the brain that allows communication between the various parts of the brain. The brain contains over 100 billion *neurons*, or nerve cells. Each neuron consists of a cell body and conducting fibers called branches (Figure 1.8), similar to the vast network of roads that enable us to travel

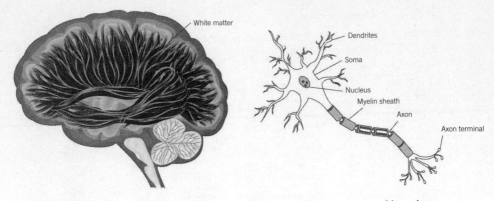

Figure 1.7. *The white matter.*

Figure 1.8. *The neurons and branches.*

from one place to another. These branches can be as short as a fraction of an inch or as long as several feet and connect to a trillion other branches through specific hubs. As a comparison, consider a dirt road that leads to a cul de sac, or a superhighway that can take us across the country. The electrical impulse travels toward the end of a nerve fiber, also called the axon. Between the ends or along the sides of each branch are tiny gaps called *synapses* (Figure 1.9). Most synapses are at the end of a nerve, though there are additional types (Figure 1.10).

When working properly, a neuron transmits electrical impulses to adjacent nerve cells at speeds of up to several hundred miles an hour. The electrical signal

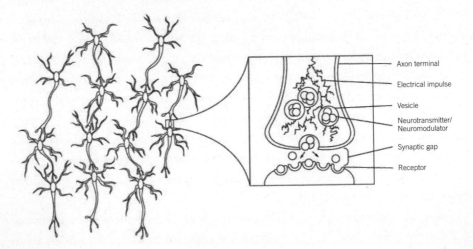

Figure 1.9. *A synapse.*

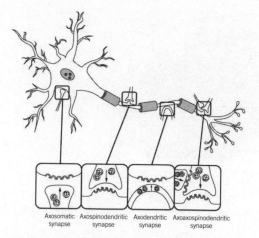

Axosomatic synapse   Axospinodendritic synapse   Axodendritic synapse   Axoaxospinodendritic synapse

Figure 1.10. Additional types of synapses.

that is formed pulses at differing rates of speed, creating a push/pull effect similar to the ebb and flow of the ocean. These electrical signals are called brain waves, and their speed is measured in electrical units called hertz (Hz). In 1940, W. Gray Walter was the first to identify that different brain waves have different effects on how we function. Table 1.3 shows different brain waves, their frequencies, and what they do. Individual brain waves work together as a team to send signals to different parts of the body, operating much as your car does when all the wheels are in alignment.

The synapses play a critical role in how the brain enables us to function, similar to the activity at a busy toll plaza. The brain's nerves are not in direct contact with one another, and the synapse between each nerve regulates functioning through a burst of chemicals called neurotransmitters (Table 1.1) and neuromodulators (Table 1.2), each of which has a specific task. Neurotransmitters are similar to traffic lights that signal electrical impulses to stop (inhibit) or go (activate), controlling whether the impulses continue. Neuromodulators are similar to police officers controlling traffic at busy intersections, overseeing a gradual flow of traffic in all directions.

These electrical impulses combine with the chemicals to connect one branch to another, forming vast networks of neurons in the brain's white matter. These networks meet at specific hubs to enable particular brain functions. For example, there is a hub for attention, and another for memory (Figure 1.11).

Many factors influence the push-and-pull activity of brain waves, including the aforementioned blood flow, quality of the nerve fiber, and impact of neurotransmitters, neuromodulators, and hormones. In 1929, Hans Berger first identified and named Alpha and Beta waves, while E. D. Andria and Brian Matthew named Delta and Theta waves in 1930. Since then, many others have identified additional waves seen below. Figure 1.12 illustrates a brain wave and shows its

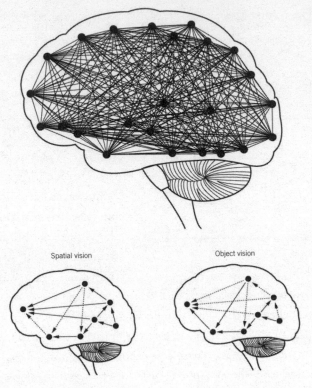

Spatial vision

Object vision

Figure 1.11. White matter with various hubs.

TABLE 1.1. NEUROTRANSMITTERS

Neurotransmitters are chemicals that allow the movement of information across the synapse, or gap, between one neuron and an adjacent neuron. A neurotransmitter functions similarly to a traffic light, or a driver putting a foot on either the accelerator or the brake in a car.

NEUROTRANSMITTER	BEHAVIOR	PURPOSE
Glutamate	This chemical acts like a green light or a car's accelerator, telling the system to go. It permits the electrical signal and its purpose to communicate to the next nerve. Glutamate is called the excitatory neurotransmitter and . . .	Is involved in most aspects of normal brain function including cognition, memory, and learning Mediates a good deal of information, including that which regulates brain development and that which determines cellular survival
Gamma-Aminobutyric Acid (GABA)	This chemical acts like a red light or a car's brakes, telling the system to stop. It stops the electrical signal from continuing to the next nerve. GABA is called the inhibitory neurotransmitter and . . .	Contributes to motor control, vision, and many other cortical functions Regulates anxiety Helps stimulate relaxation and sleep Stabilizes the brain by preventing overexcitement

TABLE 1.2. NEUROMODULATORS

Neuromodulators are chemicals that do not directly activate or inhibit; rather, they are similar to the police officer who regulates and coordinates traffic flow. Neuromodulators work together with neurotransmitters, enhancing the excitatory ("go," or "go with caution") or inhibitory ("stop," or "slow down") responses of the receptors. Each of the neuromodulators has specific functions, as seen below.

NEUROMODULATOR	FUNCTION
Dopamine	Regulates and limits cortical and subcortical signals to the brain
	Can either activate or inhibit
	Controls arousal levels in many parts of the brain
	Is vital to the provision of physical motivation
	Governs internal control of sustained attention
	Modulates attention to sensory input
Serotonin	Acts as a feel-good chemical
	Influences sustained arousal and electrical impulses in the brain, and controls the feeling of well-being
	Has multiple roles regarding sleep, temperature regulation, sexual behavior, appetite, learning, memory, anxiety, mood, and endocrine, muscular, and cardiovascular function
	Impacts the regulation of one's pain threshold
	Is not connected to sensory input
Acetylcholine	Activates motor neurons that control skeletal muscles
	Controls activity in the brain area connected with attention, learning, and memory
	Is involved in central nervous system responses, including wakefulness, attentiveness, anger, aggression, sexuality, and thirst
Histamine	Helps regulate and modulate the activation of electrical signals
	Is involved in the body's inflammatory response
Noradrenaline (also called norepinephrine):	Helps regulate and modulate the activation of electrical signals
	Is active in the startle response
	Enhances emotional memory
	Contributes to the modulation of mood and arousal
	Is critical to attentiveness, emotions, sleep, dreaming, and learning
	Is released as a hormone into the blood, where it causes contraction of blood vessels and increased heart rate
Aspartate	Helps regulate and modulate the activation of electrical signals
	Regulates the metabolism of amino acids for kidney and central nervous system function
Glycine	Helps regulate and modulate the inhibiting of electrical signals
	Helps regulate the central nervous system, especially the brain stem

height and cycle duration. The height is the quantity of the wave being produced, or the amplitude. The duration reflects the time the cycle takes to repeat itself. The wave's frequency, or number of cycles per second, is the inverse of the duration of one cycle in units of hertz.

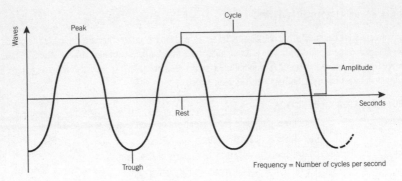

Figure 1.12. *A brain wave.*

The brain and body systems are also strongly affected by hormones, chemicals that are released from cells and glands. These effects include:

- Stimulation or inhibition of growth
- Mood swings
- Sleep
- Induction or suppression of *apoptosis*, or programmed cell death
- Activation or inhibition of the immune system
- Regulation of metabolism
- Preparation of the body for mating, fighting, fleeing, and other responsive activity
- Preparation of the body for a new life phase, such as puberty, parenting, and menopause
- Control of the reproductive cycle
- Hunger cravings
- Sexual arousal

For instance, melatonin is a chemical that helps you sleep at night. If your electrical system is working properly, it sends a message for this chemical to be released when it is dark and you are fatigued, thereby helping you sleep. As expected, there is ebb and flow present. If the electrical impulse can't reach the cell or the melatonin can't reach the proper area, the system doesn't work properly and sleep patterns are disturbed.

Now that you know how the brain functions under normal circumstances,

TABLE 1.3. BRAIN WAVES AND THE EFFECTS OF THEIR FREQUENCIES ON BRAIN FUNCTION

BRAIN WAVE	EFFECTS ON BRAIN FUNCTION
Delta (0.5 to 4 Hz)	Are predominant during sleep
	Should be low while awake
	Repair the brain
	Serve as emotional radar
	Are responsible for intuition and unconscious thought
	In abundance, can interfere with emotional or cognitive processing
Theta (4 to 8 Hz)	Present during pre-sleep or trance state
	Promote insight and meditation
	In abundance, can create inattentiveness, distractibility, and lack of focus
Alpha (8 to 12 Hz)	Promote relaxation
	Serve as gateway for restorative sleep
	In abundance, can make you spacey, unmotivated, inattentive, and depressed
SMR (12 to 15 Hz)	Are related to calm external attention
	Regulate impulsivity and hyperactivity
	Promote body awareness
	Help control anxiety and anger
	Promote the inhibition of movement
Beta (15 to 20 Hz)	Are related to active external attention
	Enhance cognitive processing
	Improve concentration, attentiveness, and focus
High Beta (20 to 36 Hz)	Are related to body tension
	Promote a high state of arousal
	Result in excitement, anxiety, and stress
	Related to post traumatic stress disorder (PTSD)
Gamma (36 to 64 Hz)	Are linked to intellectual comprehension
	Are related to creativity
	Promote integrative thinking

we can look at what happens when a concussion causes dysregulation in the brain. Whether structural damage to the brain's gray or white matter is apparent or not, the aftermath of a brain injury results in dysregulation in the function of the lobes, hormones, neurotransmitters, neuromodulators, or hub activity. This dysregulation is the underlying cause of the problems seen in *post concussion syndrome* (PCS) in areas such as mood, behavior, sleep, fatigue, or intellect. The following chapters explore the various causes of concussion and how the resulting dysregulation of the brain is diagnosed. In addition, information is provided on approaches to treating the symptoms of PCS.

CHAPTER 2

SYMPTOMS OF CONCUSSION/MILD TRAUMATIC BRAIN INJURY

■

A S MENTIONED EARLIER, INJURY TO THE BRAIN FROM AN OUTSIDE FORCE IS called a traumatic brain injury, or TBI. Most people who experience severe brain trauma display language, motor, or perceptual problems that can be traced to a particular incident or event that caused a specific type of brain damage. *Mild traumatic brain injury* (mTBI), also called concussion, is characterized by a loss of consciousness ranging from negligible up to an hour in length, along with a loss of memory of events before and/or after the time of injury. Concussion can occur from a variety of causes. Automobile accidents account for the majority of cases, followed by, in order of prevalence, falls, assaults and other violence (including physical abuse), sports- and recreation-related accidents, and blast injury. The last three causes weren't linked to TBI for years; thus, diagnosis and treatment have been almost completely overlooked until recently. Now it is clear that even a small dysregulation of the brain can have an enormous effect on one's life.

Some people suffer no ill effects at all following a concussion, while others encounter persistent problems and feel the effects of their injury in every aspect of life. In addition to suffering from head or neck pain, many people feel disoriented and experience memory loss immediately after the blow. These complaints often resolve within a few minutes, but over the next several hours it is common to experience an onset of dizziness, nausea, headache, and fatigue. Depending on the number of concussions experienced by an individual and the location of the brain injury, symptoms are frequently misdiagnosed or missed altogether.

However, a week or two later, as the person attempts to resume normal responsibilities at home, school, or work, he or she may encounter another group of symptoms that have collectively come to be called *post concussion syndrome* (PCS). These complaints include persistent headaches; fatigue; impaired attention, concentration, and decision-making ability; sleep disturbances; dizziness;

gait imbalance; loss of taste and smell; loss of sex drive; intolerance for alcohol; reading and communication difficulties; and emotional or behavioral problems. These symptoms may appear alone or in any combination. A concise list of common concussion aftereffects is presented in Table 2.1.

In 2009, the International Symposium on Concussion changed its labels of *simple* and *complex concussion* to *acute concussion* and *post concussion syndrome.* Despite the change in terms, the core features of these conditions remain the same.

ACUTE CONCUSSION

An acute concussion is a temporary disruption of brain function that results in an alteration or loss of consciousness, and one or more of the memory symptoms contained in Table 2.1. Acute concussions spontaneously resolve within a week or two with rest and proper diet. This occurs due to spontaneous healing, a re-regulation of brain and nerve tissue, or the formation of new nerve-cell pathways that bypass damaged circuits (which characterizes the brain's neuroplasticity, or ability to change itself). With this type of concussion, symptoms can be treated by your primary care physician (PCP) or by a certified athletic trainer or coach working in conjunction with your PCP.

POST CONCUSSION SYNDROME (PCS)

When concussion symptoms do not resolve within a week or two of disrupted brain function, the label *post concussion syndrome* (PCS) is applied. Along with the various symptoms contained in Table 2.1, PCS can also include convulsions. With this type of condition, it is important to be seen by a neurologist who has expertise in treating concussion.

MULTIPLE CONCUSSIONS

When an individual has had multiple concussions due to repeated impact to the brain, natural and spontaneous healing and regulation are unlikely. This phenomenon affects nearly 90 percent of people who experience a concussion. Repeated brain injuries, including multiple concussions, can have severe or even fatal outcomes, especially when the second injury occurs soon after the first and before recovery from the first has taken place.

TABLE 2.1. SYMPTOMS OF CONCUSSION

PHYSICAL DIFFICULTIES	Fatigue
	Sleep disturbances
	Sensitivity to light and/or sound
	Headaches
	Falling asleep unexpectedly
	Dizziness
	Nightmares or flashbacks
	Nausea and vomiting
	Alertness upon waking, followed by exhaustion
	Blurred vision
	Hand or leg tremors
	Sexual dysfunction or loss of sex drive
	Gait imbalance
	Ringing in the ears
	Loss of taste and smell
COGNITIVE (THINKING) PROBLEMS	Distractibility
	Disorientation
	Temporary amnesia
	Long- or short-term memory problems
	Poor judgment
	Slow thinking
	Inability to focus attention
	Problems with speaking
	Word-finding problems
	Feelings of confusion
EMOTIONAL DIFFICULTIES	Depression
	Agitation
	Apathy
	Irritability
	Fear of "going crazy"
	Frustration or anger
	Guilt or shame
	Feelings of helplessness
	Anxiety
	Frequent mood changes
BEHAVIORAL PROBLEMS	Confrontational demeanor
	Explosive temper
	Fearfulness
	Impatience
	Thoughtlessness
	Hypervigilance

Each repeated injury causes further dysregulation and exponential exacerbation of symptoms. This means that each injury is not simply an additional injury, as in 1 concussion + 1 concussion = 2 concussions. Instead, each injury is a multiple of the others. Thus, the effects of a third concussion are many times worse than those of the original concussion. That is why a slight blow to the head months after an initial injury can result in more, more severe, and longer-lasting symptoms than accompanied the first concussion.

Multiple concussions can result from many causes that may seem subtle or incapable of injuring the brain. Multiple concussions are divided into two categories: second impact syndrome and chronic traumatic encephalopathy.

SECOND IMPACT SYNDROME (SIS)

Second impact syndrome, or SIS, has been reported when a second concussion occurs within hours, days, or weeks of a previous brain injury. This happens frequently in sports and recreation participation, when a player suffers a concussion and resumes physical activity days later, only to receive another such injury. Yet many players, parents, and coaches have long felt that a concussion need not restrict continued involvement in a sport. Fortunately, this belief has changed with better understanding of brain injury's long-term consequences, such as chronic headaches, fatigue, and difficulty concentrating.

CHRONIC TRAUMATIC ENCEPHALOPATHY (CTE)

Chronic traumatic encephalopathy, or CTE, is a progressive neurodegenerative brain disease that appears to be caused by brain trauma (Figure 2.1). CTE evolves slowly over decades. Research has shown that the protein tau, necessary to the integrity of nerve fibers, gradually falls apart and destroys both the white and gray matter of the brain. There are three stages of CTE:

Stage 1. Includes changes in mood, behavior, and cognition. An individual may become moody, angry, or combative, while his or her thinking doesn't seem to make sense.

Stage 2. Includes problems with maintaining social activity, erratic behavior, and memory loss, as well as symptoms of Parkinson's disease that include a mask-like look to the face and movement problems.

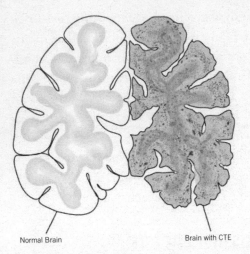

Normal Brain

Brain with CTE

Figure 2.1. *A look at CTE.*

Stage 3. Characterized by progressive deterioration into dementia.

CTE is most prevalent in boxers and football players who have suffered repeated blows to the head over an extended time period. CTE is also seen in individuals who served in the military. An in-depth explanation of sports, recreational, and blast injuries will be presented in Chapter 4.

ADDITIONAL SYMPTOMS

The various physical, emotional, and behavioral symptoms that can follow a concussion are likely to be compounded by social and psychological factors. Because post concussion problems are often invisible to the casual observer, the injured person often hears such comments as "You look wonderful!" or "Thank goodness it was only a concussion!" or even "It's great that you're already back in the swing of things!" Of course, the person isn't feeling wonderful at all and is painfully aware of not functioning as he or she used to. This causes many people with a concussion to feel anxiety and a loss of confidence, both of which can reveal themselves in out-of-character behavior such as self-involvement and extreme vulnerability to stress. Worse still is the fact that by the time concussion consequences begin to disrupt an individual's life, he or she may not even connect the symptoms to the accident that caused them. It is no wonder, then, that after weeks of seeing little or no improvement in their symptoms, many people with a concussion find themselves facing another roadblock: persistent depression and underlying grief from the loss of self.

Perhaps the greatest impact of concussion is psychological. An unexpected, unexplained inability to function can shake you to the core. Consider the insurance agent who suddenly struggles to remember clients' names and navigate the office complex, or the student who can no longer stay focused on class work and note-taking, or the mechanic who can no longer reassemble an engine. None of these people look any different from before, but all are having difficulty at work or school and are quite likely also struggling to cope with everyday chores and concerns at home. Many people with PCS begin to second-guess their every move in an attempt to avoid failure and embarrassment. This sort of anxiety can easily initiate a vicious cycle, building to such proportions that it actually contributes to cognitive problems, which in turn make the anxiety worse, and so on. It is reassuring to know that there are methods of treatment that can help you recover from your symptoms.

CHAPTER 3

TYPES OF CONCUSSION/MILD TRAUMATIC BRAIN INJURY

■

THERE ARE TWO TYPES OF TRAUMATIC BRAIN INJURY: INJURY ACCOMPANIED BY visible external damage, and injury without visible evidence. In what was formerly called an *open head injury*, the skull is penetrated. Brain damage takes the form of a *focal injury*—that is, injury to a specific area of the brain— such as that from a gunshot wound or severe external trauma that causes the brain to swell. In a concussion without visible evidence, once called a *closed head injury*, the skull is not penetrated. Brain damage occurs as a result of an external force that causes the brain to move within the skull, producing any combination of the following: focal (direct contact), diffuse, rotation, sound pressure, or generalized injury.

The human skull and the underlying fluid-filled membranes rarely sustain damage during a concussion (also called *mild traumatic brain injury*, or mTBI). Any time the head is subjected to violent force, sound, or motion, however, the soft, floating brain is slammed against the skull's uneven interior. Sometimes it rotates in the process. When this happens, the brain's threadlike nerve cells are stretched, strained, and even torn at the point of impact (focal injury, or direct contact) or in a widely scattered fashion (*diffuse injury*) or both. Many times, such an accident causes both stretching and tearing of nerve fibers. While this nerve-cell damage is usually microscopic, the effect on the brain's neurological circuits is significant, causing dysregulation of specific areas or hubs or throughout the entire system.

DIRECT CONTACT FORCE CONCUSSIONS

Impact injuries, or *direct contact force concussions*, result in observable tissue damage in a particular area of the brain. One common type of direct contact force injury occurs during car accidents and sports collisions that involve acceleration followed by rapid deceleration—that is, when the forward-moving head comes to a sudden stop after striking a stationary object. When this happens, the brain keeps moving forward until it collides with the front of the skull. This acceleration/deceleration impact causes *fronto-temporal lesions*, or bruising of the *frontal* and/or *temporal lobes* of the brain, as shown in Figure 3.1. This type of injury generally affects a person's ability to memorize, plan, concentrate, and/or control behavior—skills that are largely regulated by the frontal and temporal lobes. You may have sudden difficulty storing and retrieving new information, be unable to organize your thoughts, be highly distractible, or have problems modulating your behavior. These impairments result from disruption of the nerve connections between the *cerebrum* and the inner brain, which is in effect a neurological short circuit.

A second type of direct contact force brain injury is the *coup/contrecoup* (literally, "blow/counterblow") injury. Generally, this trauma occurs when a moving object makes contact with the head, briefly denting the skull inward. The brain beneath is bruised first at the point of impact and then is thrown against the opposite side of the skull, where additional bruising takes place, as shown in Figure 3.2. In coup/contrecoup injuries, the site of bruising and the resulting impairments depend on where the initial blow landed. You may encounter one or more of a range of problems, including personality changes, perceptual and sensory problems, difficulty expressing yourself, and balance and motor problems.

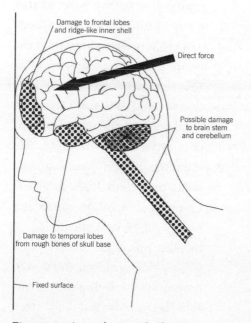

Damage to frontal lobes and ridge-like inner shell

Direct force

Possible damage to brain stem and cerebellum

Damage to temporal lobes from rough bones of skull base

Fixed surface

Figure 3.1. An acceleration/deceleration injury.

DIFFUSE AXONAL INJURY (DAI)

A mild blow to the head that causes momentary alteration or loss of consciousness with no observable disruption of nerve impulses is called a *diffuse axonal injury* (DAI), shown in Figure 3.3. DAIs are

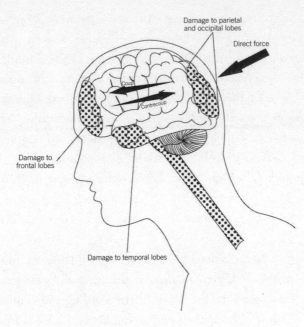

Figure 3.2. A coup/contrecoup injury.

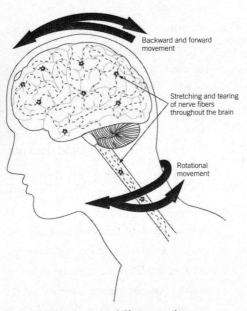

Figure 3.3. A diffuse axonal injury caused by whiplash.

commonly caused by whiplash injury. It was long believed that diffuse axonal injury caused only a brief short-circuiting within the brain. However, it is now known that the stretching of nerve cells due to brain movement in multiple directions simultaneously interferes with their ability to fire impulses, thereby causing dysregulation. This leads to alteration or loss of consciousness and in turn a general disruption of mental processes. People with DAIs process information slowly, have trouble splitting their attention between tasks, and often find themselves struggling to

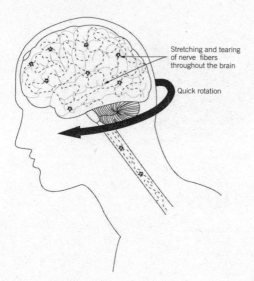

Stretching and tearing of nerve fibers throughout the brain

Quick rotation

Figure 3.4. *A rotation injury.*

organize and sort the details of incoming information. Abstract thinking may be impaired, as may the ability to express thoughts accurately and clearly. DAIs can occur either alone or in conjunction with a direct contact force brain injury.

ROTATION INJURY

Sudden rotation of the brain in the absence of a direct blow or whiplash movement can cause symptoms of dysregulation of connections and circuitry known as *rotation injury*. This type of injury occurs from violent movement of the head with or without contact, commonly occurring during recreational activities or sports. Figure 3.4 illustrates rotation injury.

BLAST INJURY

The explosion of a bomb or improvised explosive device produces a sound wave called a supersonic wave. The movement, amplitude, and duration of this sound wave result in sufficient pressure within the brain to cause actual tissue damage along with dysregulation of connectivity and brain waves. An individual does not have to be physically moving or in contact with the blast for the injury it causes to be enormous. This damage to the brain is called *blast injury*, illustrated in Figure 3.5.

Most of the brain cells, branches, hubs, neurotransmitters, neuromodulators, and hormones affected by a concussion receive only minor damage and eventually return to normal functioning. It is the parts of the brain's neuroconnectivity that are damaged or destroyed by overstretching, tearing, bleeding, and/or swelling that ultimately shape an individual's post-injury experience, because the resultant dysregulation results in *post concussion syndrome* (PCS), as described in

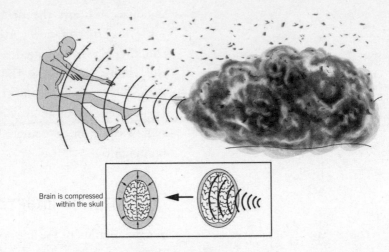

Brain is compressed within the skull

Figure 3.5. A blast injury.

Chapter 2. If there are cumulative injuries, the effect of these minor blows, rotations, or falls becomes a foundation for ongoing symptoms and determines the severity and duration of recovery from PCS. Chapter 4 addresses the issue of multiple concussions in more detail.

LEADING CAUSES OF CONCUSSION/ MILD TRAUMATIC BRAIN INJURY

■

WHEN CONSIDERING THE CAUSE OF A CONCUSSION, ALSO CALLED *MILD traumatic brain injury* (mTBI), it is important to recognize the significance of age, gender, and the circumstances surrounding the injury, such as a motor vehicle accident, fall, assault or violent shaking, recreational activity, blast injury, or sports collision.

Age and gender have a surprising effect on one's risk of concussion. Until the age of 15, males and females have an equal risk. Between the ages of 15 and 24, males are at higher risk of this type of injury. A male's risk remains slightly higher during the working years, due to the greater likelihood of participation in physical occupations. After age 64, the risk of concussion for males versus females is again equal.

INFANCY AND CHILDHOOD

In infancy, the number-one cause of concussion is shaken baby syndrome, followed by falls and motor vehicle accidents. In childhood, the leading causes of concussion are domestic violence, motor vehicle accidents (even when restrained in a safety seat), and being struck by a car while walking or riding a bicycle or scooter. Seemingly benign amusement park rides also increase a child's risk. The sudden acceleration and deceleration of roller coasters and other rides are known to cause concussion, particularly if this impact is preceded by other concussions.

It is likely that concussions related to riding toys are underreported, because the parent or caregiver may focus on external injuries such as scrapes or bruises. It is easy to overlook a child's appearing dazed and shaken if her knee is bleeding or his arm is injured. Even when an injury is serious enough to warrant a trip to the emergency room, the focus tends to be on the visible. Medical personnel may overlook that a child seems to be dazed or not thinking clearly, which is why concussion is called "the Silent Epidemic."

Increasing numbers of children now engage in sports activities at early ages when their brains are still developing. It is not uncommon to see 4- and 5-year-olds on skis or snowboards, horses, rock-climbing walls, or snowmobiles. In addition, small children are increasingly encouraged to participate in organized sports. Along with these pastimes is time spent in classic recreational settings such as playgrounds and climbing areas, all of which carry the risk of concussion from a fall that can occasionally happen despite supervision and safety precautions.

By the age of 10, many children are involved in one or more organized sports, whether played on a court, rink, or field. Individual sports such as figure skating, gymnastics, dance, and karate are strongly in play by this age as well. A pre-teen's choice of recreational activity also impacts his or her risk of concussion, be it skateboarding, roller- or ice-skating, diving, or just wrestling with a friend.

THE TEEN AND YOUNG ADULT YEARS

Between the ages of 14 and 25, most athletes work at increasing their skill level in order to remain competitive with peers, making sports participation more risky. Along with this comes an increase in gym workouts and aggressive recreational activities such as trampoline, racquetball, and bungee jumping. Table 4.1 presents some of the leading recreational activities pursued by teenagers. During the teen years, nutrition frequently becomes worse as parental regulation decreases and the temptation increases to use energy drinks, bodybuilding supplements, alcohol, and drugs. All of this puts the developing brain at risk, because the connective *myelin* in the prefrontal lobe, which helps regulate how we think, behave, and feel, is just beginning to grow. Yet it is during this time of life that many youths are involved in hard-hitting or risky athletic pursuits.

Because concussion is so often invisible before the age of 16, it is thought that most children suffer at least one concussion that is either never identified or is misdiagnosed. Parents, doctors, and coaches often dismiss the fact that a child cannot remember the score of a game or seems distracted. In fact, these symptoms of concussion are often seen as attention deficit disorder (ADD) or attention deficit/hyperactivity disorder (ADHD). Then, when there is an obvious knock-out from an auto accident or sports injury and the child complains of seeing stars, hearing bells ring, or having a severe headache, a diagnosis of concussion is finally made and rest is recommended. Because everyone thinks this is the child's first concussion, however, they are puzzled when the symptoms of fatigue, confusion, chronic headache, and light and noise sensitivity persist weeks after a seemingly minor incident. In truth, the majority of most first-known and diagnosed concussions have been preceded by numerous others that have gone unnoticed, again characterizing "the Silent Epidemic." This is why a child's concussion symptoms may persist.

As mentioned previously, males between the ages of 16 and 24 have historically had a higher incidence of concussion than females, most through participation in regular and extreme sports, recreational activities, auto accidents, and military duty. One of the symptoms of concussion is aggressive behavior, which, along with the male hormone testosterone, causes more risk-taking and aggressive behavior that in turn can result in additional concussions from blows to the head. Some examples are skateboarding without a helmet, and getting into physical fights in which punches are thrown to the face or head. A recent trend is toward females in this age bracket also being diagnosed with multiple concussions by the age of 24 through athletic participation and blast injuries incurred during military duty.

Statistics show a higher incidence of drinking among teens and young adults, as compared with adults (35 to 65) and seniors (65 and older). The resulting impaired thinking leads to an increase of sports, recreational, and automobile accidents. It is following these incidents that a concussion is likely to be reported; however, the injury is usually seen as an initial concussion rather than the latest in a series. As with younger athletes, prior concussions may have been dismissed or minimized, either purposefully or because the person truly doesn't remember having been knocked out. Or there may have been a misdiagnosis on a medical professional's part. Chapter 5 addresses the various methods for accurately diagnosing and assessing concussion.

Please note that the above list does not include recreational activities that can cause concussion but often do not involve a visit to a doctor's office or hospital. Also, activities and the frequency of related injury may vary according to recreational trends, locale, and time of year.

TABLE 4.1. 24 LEADING SPORTS AND RECREATIONAL PURSUITS THAT CAN CAUSE CONCUSSION

1. Cycling	12. Winter sports, including skiing, sledding, snowboarding, and snowmobiling
2. Boxing	13. Horseback riding
3. Football	14. Gymnastics, dance, and cheerleading
4. Wrestling	15. Karate
5. Baseball and softball	16. Golf
6. Basketball	17. Roller and ice hockey
7. Water sports, including diving, scuba diving, surfing, swimming, water polo, waterskiing, and water tubing	18. Tennis
	19. Racquetball
8. Powered recreational vehicles, including ATVs, dune buggies, go-carts, gas-powered scooters, minibikes, and dirt bikes	20. Other unspecified ball sports
	21. Trampolines
9. Soccer	22. Rugby and lacrosse
10. Skateboards and nonpowered scooters	23. Roller- and inline skating
11. Fitness, exercise, and health club participation	24. Ice-skating

THE ADULT YEARS

By the age of 24, all of a person's myelin connections are formed and connected to the frontal lobe, allowing for clear thought and optimum control of behavior and emotions, which leads to decreased impulsivity and recklessness. Of course, major illness and one or more concussions can play havoc with this balance in behavior. Between 24 and 64 years of age, engagement in contact and competitive sports decreases while the pursuit of recreational sports remains about the same. Auto accidents and falls are fewer in this age bracket as well, with the exception of occupational mishaps and incidents of domestic violence. The incidence of first-time concussion is lower; but, as previously mentioned, the probability of such an injury actually being a first-time event is smaller than most people think. The chapters that follow will demonstrate the importance of considering not only the number of concussions a person has had, but also how often and how close together they occurred. These factors are very important to eventual recovery.

After the age of 64, the frequency of concussion from sports, occupational, and blast injuries naturally decreases. However, people in this age group face a greater risk of concussion from auto accidents, falls, illness, elder abuse, assault, improper use of medication, and substance abuse.

SECONDARY CAUSES OF CONCUSSION

Along with focal and diffuse nerve damage and rotation and blast injuries, the neuroconnective damage that characterizes a concussion can also result from factors that may be deemed secondary causes. These include:

- Anoxia, or a lack of oxygen
- Bypass surgery
- Substance abuse
- Diabetes
- Lyme disease
- Contusion, or a bruise that can go undetected during conventional testing
- Edema, or swelling due to an accumulation of fluid in brain tissue
- Hematoma, a localized brain swelling due to an accumulation of blood from a break in a blood vessel
- Hemorrhage, or bleeding, in which a torn vessel releases blood into the brain tissue

The symptoms of *post concussion syndrome* (PCS) from secondary causes are often not observed or treated, because the medical specialist's focus is on the specific disease, such as diabetes or Lyme disease. The emphasis in these cases is on regulating the body's sugar levels or treating the bacterial infection, not on how the disease causes dysregulation to the brain. No matter how careful one may be, there are circumstances and pastimes in life that carry the risk of concussion. It is certainly beneficial to be aware of the physical consequences of such an injury and to understand the signs and symptoms to look out for. Chapter 5 provides important information about steps to take when you suspect a concussion has occurred.

DIAGNOSING AND ASSESSING CONCUSSION/ MILD TRAUMATIC BRAIN INJURY AND POST CONCUSSION SYNDROME (PCS)

∎

THIS BOOK IS DEVOTED TO THE PROPER DIAGNOSIS AND TREATMENT OF concussion (also known as *mild traumatic brain injury*, or mTBI) and *post concussion syndrome* (PCS), as well as the consequences of multiple concussions. If you are just beginning the process of recovery from a concussion, please realize that it is common to feel afraid and to feel, perhaps, that you are losing your mind. After all, time has passed since your injury, you look just fine, and your diagnostic tests have all yielded normal results. Yet, clearly, all is not well. It will likely take a sympathetic doctor's referral and a neuropsychological workup—a diagnostic process designed to reveal problems with reasoning, memory, and other brain functions—to finally pinpoint the source or sources of your difficulties. Once that is accomplished, you will almost certainly feel an overwhelming sense of relief that someone understands what you have been going through. This affirmation, along with support from medical professionals, friends, and family, can help to head off many of the debilitating psychological responses to a concussion.

Overall, the outlook for recovery from a concussion is brightest with the early diagnosis and treatment of symptoms. Optimally, you can hope for slow, steady progress toward normalcy in the months after injury. If it is determined that long-term or permanent cognitive, physical, or emotional deficits exist, you can best help yourself by understanding the nature of your problems, acknowledging your limitations, and making necessary accommodations at home, school, and work. The following two chapters will provide you with information about assessment techniques and the most successful approaches to lingering problems that can follow a concussion.

Chapter 1 explained how the brain is composed of vast interconnectivity networks similar to the telecommunications or airline networks. In those industries, when a major hub is disrupted, it can result in chaos and shutdown in many areas. The disruption of a major hub can come from a single event, such as a workman flipping a wrong switch that eventually causes a blackout across all of southern California, or it can stem from multiple events (the domino effect). In either case, it is extremely important to discover the source of the disruption in order to be able to fix it.

This is also the case with a concussion, whether caused by an automobile accident, assault, or sports injury, since most people appear quite normal within hours of the impact. Thus, even if symptoms are observed by a coach, trainer, or physician, rest and relaxation is often the initial suggestion. It is only when new or lingering symptoms occur that a person may be compelled to seek additional medical assistance. As discussed in Chapter 4, a concussion may not be your first, and the continued cluster of symptoms that follow, called post concussion syndrome (or, in some parts of the world, post concussion disorder), must be correctly diagnosed for accurate and appropriate treatment to follow.

In the past, such a definitive diagnosis was elusive. However, in recent years, both the understanding of the workings of the brain and the technology used in brain imaging have advanced greatly. Where before only major damage to the gray matter or vascular system could be seen, today minute and subtle structural injuries can be seen in both the gray and white matter as well as the vascular network. In addition, there have been diagnostic advances in the area of brain functioning, including specific tests for evaluating the ability to perform in sports.

In this chapter, we will explore the various professionals and methods involved in evaluating a concussion and PCS. Along with medical and neurological evaluation and functional testing, we will discuss imaging and diagnostic methods, including structural, sports, and online tests. Included is discussion about the mode of evaluation; that is, whether blood flow or electrical activity is being measured. Such testing can locate the reason for the dysregulation being experienced, point out specific areas that are not working properly, and guide the course of treatment needed for recovery.

It is important to understand that conventional medical techniques are the only means of evaluating brain injury. No matter where your health care preferences lie, treatment of concussion symptoms should always be preceded by a traditional diagnostic workup so that preexisting or potentially life-threatening conditions can safely be ruled out. Only with the most accurate possible diagnosis in hand can you make informed decisions about your post-injury health care.

THE CHALLENGE OF IDENTIFYING A CONCUSSION AND PCS

Not all people who suffer head trauma, whiplash, sports injury, or blast injury lose consciousness or receive medical attention immediately after injury. However, concussion professionals view an evaluation by an emergency room physician as the best course of action after any blow to the head, because even momentary loss of consciousness can foreshadow impaired judgment and improper reporting of the incident. In addition, headaches, confusion, and blurred or double vision, also characteristic of concussion, may place a person in jeopardy if he or she chooses to drive, perform delicate tasks, or return to the activity that resulted in the injury. Moreover, in a small number of cases, the individual's condition actually deteriorates in the hours after the accident because of brain swelling or bleeding. It is therefore wise to have any head trauma evaluated as quickly as possible.

Parents and others who care for children need to know that if a child suffers a blow to the head, his or her condition immediately afterward is not a reliable indicator of how seriously the brain has been injured. With increased awareness of the repercussions of sports injuries, some high school and most college and professional coaches and athletic trainers now use computerized assessments to provide pre-injury baselines that help assess the possibility, severity, and cognitive profile of a concussion.

About 12 percent of people who experience a concussion are hospitalized overnight for observation after injury. Most people, however, are sent directly home from the emergency room or doctor's office with nothing more than a prescription for rest and painkillers. Other times, as in the case of Lynn, the dental hygienist whose story introduced this section, the injured parties themselves see no need for medical attention and dismiss their accidents completely until symptoms start to play havoc with their day-to-day functioning. A visit to a primary health care provider or hospital emergency room may then lead to a skull X-ray, electroencephalogram (EEG), or computed tomography (CT) scan to check for a skull fracture or brain injury. Pain medication may be ordered for headaches or neck pain. Finally, the patient may be referred to a behavioral neurologist, sports medicine doctor, or other specialist for evaluation of persistent or additional symptoms.

"Your test results are negative. Go home, rest for a few days, and you'll be just fine."

For years, pronouncements like this were what people with a concussion typically heard after seeking medical help for symptoms such as dizziness, fatigue, headaches, light or sound sensitivity, memory loss, chronic pain, sleep problems, or distractibility. Doctors routinely disputed or dismissed the notion of structural damage to the brain after a concussion because the diagnostic tools at their disposal were not sensitive enough to detect the dysregulation of brain neuroconnectivity and nerve-cell damage that we now know can lead to a wide range of complaints. Traditional psychological testing also failed to pinpoint a problem, because the level of dysfunction of people with a concussion is subtle and their complaints are often nonspecific.

In addition, as mentioned in Chapter 4, the injured party's age and gender can also affect how symptoms present and are interpreted. For instance, the aggressive behavior of a 16-year-old football player after a concussion may be seen as just youthful acting-out behavior. In the past, if the possibility of an organic problem was dismissed and psychological tests were interpreted as inconclusive, many people with a concussion were told that their symptoms were psychosomatic. Worse, some people were accused of faking their problems for insurance or sick-leave purposes.

Unquestionably, concussion has a psychological component. After all, the overall disruption of mental processes so common to this type of injury, combined with lingering physical complaints, can easily lead to out-of-character behavior and emotions. However, as presented in Chapter 1, there is now clear evidence that symptoms following a concussion have a physical cause. The confirmation of actual dysregulation or neuroconnectivity and/or brain damage not only helps to steer people toward appropriate treatment, but also it affirms that their experience is real and frees patients from the accusation that they are just being lazy or making things up—an experience common to victims of automobile or occupational accidents in which the opposing side must disprove the reality of a physical cause in order to avoid liability. Not surprisingly, then, the goal of proving that the brain has suffered physical damage and/or neuroconnectivity dysregulation is usually shared by the victim's family, and is also critically important to professionals who specialize in diagnosing, assessing, and treating brain injury.

The list of professionals who are trained to diagnose and/or assess concussion includes the following: an emergency medical technician (EMT), certified athletic trainer (ATC), team physician, emergency department physician (EDP), primary care physician (PCP), nurse practitioner (NP) or advanced registered nurse practitioner (ARNP), and physician assistant (PA) or certified physician assistant (PA-C).

SPECIALISTS IN THE FIELD OF CONCUSSION DIAGNOSIS AND ASSESSMENT

Behavioral neurologist. A neurologist with a sub-specialization in the branch of neurology pertaining to changes in a person's behavior, personality, or intellect because of brain damage. Injuries that can lead to this type of brain damage include head trauma and concussion.

Neuropsychologist. A licensed psychologist with specialized training and/or board certification in the assessment of brain function.

Neurosurgeon. A neurologist with specialization in the areas of brain trauma and surgery.

Physiatrist. A physician who specializes in physical medicine and rehabilitation.

Sports medicine physician/doctor. A licensed medical doctor with specialized training focused on sports injuries.

DIAGNOSTIC METHODS

Glasgow Coma Scale

For years, the first tool used to determine a diagnosis of concussion, regardless of cause, was the Glasgow Coma Scale, which measures an individual's overall responsiveness and potential for recovery. This was and still is primarily used at the scene of an accident or injury as well as in emergency rooms and intensive care units. The scale measures awareness, assesses motor and verbal function, and pinpoints coma level (see Table 5.1). A score of 13 to 15 on the Glasgow Coma Scale is considered indicative of concussion. A person who scores lower than 13 is considered to be moderately or severely injured.

Interestingly, the Glasgow Coma Scale has been criticized by neurologists because it assesses a patient's condition at the time help arrives rather than immediately after injury. Many accident victims have already emerged from an unconscious or semiconscious state by the time police or medical personnel arrive. It is therefore easy to imagine that many brief blackouts—and the nerve-fiber damage that causes them—may be overlooked in the treatment of accident victims. As a result, a brain-injured person may be discharged from medical care with

TABLE 5.1. THE GLASGOW COMA SCALE

The Glasgow Coma Scale uses an individual's reactions to outside stimuli to assess the severity of brain injury. Medical personnel look for the level of response in three different categories, as detailed in the table below.

BEST RESPONSE	STIMULUS	SCORE
Opens eyes	Spontaneously	4
	In response to voice	3
	In response to pain	2
	Does not open eyes	1
Moves	In response to commands	6
	Examiner's hand away from pain site	5
	Body part away from pain site	4
	By flexing in response to pain	3
	By becoming rigid in response to pain	2
	Does not move	1
Verbalizes	In an oriented manner	5
	In a confused or disoriented manner	4
	Using inappropriate words or phrases	3
	Using incomprehensible sounds	2
	Does not verbalize	1

A person's total score equals the sum of the responses in each category, as assessed by a trained specialist. The score is then used to determine the severity of brain trauma as follows: 13 to 15, mild injury; 9 to 12, moderate injury; 3 to 8, severe injury.

more severe neurological problems than anyone realizes at the time. Further inaccuracy may come from the person evaluating the patient, whether this is being done by a neurosurgeon, emergency room physician, or someone with less training. The score may also be impacted by observations being made before or after hypotension (low blood pressure that can cause dizziness) or oxygenation (a need for increased oxygen) has been corrected. Finally, intoxicated or drug-impaired patients at first have very low Glasgow scores that correct very rapidly over the ensuing hours. Toxicity levels taken from initial blood work usually arrive long after the Glasgow evaluation is done.

Sports and Recreational Assessment Tools

With increased awareness and incidence of concussion resulting from sports and recreational activity, there has emerged a variety of assessment tools that gather pre-injury baseline information used to determine whether an athlete has sustained a concussion and whether or when he or she can return to that activity.

SPORTS CONCUSSION ASSESSMENT TOOL (SCAT 2)

This standardized assessment, also called the Sideline Concussion Assessment, was developed by the International Consensus Conference on Concussion in Sports. This tool has numerous steps, including, but not limited to, the following:

1. *Physical signs.* Was the person unconscious? If so, for how long? Has the person had a memory loss or problems with orientation?
2. *Balance assessment.* Was there a problem with balance or steadiness? One tool to assess this is the Balance Error Scoring System (BESS).
3. *Glasgow Coma Scale.* How does the victim rate?

NEUROPSYCHOLOGICAL COMPUTERIZED ASSESSMENTS

Aside from sideline assessments, there are several computerized assessments that are used post-injury in a clinic or office setting. The most frequently used assessments are:

- *Immediate Post-Concussion Assessment and Cognitive Testing (ImPACT).* This assessment tool helps doctors, trainers, and other professionals to determine an athlete's ability to return to play after suffering a concussion.
- *Concussion Resolution Index (CRI), also called HeadMinder.* This index involves a pre-season baseline measure of reaction time, memory, and other neurocognitive functions. If a concussion is suspected, a post trauma test gives the ability to statistically compare results with the athlete's baseline.
- *Axon Sports, by CogState.* This computerized tool allows team management and doctors to monitor a concussed athlete's cognitive abilities against a baseline measure taken prior to injury.

In addition, there are online methods available to a PCP or neuropsychologist for quick assessment. An example is CNS Vital Signs (CNSVS-V57). This computer-based assessment is a rapid and immediate read of a patient's neurocognitive status, or thinking ability. Another method is BrainTrain. This program's main function is as a cognitive training tool; however, it includes a quick cognitive assessment that is often helpful in evaluating a concussion.

Neurological Examination

A neurological examination is a workup done to assess a person's neurological functioning and look for signs of neurological injury. An in-depth neurological evaluation has several parts. The first step is to obtain detailed information about the circumstances of the injury and resulting symptoms. This includes a thorough medical history, including family history, prior illnesses, injuries or infections, and information about such developmental milestones as walking, talking, and social skills. Also requested is information about alcohol and medication use, as well as use of recreational substances, and any history of psychological trauma that might lead one to embellish symptoms. The neurologist also gathers information about hearing, vision, sleeping, work- or school-related interactions, and physical appearance.

Next comes a test of the cranial nerves. This provides information about vision, taste, facial expression, chewing, swallowing, balance, and the ability to speak. You may be asked to smile, follow the doctor's finger with your eyes, or listen for certain sounds during this part of the exam. Components of motor function will then be assessed, including walking, the ability to stand on one foot, blinking, mouth movements, and eye-hand coordination.

If the results of the in-depth neurological evaluation indicate that you have PCS, information will be compiled regarding your alertness, attention, memory, reasoning, judgment, and understanding. In addition, the evaluator may request specific diagnostic tests to determine the nature of the suspected brain injury. He or she may also refer you to a neuropsychologist (a psychologist with special training in the relationship between behavior and the brain) for an evaluation of your current level of functioning.

Neurodiagnostic Testing

Your physician's decision for or against neurodiagnostic testing will probably depend on such factors as the length of time you spent unconscious and the severity of your head pain, disorientation, and memory deficits. Tests can be used to pinpoint the cause of post-accident symptoms and damage to specific parts of the brain, giving both you and your doctor a better idea of what to expect in the way of a recovery process.

There are two vital components to evaluating the brain: its structure and how it is functioning. Tests that evaluate the structure of the brain look at the location of injuries to the brain, such as the gray mater, white matter, or vascular system. Tests of function, on the other hand, provide information on how well the brain is able to perform any given task, from walking and talking to communicating to adjusting blood pressure and heart rate. The following are some of the neurodiagnostic measures most frequently used with concussion patients. These are divided into tests based on blood flow in the brain and tests based on the neuroelectrical system and neuroconnectivity. The descriptions provide a brief introduction to the various methods. For more in-depth information, it is important to consult with your primary care physician (PCP) or neurologist about the diagnostic method best suited to your circumstances.

STRUCTURAL MEASURES

Skull X-Ray

This two-dimensional picture of the head is usually taken from several angles to check for the presence of a skull fracture after a head injury. This test photographs waves of low-level radiation as they pass through the affected area. The rays' passage is blocked by solid bone, which shows up as a white area on the developed film. However, X-rays easily pass through splits and cracks, so if there is a fracture, it appears on the film as one or more irregular dark lines.

The procedure is brief and painless—not unlike dental X-rays, except that the camera angle is different and you lie in a prone position to have it done. The disadvantage of a skull X-ray is that the test assesses only the brain's bony covering and yields no information about the functioning of the brain itself.

Computed Tomography (CT) Scan

This test, sometimes called a computerized axial tomography (CAT) scan, is based on X-ray technology. It is a three-dimensional imaging technique that shows much more detail than older techniques such as ultrasound and X-rays. A CT scan examines cross-sectional "slices" of the area in question and generates a series of screen images that can reveal masses, swelling, and/or bleeding within the brain.

The CT scan procedure takes less than a minute to do and uses a small amount of radiation. You lie on a half cylinder, which moves slowly into camera range with a series of brief clicks. Dye is sometimes injected to provide a clearer image of the brain, and this occasionally leads to allergic reactions. If there is a question that you may be allergic to the dye, you have two choices: ask your doctor to prescribe prednisone to prevent a reaction, or request the use of nonallergenic dye if

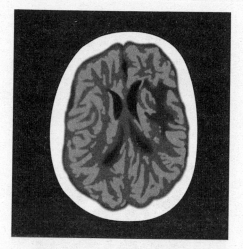

Figure 5.1. *A computed tomography (CT) scan.*

available. It is important to note that non-allergenic dye is quite costly and may not be covered by insurance. If you are highly allergic, your doctor may prefer to skip this test, since most people with a concussion do not sustain injuries severe enough to be detected by this technique. Common reasons to use a CT scan of the head are bleeding, brain injury, swelling, and skull fractures in a patient with a head injury, or bleeding caused by a ruptured or leaking aneurysm in a patient with a sudden, severe headache.

Magnetic Resonance Imaging (MRI)

Magnetic resonance imaging (MRI), a three-dimensional imaging technique, outperforms the CT scan in detecting microscopic structural changes and other abnormalities of the brain. The MRI is one of the tests most frequently used to evaluate people with a suspected concussion. It uses computer technology and an intense electromagnetic field that acts on water protons in bodily tissue to project detailed images of the area under examination.

For an MRI, you lie horizontally in a metal cylinder for between forty and ninety minutes while the imaging is done. It is not unusual for the confinement, forced motionlessness, and external machine noise to cause anxiety, so you can usually opt to take a mild sedative before the test is begun. A so-called open MRI is available that all but eliminates the claustrophobia problem.

It is important to note that there are various types of MRIs. Unfortunately, the incorrect type is often used to assess concussion. The T3/T4 MRI scan (Figure 5.2a) may be only marginally effective in detecting problems in nerve-cell tissue and body areas that contain little or no water. In contrast, susceptibility weighted imaging (SWI) provides high detail of the minute and subtle damage that is seen in a concussion. At the First International Conference of Mild Traumatic Brain Injury, in 2009, the consensus was that the SWI MRI was the imaging technique of choice for detecting structural damage of the gray matter that characterizes a concussion. (See Figure 5.2b.)

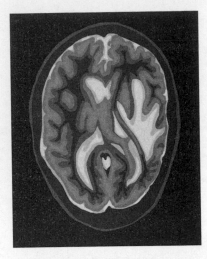

Figure 5.2a. *A T3/T4 magnetic resonance imaging (MRI) scan.*

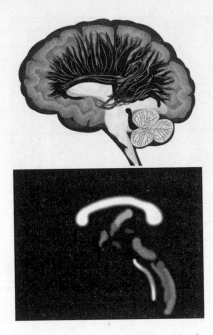

Figure 5.2b. *A susceptibility weighted imaging (SWI) MRI.*

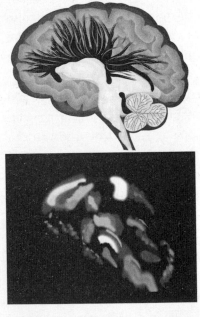

Figure 5.3. *A diffusion tensor imaging (DTI) MRI.*

Diffusion tensor imaging (DTI) is another form of MRI that is able to assess minute and subtle structural damage to and lesions of the white matter, including damage to neuroconnectivity. (See Figure 5.3.)

The DTI shows the intricate white matter neuroconnectivity along with any subtle weakened links or damage.

Magnetic Resonance Angiogram (MRA)

This imaging test is a form of MRI that uses magnetic waves to assess the structure of the vascular system and blood flow in the brain.

Cerebral Angiogram

This is a type of X-ray procedure that examines the structure of blood vessels and assesses blood flow to and within the brain. It is often done after a positive MRI or MRA, to determine the type of structural damage present in the brain.

In this technique, you are placed in restraints to ensure that your head does not move. A thin catheter is inserted in a major artery and threaded through the arterial system to the starting point of the carotid arteries; then dye can be injected selectively to one or both arteries. X-rays are taken as the dye makes its way to and through your brain. The procedure involves some discomfort, including soreness and bruising at the site of the catheter insertion and a burning sensation from the movement of the dye. As with all diagnostic tests involving dye, allergies can occasionally pose a problem. In addition, there is a small risk that a bit of plaque dislodged by the catheter may travel to the brain and cause a blockage or stroke.

FUNCTIONAL MEASURES USING BLOOD FLOW OR CEREBRAL METABOLIC RATE (CMR)

Functional Magnetic Resonance Imaging (fMRI)

As is the case with other MRI assessments, functional magnetic resonance imaging (fMRI) uses magnetic waves to make assessments. However, this test measures tiny metabolic changes that take place in an active part of the brain. It examines where and how the brain is functioning during any given task. It also determines precisely which part of the brain is handling critical functions such as thought, speech, movement, and sensation. Brain mapping is produced in color pictures of the brain's structure and function. (See Figure 5.4.)

Positron-Emission Tomography (PET) Scan

This technique also produces colored pictures of the brain's structure and function. It examines biochemistry and metabolism along with different areas of thinking activity, pinpoints the origins of seizures and other neurological problems, and evaluates any existing brain masses.

For a positron-emission tomography (PET) scan, you are injected with a glucose solution that contains a radioactive tag that makes it possible to follow the speed and path of the solution as it travels throughout the brain. You lie prone on a thin table that moves slowly into a cylinder similar to that used in a CT scan. Here, however, the machine is a receiver, feeding rays into a computer that

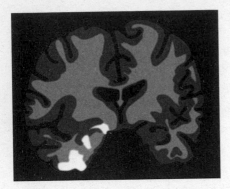

Figure 5.4. *A functional magnetic resonance imaging (fMRI) scan.*

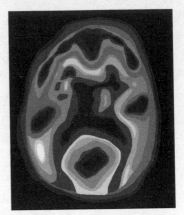

Figure 5.5. *A positron-emission tomography (PET) scan.*

analyzes data and eventually provides a three-dimensional image that is clear and precise—in effect, a picture of the brain at work. The PET scan detects irregularities in blood flow, nerve-cell activity, and the presence of oxygen. The test takes approximately one hour. (See Figure 5.5.)

Single Photon Emission Computed Tomography (SPECT) Scan

This procedure is similar to the PET scan in that it produces a three-dimensional image of the brain, although it is neither as expensive nor as precise. However, the single photon emission computed tomography (SPECT) scan does provide ready information about abnormalities and circulation within the brain. It creates an image whose color and intensity reflect the amount of circulation activity present in that area of the brain, which can be compared with scans of other brain regions. Areas of damage show less or abnormal activity compared with that in the corresponding area of the opposite hemisphere. The SPECT scan can also be used to correlate the results of other procedures, including the MRI and neuropsychological tests. Together with the MRI and neuropsychological testing, the SPECT scan is one of the procedures most frequently used to evaluate people with a suspected concussion. (See Figure 5.6.)

Magnetic Resonance Spectroscopy (MRS)

Magnetic resonance spectroscopy (MRS) uses magnetic waves to detect subtle differences and alterations in the way the brain metabolizes various chemicals to allow for neuroconnectivity. Because the subtle changes in the functions of

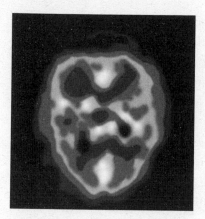

Figure 5.6. *A single photon emission computed tomography (SPECT) scan.*

neuroconnectivity can cause long-term havoc after a concussion, the focus on brain regulation is extremely important.

FUNCTIONAL MEASURES USING ELECTRICAL ACTIVITY

Electroencephalogram (EEG)

An electroencephalogram (EEG) utilizes electrodes placed on the scalp to measure the electrical activity of the brain. At the other end, they are attached to a machine that displays and prints out results. A visual inspection of the EEG printout is done to assess the frequency and distribution of brain wave forms through various areas of the brain.

In concussion cases, EEGs are used primarily to rule out such factors as seizure disorder or brain wave slowing as the cause of neurological problems (or of the injury itself). The presence of abnormal brain wave patterns or slower than normal wave movement at any point during the test signals brain damage. Different versions of this test can be done on an outpatient, inpatient, overnight, or ambulatory basis. The test takes about twenty minutes and is completely painless. However, most people with a concussion have normal EEG results, so while the test may rule out certain conditions as the cause of your problems, it probably will not bring you any closer to a specific diagnosis.

Polysomnogram

A polysomnogram is an EEG recording that is performed while you are asleep, to determine neurological changes, such as alterations in rapid eye movement (REM), frequent awakenings, or lack of dreaming. This test also provides information about restless leg syndrome, post traumatic nocturnal seizures, and narcolepsy, conditions that can disrupt sleep/wake patterns, thereby causing fatigue and making other post concussion symptoms worse.

Quantitative Electroencephalogram (qEEG)

This evaluative test is a computerized EEG that not only can detect dysregulation of neuroconnectivity, but also can determine how the brain is communicating in the various hubs, the level of communication between the hubs, and the level of function. More sophisticated and informative than an ordinary EEG, the quantitative electroencephalogram (qEEG) involves recording brain waves as signals played into a computer. The technician measures the time delay between nerve impulses moving about the brain, as well as the time it takes for signals to be transmitted from one region to another. By comparing this information with certain standards, a specialist can often detect a neurological basis for concussion symptoms, linking brain injury to brain behavior.

One of the fascinating applications of qEEG data is the Low Resolution Electromagnetic Tomography (LORETA) program, which reconfigures the data into a deep image of the brain and reveals the area of dysfunction. It displays damage due to shearing and tearing of individual neurons as well as the changes in the timing and disorganization of brain rhythms following trauma that do not show up on X-rays and are not detected by visual examination of a standard MRI. Also, the results of this evaluative test are seen as viable evidence in a court of law. The procedure takes about two hours and is painless. (See Figure 5.7.)

Other Diagnostic Procedures

In addition to the various tests described above, there are a number of other less often used tests that may be helpful in the diagnosis of concussion. The modal evoked potentials (MEP) test, an electrophysiological study of the capabilities of the brain stem (see Chapter 1), is occasionally suggested, though it is more effective in screening more serious head injuries. The transcranial Doppler (TCD) test diagnoses brain injury by viewing and assessing the flow of blood through six intracranial arteries. Magnetoencephalography (MEG) combines EEG and MRI techniques in assessing brain wave movement and brain structure. Additional, more commonly used tests are described below.

AUDIOGRAM TESTING

This test evaluates hearing loss and the ability to hear specific sounds, sensitivity to specific sounds, and the ability to hear various sounds in different environments. In addition, this test measures your ability to hear and comprehend conflicting sounds, such as two or more people talking. Difficulties in the area, also called figure/ground or auditory processing, are a common symptom of PCS.

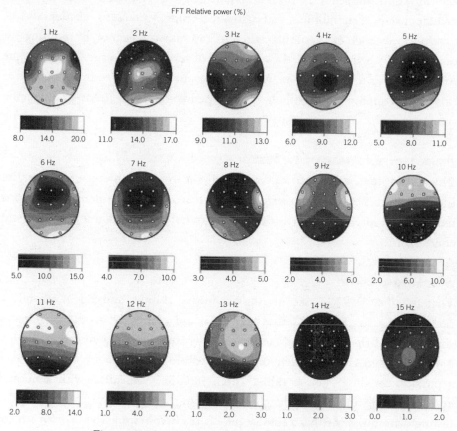

Figure 5.7. *A quantitative electroencephalogram (qEEG).*

ELECTROMYOGRAM (EMG)

This test measures the electrical activity of a muscle or a group of muscles. An electromyogram (EMG) can detect abnormal muscular activity that is caused by disease or neuromuscular conditions.

VESTIBULAR TESTING

Dizziness and a feeling of imbalance is one of the most common symptoms of PCS. Vestibular testing provides needed information on the specific cause of such symptoms. The *vestibulo-ocular reflex* (VOR), a reflex that generates eye movements that compensate for head rotations, to preserve clear vision during walking and running, is the most accessible gauge of vestibular function, which includes balance, equilibrium, and spatial reasoning. Evaluating a patient's VOR requires application of a vestibular stimulus and measurement of the resulting eye movements. There are other frequently used vestibular measures, such as the rotational chair test, where you are placed in a chair and moved in various directions. The appropriate vestibular test depends on your needs and specific symptoms.

VISUAL EVOKED POTENTIAL (VEP) TEST

This test evaluates the electrical activity of the visual pathways of your brain. Electrodes are placed on your scalp and detect electrical responses to what is seen on a monitor. This test is used to evaluate blurred vision, eye injury, and concussion.

VIRTUAL REALITY (VR)

Virtual reality (VR) is used to assess cognitive abilities and aid in rehabilitation training strategies. VR uses a camera and computers to create graphics that surround the subject and create a visually immersive environment. Participants are given the sense that they are involved in a situation that provokes a physical response, such as riding a roller coaster. VR carries with it normal and predictable results. Whether deviation from the norm is detected during VR testing determines whether a combat pilot is ready to resume flying or an athlete can return to the playing field. Delayed reaction times and abnormal motor coordination are often seen after a concussion, often corresponding to differences in brain waves when compared with the subject's baseline readings taken before injury.

One form of VR testing uses the patented KINARM product line to enable researchers to explore sensory, motor, and cognitive performance. The robotic and software tools create complex mechanical and visual worlds that can detect specific symptoms of PCS and offer recommendations for treatment.

VISUAL FIELD TEST

Visual problems are another common symptom of PCS. You may have blurred or double vision, be unable to focus, or be unaware of things around you. The visual field test can detect dysfunction in central and peripheral vision, while a vision test can detect changes in your ability to see, determine how well you focus, and measure whether you have double vision and how you see objects.

NEUROPSYCHOLOGICAL TESTING

In some cases, an exhaustive battery of neurodiagnostic tests fails to yield hard evidence of structural damage to the brain after a concussion. In other cases, repeat testing shows that signs of physical damage to the brain are improving, yet symptoms persist. At this point, it is often best to change directions—that is, to evaluate the extent, rather than the cause, of brain dysfunction. After all, you may have to live with your new limitations for some time. And regardless of the diagnosis (or lack of one), helping you cope with the injury's aftereffects should be the ultimate goal of all concerned.

A neuropsychological workup evaluates the effect of brain dysfunction on your emotional state, behavior, and mental functioning, and assesses discrepancies between your current and former skills and behavior. This evaluation provides a great deal of information about specific neurological deficits and the prognosis for recovery. The testing is done by a neuropsychologist who specializes in the emotional, behavioral, and cognitive problems that stem from brain dysfunction, and it involves a careful review of your medical history and school and employment records. This is followed by a series of tests that measure a variety of cognitive and other skills, as well as various aspects of your personality and social behavior, under conditions that mimic those of normal living—that is, in the presence of constant new information and potentially distracting outside stimuli. A comprehensive neuropsychological examination takes between six and eight hours. Some of the tests that may be used include:

- *Intelligence tests.* These tests measure verbal and nonverbal abstract reasoning and general intellectual capability. Examples include the Wechsler Adult Intelligence Scale (WAIS) and the Wechsler Intelligence Scale for Children (WISC-R).
- *Sensory perceptional function tests.* The ability to perceive sensory information can be assessed by the Halstead-Reitan Neuropsychological Battery (HRNB) subtests, the Tactual Performance Test, and the Sensory Perceptual Examination.

- *Academic skills tests.* These survey basic academic skills and reading comprehension. Examples include the Nelson-Denny Reading Comprehension Test and the Wide Range Achievement Test.
- *Language skills tests.* These tests are designed to measure your ability to understand and use language. Examples include the Peabody Picture Vocabulary Test and the Boston Naming Test.
- *Nonverbal reasoning tests.* These tests measure the ability to establish, shift, and maintain thought processes. An example is the Wisconsin Card Sorting Test.
- *Visual perception skills tests.* These tests are done to evaluate the ability to perceive visual information. An example is the Hooper Visual Organization Test.
- *Memory tests.* These tests assess verbal and nonverbal memory skills. Examples include the Wechsler Memory Scale and the California Verbal Learning Test.
- *Personality tests.* These assess personality issues related to depression and anxiety. Examples include the Beck Depression Inventory and the Minnesota Multiphasic Personality Inventory.

The results of these tests are compared with your estimated level of functioning before injury and matched with your reported neurological symptoms. The relationships among the various deficits revealed during testing are also examined. This helps the neuropsychologist to separate the effects of secondary problems, such as depression, from symptoms that are a direct result of brain trauma. Most important, this kind of evaluation can lead to specific suggestions about the treatment of symptoms—information that is much more useful than the general reassurances typically heard after a diagnostic workup. Neuropsychologists are perhaps the best source of information about rehabilitation and coping techniques, and can suggest approaches to recovery that are tailored to your particular needs.

DISSENT AMONG DIAGNOSTICIANS

Unfortunately, while today's technology and improved testing procedures have yielded welcome evidence that there *is* a physical cause behind the symptoms of

PCS, doctors and scientists still disagree on diagnostic procedure. One of the reasons for this is the small, but nevertheless significant, number of cases in which recovery from a concussion fails to correlate with test results and follow-up procedures. Sometimes, for instance, memory loss persists despite an improvement in the results of a patient's MRI. Or word-finding problems fail to fade at the same rate as signs of injury to the brain's speech centers. Circumstances like these lead to professional debate about many issues, among them the following:

- Are CT scans always a logical first step in the diagnosis of a concussion?
- Should MRIs and electrophysiological tests be used routinely, and if so, which type is best: the T3/T4, SWI, or DAI?
- How far should diagnostic procedures be pursued when early exams are negative?
- How valid are the various tests as prognostic and follow-up tools?
- Do alternative practices like chiropractic, acupuncture, and natural remedies have a place in the evaluation and treatment of a concussion?

The newest diagnostic techniques, such as brain imaging and electrophysiological tests, are time-consuming, costly, and available at only a relatively small number of hospitals. In today's tight financial climate, health care professionals look carefully at the cost-effectiveness of such tests, which often involve not only the use of expensive equipment but also the transporting of the patient to a private facility some distance away. Particularly if you seem to be recovering at a more or less normal pace, your doctor may be unable to justify the expense of pursuing a specific diagnosis. He or she may also be hesitant about recommending alternative approaches, such as chiropractic, acupuncture, or herbology, the effectiveness of which varies, and which have been subject to limited documentation and research.

Some medical professionals also question the effect on patients of doing every test available. There is a significant stress factor involved in many diagnostic procedures—they may be uncomfortable, and they raise the possibility of a discouraging diagnosis. For better or worse, therefore, physicians often guard against doing more testing than is absolutely necessary. Some practitioners may even hesitate to pursue testing that will spell out the precise causes of concussion-related symptoms because of concerns that graphic descriptions of brain injury may lead to psychosomatic complaints that will hinder a patient's recovery.

DIAGNOSTIC AND ASSESSMENT SUMMARY

With increased awareness of the dangers of concussion, coaches, trainers, and parents no longer brush off or minimize the fact that a child has been knocked out briefly during play. While in most such cases, children recover quickly and are perfectly fine, it is possible for a child to experience residual PCS from a seemingly minor blow to the head. If there is any doubt, or if a child exhibits behavior changes after injury, he or she should be seen promptly by a doctor with a background in concussion.

If you or a family member has symptoms of PCS, the proper diagnostic test often depends on the cause of injury. If the concussion is from a motor vehicle accident, fall, or occupational injury where it may be legally necessary to prove your injury, it is important to have the following tests done to evaluate the brain both structurally and functionally:

- CT scan, SWI MRI, and DTI MRI
- Neuropsychological testing
- Evaluation by a neurologist and a psychologist
- qEEG

Each of the above tests holds up as evidence in a court of law and is needed to prove the existence of a concussion and the extent to which it is affecting your life.

If your injury occurred during sports or recreation, the following methods can measure your current ability and help determine when you can safely return to that sport or activity:

- SCAT 2
- Evaluation by an athletic trainer, PCP, sports medicine doctor, neurologist, and/or neuropsychologist
- Neurocognitive testing such as ImPACT, HeadMinder, etc.
- CT scan and T3/T4 MRI
- Neurological evaluation

If ongoing symptoms occur, an SWI MRI may be needed; however, this is usually not necessary if the existence of injury is not being questioned.

Only when the source of dysregulation of the brain's neuroconnectivity has been identified, both structurally and functionally, can a proper treatment program be developed. The chapter that follows will describe the various professionals, methods, and approaches for the treatment of concussion.

CHAPTER 6

APPROACHES TO TREATING POST CONCUSSION SYNDROME (PCS)

C HOOSING AN APPROACH TO TREATING *POST CONCUSSION SYNDROME* (PCS) can be a daunting challenge. Your primary care physician (PCP), neurologist, sports medicine doctor, trainer, family members, or friends can offer advice, and you may spend hours on end searching the Internet for information and help. An added challenge is whether or not a definitive diagnosis can be made to pinpoint the cause of lingering symptoms that change your life for as long as they persist. You and your family will sense major differences in how you think and react, and it may soon become apparent that recovery will likely be a long, tedious process.

Fortunately, there are many different treatment approaches that may be helpful. In addition to a wide range of conventional medical therapies typically covered by insurance, such as medication and physical therapy, there are also complementary treatments, which may or may not be covered by insurance, as well as alternative approaches that are not covered but may nevertheless be very beneficial. It is extremely important to keep in mind that each person is unique and that the circumstances and conditions are different for each case of PCS. The method of treatment that may work for one person may not necessarily be helpful to another; in fact, it may even be harmful in some cases. The methods or treatments that are right for you depend on the nature of your symptoms, your personal health care preferences, and other factors. It is worth noting that no single treatment, whether conventional, complementary, or alternative in nature, relieves every symptom for every person with PCS. Nor does any particular combination of approaches guarantee a faster recovery from long-term problems with thinking, reasoning, and understanding. However, thorough and proper diagnosis, evaluation, education, a strong will to recover, and the development of a strong support system, combined with restorative sleep, exercise, proper nutrition, and stress reduction are vital components of progress in the months after injury.

To maximize your chances for successful recovery, you will want to ally yourself with a neurologist or other practitioner who specializes in treating brain injury, and who is non-intimidating, sympathetic, and, above all, willing to coordinate rehabilitation efforts with other health care professionals. Once you have found such a professional, you and your family can turn your attention to choosing an approach or combination of approaches to wellness. As you do so, you should keep in mind that there are many dimensions to the aftereffects of PCS. That is why I developed a Five-Pronged Approach for my patients that, regardless of the presenting problem or situation, helps me to see every individual as unique from five distinct perspectives:

Physical
Psychological
Emotional
Spiritual
Energy

Often, these five areas intertwine, and each needs to be addressed during the journey to recovery. I usually look for a core issue that becomes the vantage point to choosing a path to overcoming life's challenges and returning to wellness. Along with my Five-Pronged Approach, I believe in pursuing an integrative brain rehabilitation where there is acceptance of and openness to a balance of conventional, complementary, and alternative approaches to treatment. Slowly but surely, professionals in the field are arriving at the same conclusion; in fact, in many major cities, it is common to find a department of complementary or integrative medicine as part of a rehabilitation hospital, or to see classes that include such alternative approaches as Reiki.

Regardless of approach, it is imperative to treat not only an individual's physical condition, but his or her cognitive (mental) function and emotional state as well. Treating the whole person appears to be the surest route to overall wellness.

BRAIN REHABILITATION

Brain rehabilitation aims to return the person with a concussion (also called *mild traumatic brain injury*, or mTBI) or PCS to his or her former levels of functioning. Various types of practitioners provide rehabilitative services, including physical, occupational, and vocational therapists; speech/language pathologists; and special education professionals. Brain rehabilitation can involve cognitive retraining—the relearning of skills in ways that make allowances for your limitations—or the approach can be educational, involving practice and exercises to gradually improve memory, visual and motor ability, concentration, and academic skills. Commonly recommended types of rehabilitative work include medication, physical therapy, craniosacral therapy, massage, occupational therapy, vocational therapy, speech therapy, cognitive remediation, nutrition counseling, acupuncture, Reiki, and special education. In addition, hyperbaric oxygen therapy is often recommended.

Conventional Approaches

The appropriate means of treating your symptoms from PCS depend on the kinds of difficulties you are experiencing and on your perspective on health care. There are several approaches to recovery that are commonly recommended by physicians. These techniques may be used individually or in conjunction with other treatments. Rehabilitative medicine and psychotherapy are two major approaches in this area.

MEDICATION

The Food and Drug Administration–approved prescription or over-the-counter medication most appropriate for your symptoms needs to be thoroughly discussed with a behavioral neurologist, sports medicine doctor, or physiatrist (a medical doctor specializing in rehabilitation medicine). When treating a concussion, medication can also be used to improve motor function, depression, cognition, and memory, along with helping a patient with pain management. Once again, each person requires therapy tailored to suit his or her specific needs.

It is extremely important to avoid taking medication someone else might be using for the same symptom, because each patient is unique, and the wrong medication can possibly cause your symptoms to become worse. Also, it is important to note that once you have had more than one concussion, any medication that affects the central nervous system (CNS) can have detrimental effects and can cause additional symptoms you did not have before. It is very important to check the potential side effects of any medication before you take it.

There are also behavioral aspects to each patient that should be carefully observed by the treating physician. An understanding and thoughtful clinician has more to do with the effectiveness and outcome of treatment than the number of credentials the doctor possesses. The following are examples of concussion medications best selected by symptoms.

Treatment of Severe Agitation

- *Antipsychotic agents.* These are reluctantly used and generally avoided unless agitation is so severe that the patient cannot rest or sleep and leaving the patient in this state could be more adverse than treatment. These agents exert potent effects, but have powerful side effects as well. Particular caution should be used in the elderly and those patients with disturbances of heart rhythm. Examples of currently used agents include quetiapine (Seroquel), olanzapine (Zyprexa), and aripiprazole (Abilify). Older antipsychotics such as haloperidol (Haldol) are still used in the hospital setting but should be avoided whenever possible. Antipsychotic agents carry warnings that prolonged use can cause movement disorders and can lead to paradoxical rebound agitation in the TBI patient, which means that the medication designed to calm a person can actally have the opposite effect and cause the person to feel more anxious, jittery, and fearful than before.

- *Benzodiazepines.* This class is the Valium family of medications. They are used to produce sedation in anxious patients and somnolence when patients can't sleep. Benzodiazepines can also treat vertigo and tremors. They should be used cautiously with the TBI patient because they can induce rebound agitation after a short period of sedation, along with contributing to cognitive impairments. Generally speaking, both antipsychotics and benzodiazepines are avoided as first-choice treatments. There are alternative methods, such as the use of a Vail Bed, which is totally enclosed, that assist the treating staff during the recovery of a very severely agitated TBI patient.

- *Anticonvulsants.* These were originally employed to treat seizures but are very useful in the treatment of head injury. They are particularly useful in the treatment of aggression, the promotion of mood stability, the improvement of cognition, and the treatment of bipolar disorder. Commonly used examples are valproic acid (Depakote), oxcarbazepine (Trileptal), levetiracetam (Keppra), and topiramate (Topamax). Older examples include phenytoin (Dilantin) and carbamazepine (Tegretol). Side effects of anticonvulsants may include nausea, vomiting, lack of coordination, slowness of thinking, insomnia, somnolence, weight gain or loss, mild to severe rashes, and rapid involuntary eye movements. Skilled clinicians watch keenly for side effects. Good communication among patient, family, and physician is very important when this medication is prescribed.

PHYSICAL THERAPY (PT)

Physical therapy (PT) is often suggested for injury-related neck pain and whiplash injuries. A therapist trained in muscle rehabilitation guides you through a series of exercises designed to improve motion, reduce pain, and prevent disability. Craniosacral treatment, massage, and water therapy, in which water keeps the body buoyant and keeps pressure off the neck, are three popular techniques. Other treatments used by physical therapists include hot packs, ice massage, ultrasound, and therapeutic exercises. Also, many rehabilitation hospitals now include hyperbaric oxygen therapy in patients' recovery from brain trauma.

- *Craniosacral therapy.* Developed by Dr. John Upledger, this therapy employs the concept of dynamic activity and relationship within the craniosacral system that includes cerebro-spinal fluid (CSF), which surrounds the brain and supports and lubricates the spinal nervous system as it flows down the back through a sheath around the spinal cord. Craniosacral therapy is a technique based on cranial osteopathy; therapists believe that the natural movements of the skull bones come from the membrane that lines our nervous system structures leading to the brain and spinal cord. Improving the natural rhythmic movement helps to improve brain functioning.
- *Massage therapy.* Neuromuscular massage is a form of deep tissue massage that is applied to individual muscles. It is used to increase blood flow, reduce pain, and release pressure on nerves caused by injuries to muscles and other soft tissue. Along with neuromuscular massage, there are two other methods that improve the symptoms of PCS. One is reflexology, an ancient form of Chinese massage that is done on the feet and/or hands, activating acupressure points by applying pressure to reflex areas that correspond to specific organs and other parts of the body. This stimulates the release of endorphins throughout the entire body, reducing stress and returning the body to equilibrium. Another method is Structural Integrative Massage, a combination of neuromuscular massage, craniosacral therapy, reflexology, and structural alignment that works to gently realign bones, relax muscles, and increase

joint mobility to help restore harmony and regulation to the brain. Muscle Release Technique is another extremely beneficial massage approach.

- *Water therapy (aquatic therapy).* Water is a great healer and is the ideal medium for rehabilitation, conditioning, and training. The hydrostatic (passive) and hydrodynamic (active) properties of water provide an optimal environment for safe, effective therapy and conditioning. Bearing little or no weight in the water, an injured patient is able to return to desired activities quickly and safely. Among many forms of water therapy (also known as aquatic therapy), a standout is the Burdenko method, developed by Dr. Igor Burdenko, who is known worldwide and is the founder and chairman of the Burdenko Water and Sports Therapy Institute. He has worked as a rehabilitation and training consultant to numerous athletes from professional and Olympic teams, as well as top international dancers and figure skaters. Dr. Burdenko is also on the board of directors of the National Youth Sports Safety Foundation.

Physical therapy and massage services are provided by licensed therapists, (PTs, DPTs, or PTAs) and by massage therapists, or MTs. A physical therapist has a masters or clinical doctorate and national license. They work under a physician's supervision in a private, school, or hospital setting. Physical Therapy Assistants (PTAs), who have an associate's degree and national certification, provide massage, strength, mobility, and other services under the direction of a PT/DPT. An MT, who is trained in anatomy but not rehabilitative medicine, works in a private setting and applies therapeutic movements to the muscles.

OCCUPATIONAL THERAPY (OT)

Occupational therapy (OT) is designed to evaluate and address the physical, cognitive, psychosocial, sensory-perceptual, and other aspects of a patient's performance in a variety of environments. Together with the patient and family, an occupational therapist will help determine the best ways to perform daily living tasks including showering, dressing, and attending to personal hygiene. The therapist will identify equipment that can help the patient eat, dress, and bathe. In addition, OT helps an individual adapt to educational and classroom environments and the workplace. OT can also be used to help brain-injured adults to improve their fine motor and social skills and learn new techniques for managing everyday responsibilities such as shopping and household chores, as well as new ways of performing various job tasks and how to avoid re-injury.

The registered licensed occupational therapist (OTR/L) who provides this rehabilitation has an educational background similar to that of a physical therapist. A Certified Occupational Therapy Assistant (COTA), who works under the supervision of an OTR, gathers information about the patient and collaborates with the OTR to develop an intervention plan.

VOCATIONAL THERAPY

This approach is most often used to evaluate past vocational or educational performance. Unlike OT, which increases a person's overall ability to function, vocational therapy targets a person's employment prospects, teaching new or different work skills and/or identifying job alternatives for those whose skills have undergone a change.

Vocational therapy is provided by a certified vocational counselor (CVC) or certified vocational educator (CVE). Such a practitioner has a bachelor's degree plus additional course work in employment retraining. A vocational therapist can practice in either a rehabilitation hospital or a private setting.

SPEECH/LANGUAGE THERAPY

This type of therapy helps to resolve communication and hearing disorders. A speech/language pathologist, who should be licensed and state certified, provides evaluation, assessment, and treatment of speech functions, including articulation, prosody (the rhythm, stress, and intonation of speech), and rate, and well as language abilities, such as reading, writing, speaking, understanding, and proficiency in the alternative communication systems. Cognition is also evaluated and treated, as are problems with voice, swallowing, and social communication skills. Each therapist devises an individual treatment plan consisting of education, tasks, and exercises to improve concentration, memory, speech, comprehension, and listening skills. The goal of treatment is to improve skills and learn compensatory strategies that will help any individual become more independent with regard to daily tasks.

COGNITIVE REMEDIATION

The focus of cognitive remediation is to help an individual acquire tools and strategies necessary to improve thinking, executive functioning, time management, and decision-making. In cognitive remediation, you are helped to modify your environment to minimize the effects of your brain injury on everyday functioning. For instance, a job change, lighter course load, or reliance upon maps and lists might be recommended. You are also taught to remind others that you have difficulty recalling telephone numbers, screening out background noise, or whatever. This type of treatment is offered by speech/language pathologists, occupational therapists, and rehabilitation psychologists with specialized training in health psychology and rehabilitative techniques.

RECREATIONAL THERAPY (RT)

This type of therapy complements PT and OT using cognitive remediation, with a focus on enhancing emotional, social, and leisure development so the individual can participate fully and independently in chosen life pursuits. The unique feature of this therapy is the use of recreational activities. Although many treatment goals that a recreational therapist may work toward are similar to those of other therapists on the rehabilitation team, the recreational therapist incorporates the patient's unique interests in the treatment plan.

A qualified recreational therapist is nationally accredited as a certified therapeutic recreation specialist (CTRS). This is done through the National Council for Therapeutic Recreation Certification (NCTRC), which requires a bachelor's degree or higher from an accredited university, a formal internship, and the passing of a national certification examination. In addition, a CTRS must go through the NCTRC recertification process every five years in order to maintain his or her credentials.

EXPRESSIVE THERAPY

This form of therapy uses art, music, dance, and psychodrama as a means of regulating the brain. Throughout history, the fine arts have been used to benefit the brain and soul. Recently, it has been shown that specific music pieces, such as Mozart's sonata K488, can help reduce anxiety and seizure disorders. This is called the "Mozart effect."

Art, music, and dance therapy provide a productive release and a pathway to help heal the brain. Also, when the brain's language center has been dysregulated or damaged, psychodrama, art, music, or dance therapy provides a means of communication and a release of emotions along with an improvement in working memory.

An expressive therapist usually has a master's degree that entails training in art, music, dance, or drama as well as specialized training in rehabilitation therapy. He or she is knowledgeable about human development, psychological theory, clinical practice, spiritual, multicultural and artistic traditions, and the healing potential of art. Therapists use art in treatment, assessment, and research, and provide consultation to allied professionals.

Specialization in art therapy is approved by the American Art Therapy Association (AATA), with graduates eligible for certification as music therapists. Dance therapy specialization is approved by the American Dance Therapy Association (ADTA), while the psychodrama/drama specialization is currently being reviewed for approval by the North American Drama Therapy Association (NADTA).

NUTRITION

What you eat is very important to your recovery from a concussion, because diet impacts your heart/brain balance and brain regulation. Chapter 1 described the brain's vascular network and neuroconnectivity, and it is important to understand that certain foods can affect and even worsen dysregulation in these areas. Refined sugar, corn syrup, artificial sweeteners, alcohol, wine, and beer all fall into this category.

Injury to the brain causes an inflammatory response and dysregulates the hormonal and endocrine systems. What you eat eventually enters the bloodstream, affects your body's systems, and can either reduce or increase inflammation in the brain. For example, eating foods that contain omega-3 fatty acid—such as flaxseed, chia seeds, krill oil, walnuts, butter from the milk of grass-fed cows, wild salmon, sardines, and tuna—helps the brain. Coconut oil also has unique fatty acids that reduce inflammation. Conversely, consumption of omega-6 fatty acid (found in beef, for instance) should be reduced.

A good source of information on nutrition and recovery from concussion is the book *Your Healthy Brain*, by Stephen Kiraly, M.D., which has a chapter devoted to this topic. The Tufts University Friedman School of Nutrition also provides information in a pamphlet called "The Heart-Brain Diet." A book devoted solely to brain-building foods and recipes for concussion patients is *Nourish Your Noggin*, by Tina M. Sullivan.

The link between nutrition and recovery from brain injury is becoming widely known and accepted. Proof of this is the fact that the Institute of Medicine (IOM), an independent nonprofit organization that provides unbiased and authoritative advice to decision makers and the public, has been asked by the

Department of Defense and the Defense Centers of Excellence to research nutrition as it relates to concussion and post traumatic stress disorder (PTSD). Both of these conditions, of course, are of significant concern to the military.

Dietitians, nutritionists, and nutrition educators are specialists who can help you learn about the best foods to promote brain regulation. The terms *dietician* and *nutritionist* are often interchangeable. Nutrition educators may have additional training in Nutrition Response Testing.

Most of these specialists are certified or licensed and work either in rehabilitation facilities or privately. You may also wish to consider seeing an endocrinologist, a medical doctor who specializes in the hormonal and endocrine systems and understands the impact of inflammation on the brain.

Regardless of whom you choose to consult, it is extremely important to ensure that they have knowledge of and experience with brain injury and that they possess the most current information on specific foods that help with brain regulation.

HYPERBARIC MEDICINE, OR HYPERBARIC OXYGEN THERAPY (HBOT)

As discussed in Chapter 1, oxygen is the key component to a healthy brain. When there is not enough oxygen going to the brain, it causes dysregulation. An example is a frightened person who begins to pant, or hyperventilate, possibly passing out due to too little oxygen reaching the brain.

Hyperbaric medicine, now called hyperbaric oxygen therapy (HBOT), was developed as a means of dealing with decompression sickness. This therapy consists of sitting or lying in an airtight chamber while 100 percent oxygen is administered under increased and meticulously controlled conditions.

The air we breathe contains a small percentage of oxygen, and breathing 100 percent oxygen in a normal room increases blood oxygen levels by 3 to 5 percent. Breathing pure oxygen in an environment of increased pressure delivers twenty to thirty times that amount to the body's tissues. When the effectiveness of HBOT on decompression sickness was seen, other applications were tested. As an example, HBOT proved to be very effective in healing wounds quickly, because the higher-than-normal pressure and concentration of oxygen promoted more efficient absorption into body tissue. With this information, HBOT is now being used to enhance tissue affected by poor circulation, such as brain tissue damaged by stroke or head injury.

There are various forms of HBOT, and HBOT equipment can be located at a general or specialized hospital and is often covered by insurance when prescribed as part of your recovery program. There is also a form called the HBOT bag chamber, which is not approved by the Food and Drug Administration.

SPECIAL EDUCATION

Special education is often used to help children find new approaches to academic work. However, adults who need to compensate for sudden neurological deficits can also benefit from evaluation and instruction in the use of computers and other compensatory strategies. A special educator must have a bachelor's or master's degree in special education in order to be certified in most states. Special education is typically provided in schools and rehabilitation hospitals.

PSYCHOTHERAPY

Psychotherapy helps you to deal with behavioral or emotional problems and psychological reactions to life events. There are several types of, or approaches to, psychotherapeutic treatment. These include health psychology (behavioral medicine), traditional "talk therapy," and medication therapy (psychopharmacology).

For psychotherapy following a concussion, it is important to select a mental health professional (or, if needed, a team of mental health professionals) with knowledge of the treatment of symptoms of PCS, PTSD, and grief or bereavement of loss of self. Also, you may wish to consult a psychiatrist—a medical doctor who holds a state license and, in most cases, board certification in a specialty such as psychopharmacology. A psychiatrist is licensed to prescribe medication and has expertise in the diagnosis, treatment, and prevention of emotional, behavioral, and mental disorders. Alternatively, psychotherapy may be performed by a psychologist, a state-licensed professional with a Ph.D., Psy.D., or Ed.D. degree, who may also hold board certification in a specialty such as behavioral medicine—a sub-specialty of psychology dealing with factors of physical and mental health as they apply to disease prevention, health promotion, etiology or possible cause of the problem, diagnosis, treatment, and rehabilitation.

Another sub-specialty is neuropsychology, performed by a licensed psychologist (neuropsychologist) with extensive training in the anatomy, physiology, and pathology of the nervous system. A clinical neuropsychologist specializes in evaluating and treating problems with nervous system function, assessing the effect of brain dysfunction on your emotional state, behavior, and mental capacity as compared with your former skills and behaviors. A behavioral neuropsychologist applies the knowledge gained from the neurological assessment to the recommendation of various forms of treatment. A psychologist or neuropsychologist does not prescribe medication but has training in cognitive and emotional assessment and the management of attitude and behavior problems.

Other types of practitioners who offer mental health services include clinical social workers, psychiatric nurses, and marriage and family counselors. A clinical social worker (LCSW or LICSW) holds a state license and a master's degree and may also possess board certification in a specialty such as geriatric care. A social worker does not prescribe medication but has training in family systems therapy and group therapy, as well as expertise in the diagnosis, treatment, and prevention of emotional and mental disorders.

A psychiatric nurse holds a master's degree in psychiatric mental health nursing and is certified as an adult clinical specialist (MSN, RN, CS). With special certification, a psychiatric nurse can prescribe and administer medication. An MSN, RN, CS has expertise in medical issues as well as the diagnosis, treatment, and prevention of emotional and mental disorders.

A marriage, family, and child counselor; professional counselor; or marriage and family therapist needs no degree, though most have at least a bachelor's degree. The initials LMFCC, LPC, or LMFT following such a practitioner's name and degree refer to certification or licensing by state boards in that specialty. These counselors and therapists have expertise in family and marital issues.

Because it can be difficult to determine whether psychological symptoms are new or were present prior to injury—and because recommended treatments differ accordingly—psychotherapy for a person with a concussion should be provided only by a licensed mental health professional who has training in and experience with PCS and the effects of PTSD.

Psychopharmacology

This facet of the psychotherapy field, sometimes called drug or medication therapy, includes the use of medications to help change or regulate mental activity, mood, and behavior. Antidepressants and antianxiety agents are among the most commonly prescribed psychopharmacologic drugs. Among mental health professionals, psychiatrists, who have medical degrees in addition to psychological training, and psychiatric nurses can prescribe drug therapy. Psychopharmacologists are psychiatrists who specialize in the use of medications to lessen or eliminate psychological, neurological, and behavioral problems.

Traditional Psychotherapy

Traditional psychotherapy can help you to identify, understand, and cope with the symptoms and consequences of a concussion. There are various approaches to psychotherapy, each with its own theories and methods. Insight therapy, for instance, helps you to understand why things occur, while client-centered therapy provides you with an appreciation of yourself. Some therapies overlap. The use of role-playing and family counseling may be indicated as well.

The length, duration, and setting of psychotherapy depend on the individual's particular needs. As a rule, therapist/patient dialogue ("talk therapy") and stress-management training can be helpful to people with PCS. Whatever type of psychotherapy you choose, it is important to select a mental health care provider who has special training in and experience with the aftermath of a concussion.

The following types of psychotherapy have been found to be highly effective in treating the interconnected effects of PCS and PTSD symptoms:

- *Cognitive behavioral therapy* (CBT) was developed by Dr. Albert Ellis and originally called rational emotive behavioral therapy. It is a form of talk therapy. Dr. Ellis believed that our thoughts cause our reality and behavior; thus, you can either heighten or lessen the symptoms of PCS depending on how you think about them. The aim of CBT is to look at symptoms and solve problems with dysfunctional emotions, behaviors, and cognitions through a goal-oriented systematic procedure that is concerned with the here and now.
- *Dialectical behavior therapy* (DBT) is a combination of cognitive behavioral therapy and techniques for emotional regulation. This therapy, also called mindfulness therapy, was developed by Marsha M. Linehan, a psychology research professional at the University of Washington. Her therapy, which includes meditative practices, promotes the calming of the brain and helps reduce the fight/flight reaction that characterizes PTSD.
- *Eye movement desensitization and reprocessing* (EMDR) was developed by Dr. Francine Shapiro. This form of talk therapy includes an integrative eight-phase approach to disconnecting the emotional and physical reaction to a traumatic event from the thought of the event. This method of identifying the mind/body and emotional triggers that heighten PCS symptoms

provides tools to work through and sever this connection. This type of therapy is done by a mental health professional specifically trained in EMDR, or by a graduate student under the supervision of a licensed clinician.

Behavioral Medicine, or Health Psychology

This specialty deals with social, psychological, behavioral, and biomedical factors related to physical and mental health. Behavioral medicine services should be provided by a psychologist certified by the American Board of Professional Psychology (ABPP). One of the many techniques used in this field of psychology is biofeedback, which is performed by a specialist called a psychophysiologist.

Since the publication of *Coping with Mild Traumatic Brain Injury*, enormous advances have been made in the use of biofeedback, and specifically neurofeedback, to help the dysregulated brain to become regulated again. (See the "Biofeedback" section included below under "Complementary Approaches.") As mentioned in Chapter 5, the quantitative electroencephalogram (qEEG) and the qEEG/LORETA allow for a functional mapping of the brain. Another method is the Low Energy Neurofeedback System (LENS), which also assesses and maps the brain to pinpoint areas that are regulated or dysregulated. BrainAvatar, another method, allows for real-time three-dimensional images and training of the brain to achieve a state of regulation.

ADDITIONAL SPECIALISTS WHO TREAT SYMPTOMS OF POST CONCUSSION SYNDROME (PCS)

- *Neurosurgeon.* A licensed medical doctor with board certification in a subspecialty that focuses on the prevention, diagnosis, treatment, and rehabilitation of disorders that affect a portion of the nervous system, including the brain, spinal cord, peripheral nerves, and extracranial cerebrovascular system (the blood system that surrounds the brain).
- *Ophthalmologist.* A licensed medical doctor with board certification who deals with the anatomy, physiology, and diseases of the eye and who specializes in medical and surgical eye problems.
- *Neuro-ophthalmologist.* An ophthalmologist with a sub-specialization that deals with the diagnosis, treatment, and rehabilitation of disorders and issues that affect or stem from the nervous system, such as the visual symptoms of PCS.

- *Audiologist.* A licensed professional in audiology who holds either a doctor of audiology degree (Au.D.) or has supervised clinical practice as well as graduate course work in audiology that includes anatomy, physiology, physics, genetics, normal and abnormal communication development, diagnosis and treatment, pharmacology, and ethics. This professional deals with the diagnosis, treatment, and rehabilitation of disorders related to hearing and auditory processing that are common symptoms of PCS.

Complementary Approaches

Conventional medicine is certainly the most familiar approach to health care in the United States. However, there are other approaches to wellness that are based on different perspectives regarding the interaction between mind and body. Two major methods of health care are the complementary approach and the alternative approach. The distinction is in the general acceptance of these approaches by practitioners of conventional medicine and the availability of insurance coverage. As stated earlier, conventional approaches are covered by insurance, while complementary treatments may or may not be covered by insurance, and alternative approaches are not covered. Many of the alternative approaches described in our earlier book, *Coping with Mild Traumatic Brain Injury*, are now considered internationally to be complementary. Those methods and others now considered alternative do not necessarily oppose conventional medical wisdom. In fact, they are often used in conjunction with conventional approaches (for instance, Reiki can be used to increase the effectiveness of pain medication).

ACUPUNCTURE

This practice uses the principles of traditional Chinese medicine, which focuses on the flow of the body's natural energy, or *qi* (pronounced *chee*), as a key influence on health. First, an evaluation is done, which may include questions and answers, pulse-taking, abdominal palpation, and examination of the tongue, skin color, and body odor. Based on the results of the evaluation, a treatment plan is devised involving the head and scalp, ears, or other parts of the body. Hair-fine needles or topical herbal heat treatments may be used to stimulate points along the path of *qi*, thus helping the body heal through the harmonious flow of energy. One form of acupuncture, *auricular acupuncture*, involves gentle electrical stimulation of points in the ear.

The credentials of acupuncturists vary from state to state. Most states require at least a bachelor's degree, including premedical courses; some require two to three additional years of postgraduate work and a master's degree in acupuncture for a state license. The abbreviations L.Ac. or Lic.Ac. following an acupuncturist's degree indicate licensing, while Dipl.Ac. indicates board certification.

BIOFEEDBACK

Biofeedback uses information gained by monitoring skin temperature, blood pressure, heart rate, brain waves, and other body conditions to promote control over normally involuntary bodily processes through conditioning and relaxation. There are several types of biofeedback: heart rate variability (HRV), neurological (EEG), muscular (EMG), and thermal. All employ some type of computer or monitoring device along with electronic sensors to give information about what is going on in the body. Heart rate variability, or respiration, training provides feedback of information that promotes relaxation and calming, which have a positive effect on heart function. Thermal biofeedback indicates physical changes such as alterations in pulse rate, blood flow, and body temperature. Hemoencephalography measures blood flow and oxygenation. EMG biofeedback indicates changes in muscular movement, while EEG biofeedback, often called neurofeedback, shows changes in brain wave activity. These changes are usually indicated through visual graphs, sounds, or colors on a feedback display.

Using biofeedback devices is akin to looking in a mirror that shows your inner responses rather than your outer appearance. For example, you cannot ordinarily influence your brain wave activity because you have no information about it. However, when you can see instantaneous information about your brain function on a computer screen, you have the ability to positively influence that function. The appropriate type of biofeedback for treating symptoms varies according to their nature and cause. The following is a detailed list of each type, so that you and your practitioner can choose the best method for you:

- *Heart rate variability* (HRV) training is most commonly used to increase relaxation and reduce the fight/flight reaction of PCS and PTSD. A sensor or sensors are placed on your ear or finger. Through breathing techniques, you learn to control your heart rate, and this ability triggers a signal to the vagus nerve from the heart to the *amygdala* in the *limbic system* to relax. Two well-researched and effective products are the emWave, from HeartMath, and the Journey to the Wild Divine: The Passage, from Wild Divine. While both of these methods measure heart rate, the Wild Divine also uses galvanic skin response, a technique that tracks various types of activity in parts of the body.

- *Hemoencephalography* (HEG) measures brain blood oxygenation and facilitates training to provide greater blood flow to the *frontal lobes*, thereby enhancing concentration, memory, and emotion control. There are two types of HEG, near-infrared (nIR) spectroscopy and passive infrared (pIR) spectroscopy. While both types measure cerebral blood oxygenation, they vary in the way this is done. NIR spectroscopy, developed by Dr. Hershel Toomin, the developer of the HEG techniques, measures changes in the local oxygenation level of the blood. A headband is used that contains an optical sender and sensor. PIR spectroscopy, developed by Dr. Jeffrey Carmen, uses a similar sensor to detect light from a narrow band of the infrared spectrum that corresponds to the amount of heat being generated by an active brain region as well as the local blood oxygenation level. In either method, you feel nothing but are asked to perform a task and concentrate on a computer interactive presentation. For instance, in Dr. Carmen's method, you watch your favorite DVD, but when you lose focus the movie stops. HEG is used to reduce the PCS symptoms of migraine pain and depression, reduce PTSD symptoms, and improve memory.

- *Electromyography* (EMG) biofeedback measures muscle/brain electrical response. There are two basic applications of EMG recording: neurological EMG, involving the measurement of muscle response timing following artificial stimulation of a motor point, and kinesiological EMG, which involves measuring muscle activity during functional limb movements, postural tasks, and exercise training. These methods are used for pain management, mobility, and PCS problems with posture, gait, and limb movement.

- *Neurofeedback*, also known as electroencephalography (EEG) biofeedback or neurotherapy, is a technology-based learning technique that uses a computer to provide instant information about your own EEG activity. Neurofeedback helps retrain the brain, reducing problematic brain wave activity and increasing healthier activity, as discussed in Chapter 1. When the brain is dysregulated, evidence shows up in EEG activity. Neurofeedback assists you in altering brain wave characteristics by challenging your brain to reorganize and function more efficiently. Neurofeedback helps to restore the brain's more regulated, harmonious state that existed prior to injury. This is done through varied computerized methods, from graphic displays to auditory and visual feedback and electromagnetic waves. A full program of neurofeedback training takes between twenty and one hundred sessions, depending on symptom severity, time elapsed since injury, and prior medical/mental health history. Practitioners who offer biofeedback and/or neurofeedback services should be licensed health care professionals with additional specialized training. When choosing a provider, it is wise to inquire about licensing and whether the practitioner has certification from the Biofeedback Certification International Alliance (BCIA). There is a wide variety of neurofeedback methods, some of which are used alone and some of which can be used in combination with another method to produce very beneficial results. The following are descriptions of each.

Traditional neurofeedback is similar to weight training, where you work specific muscle groups. In traditional neurofeedback, you are training one or more specific brain waves in a targeted area of the brain. This method is based on *operant conditioning* to help retrain the brain waves to optimal levels. Within this type of neurofeedback are variations such as the Othmer method, developed by Dr. Siegfried Othmer and Sue Othmer, that isolates a wide variety of frequencies and trains only one specific frequency, similarly training one specific muscle. Another method, developed by Dr. Kirtley Thornton, trains only the high Gamma frequencies to work together.

There are two forms of traditional neurofeedback. One involves seeing a trained professional who can customize and adjust a program for your specific brain dysregulation, using various traditional neurofeedback methods such as low-frequency training. The other form involves prepackaged neurofeedback equipment for audio-visual entrainment (AVE), which has blinking lights that can cause seizures. Therefore, it is imperative that you not purchase AVE equipment or try to use it yourself without first consulting your neurologist.

The Low Energy Neurofeedback System (LENS) is a form of neurofeedback designed to improve brain function by locating specific areas that are stuck in dysregulation and promoting feedback to restore optimal functioning. This method is similar to using a massage therapist, who can locate where your body is stuck and then work from the least injured area to the problem area. Then, working from the least to most impacted brain locations, the brain is gradually regulated. In LENS, a map is created to assess where the brain is most dysregulated. LENS produces its effects through a tiny electromagnetic field. The feedback is only 1/400th of the strength of that received when holding a cell phone to the ear and about the intensity of output from a watch battery. Feedback travels in one-second intervals down an electrode wire while you remain still with your eyes closed, feeling nothing. Advantages of the LENS approach include the production of faster results, its suitability for very young children, and that it does not require long periods of focus on a computer screen.

Live Z-score training is similar to a fitness class where you work out with other people and compare your ability to theirs. Live Z-score training is a form of traditional neurofeedback that continuously compares your brain function to norms for average functioning at your age. This method can be very effective at returning the brain to a regulated pattern through an integrative training program. Some of the software, such as BrainAvatar, includes a real-time three-dimensional image of training, thus allowing the professional to make real-time adjustments with the patient being trained.

NeuroField is similar to LENS, because it is designed to help the brain's dysregulation. However, where LENS can be compared to going to a massage therapist, this method is like submerging your body in a hot tub. Instead of using water to produce relaxation, NeuroField uses an electromagnetic field to encourage the brain to engage its own restorative systems in returning to a balanced, *homeostatic* state. Specific amplitude and frequency changes can be measured for the purpose of guiding the brain so that it functions more effectively. NeuroField was designed to promote a healthy brain/body balance. Its electromagnetic field surrounds the brain with various frequencies that help physical and cognitive interactions to become regulated.

Personal Roshi (pRoshi) is a light/sound machine used to disrupt dysregulated patterns in the brain. Four LED lights in each visual field of a pair of glasses flash at varying speeds, helping the brain to break the pattern of current dysfunction. The glasses also emit electromagnetic frequencies. This technology provides pre-set programs to help the brain restore itself, and also helps with sleep disorders and seizures.

Thermal biofeedback is hand-temperature training that promotes relaxation and healing. This technique employs the phenomenon that our muscles retain more blood when tense; however, they allow blood to flow to the periphery of the body when we relax, thus allowing a warming of the hands.

BRAIN-COMPUTER INTERFACE (BCI)

A brain-computer interface (BCI) is a pathway of direct communication between the brain and an external device, first devised by Dr. Hans Berger, a neurologist who developed electroencephalography in 1924. Dr. Berger was the first to record an EEG, and by analyzing the results he was able to identify different waves, or rhythms, present in the brain. His first device was very simple, consisting of silver wires inserted beneath the scalps of his patients. Unlike neurofeedback, which retrains the brain, BCI operates through specially designed headgear or an electrode implant that allows a person, through the creation of a brain wave pattern, to control an external device such as a light, a computer, or an artificial limb.

CRANIAL ELECTROTHERAPY STIMULATION (CES)

Cranial electrotherapy stimulation (CES) involves a medical device approved by the Food and Drug Administration to treat insomnia, depression, and anxiety. It consists of a small box that applies pulsed electric current to the brain at a specific frequency through wires attached to your earlobes or the area behind your ears on special pads. CES has been in clinical use worldwide since the 1960s and is safe, noninvasive, nonaddictive, and has no pharmaceutical side effects. Alpha-Stim was the first to develop a product for pain frequency, while other companies, such as Mind Alive and Health Directions, produce devices for depression, sleep, and anxiety.

SELF-CONTROLLED ENERGO NEURO ADAPTIVE REGULATION (SCENAR)

This form of electrical biofeedback speaks to the body through electrical impulse signals that are modified based on changes detected at the skin's surface, such as reddening or numbness. Signals are sent to the body through the skin, based on changes within the body, and reflected back to the surface of the skin. This causes the body to move toward a more normative state. Self-controlled energo neuro adaptive regulation (SCENAR), developed by Dr. Alexander Karasev for use in the Russian space program, employs signals that are modified depending on what happened in the past—a backward-looking technology that is viewed as reorganizing. The newer Cosmodic technology of adaptive regulation looks ahead to the body's target state of response, so it is more regenerative in nature. In Russia, SCENAR is considered a conventional, rather than complementary, approach and is currently used as a principal treatment instrument.

CHIROPRACTIC

This practice is based on the premise that pressure on nerves exiting the spinal column can cause neurological and circulatory problems throughout the body. Chiropractic involves manipulation of the spine to restore free movement and nerve functioning, thereby relieving a host of disorders and symptoms. This type of treatment is performed by licensed chiropractors, who are doctors of chiropractic and who have had four years of classroom and clinical training beyond college.

In cases of PCS, a chiropractor may order an EEG, MRI, or other diagnostic test, in addition to a cineradiogram (a motion X-ray that determines the degree of trauma to the neck). This is done to rule out the possibility of structural problems that may result in further damage from certain treatments or movements. In addition to spinal manipulation, chiropractic techniques include soft tissue massage and stretching, as well as osseous (bone) treatments done with the hands or small tools. Techniques vary according to the type of injury, the practitioner's preferences and physical strength, and the patient's body type.

HYPNOSIS

This technique, also called hypnotherapy, is helpful for pain reduction and uses an altered state of consciousness to teach responses to and control over various trigger conditions. Because concentration and a peaceful mind are necessary for hypnosis to work, and because a main symptom of PCS is the inability to stay focused, this particular problem must be addressed before undergoing hypnotherapy. This technique can be used by someone who has undergone training. However, it is highly recommended that you locate a mental health professional with knowledge of PCS and PTSD, certification from the American Society of Clinical Hypnosis (ASCH), and board certification in the use of the technique.

INTERACTIVE METRONOME

This brain-based rehabilitation assessment and training program was developed to directly improve the neurological processing abilities that affect attention, motor planning, and sequencing that are central to human activity—from the coordinated movements needed to walk, to the ordering of words in a sentence. This in turn strengthens motor skills, including mobility and gross motor function, as well as many fundamental cognitive skills, such as planning, organizing, and language. The program uses neurosensory and neuromotor exercises to improve the brain's inherent ability to repair or remodel itself through neuroplasticity. Through a structured, goal-oriented process, the patient is challenged to synchronize a range of hand and foot exercises to a precise, computer-generated reference tone heard through headphones, and attempts to match the rhythmic beat with repetitive motor actions. Feedback is measured in milliseconds and a score is provided, helping the patient learn to focus attention for longer periods, increase stamina, filter out distractions, and improve the ability to monitor his or her mental and physical actions.

LIGHT THERAPY

This process, also called phototherapy, uses light waves to activate or inhibit the effectiveness of the mitochondria—the powerhouse within each of our cells. The best source of phototherapy, of course, is the sun, but its harmful side effects from ultraviolet (UV) rays led to the concept of using light and color to heal. Kate Baldwin, M.D., at Women's Hospital in Philadelphia, was among the first to use this treatment to heal wounds and restore health and body regulation. Since then, Spectro-Chrome therapy was developed, using colored lights to target a host of disorders and symptoms, as was light-emitting diode (LED) therapy, using light that spreads out with distance, and laser therapy, which employs an organized beam of light that stays consistent over distance. In addition, there are devices that combine visible and infrared light therapies to combat the symptoms of PCS, such as the Q1000 and the Quantumwave Laser. Also highly effective is Ochs Labs' LED Photonic Stimulator, which provides single-wavelength infrared light therapy and is used for depression and anxiety.

SOUND THERAPY

Stimulating the auditory pathways and the brain improves hearing and auditory processing—an area of frequent frustration in people with PCS. There are many methods and techniques used in sound therapy. The following have been shown to be very effective:

- *The Tomatis method* is the most comprehensive and well researched of all auditory stimulation programs. Developed by the French ear, nose, and throat specialist Dr. Alfred Tomatis over fifty years ago, this method uses electronically modified music to re-educate the listening system. By stimulating and improving the way a patient processes auditory information, progress is made in his or her ability to listen and communicate.

- *Bilateral sounds* is a method for helping the brain become unstuck and regulated. This method is very effective for re-educating the left and right hemispheres, as well as for relieving stress and symptoms of PCS and PTSD. A web-based company, PsychInnovations, produces some commonly used bilateral sounds for this purpose.
- *Hemi-Sync* was developed by Robert A. Monroe to help integrate and regulate the brain. Monroe observed that certain sounds create a frequency-following response in the brain's electrical activity, and he used this information to create his product. Both Hemi-Sync sounds and music are highly effective against many symptoms of PCS, including problems with restorative sleep.
- *Swingle Sounds* was developed by Dr. Paul G. Swingle, a leader in the field of neurofeedback and an authority in the field of low sound pressure psychoactive acoustics. This technique uses subliminal sounds as auditory feedback along with specific frequencies to enhance brain regulation. Dr. Swingle and his methods were instrumental in my own recovery from concussion.
- *Bio Acoustical Utilization Device* (BAUD) therapy was developed by Dr. Frank Lawlis. It uses specially designed frequencies and waveforms to quickly stimulate neuroplasticity in a targeted way. Research shows that this therapy is effective for chronic pain, depression, and other symptoms of PCS.

Alternative Approaches

Alternative approaches to wellness after a concussion are best tried after a diagnosis has been made through conventional and complementary means and after conventional therapeutic approaches have been tried. Most alternative approaches to coping with PCS are individualized treatments that focus on the natural healing of the whole person rather than correcting individual symptoms. As such, alternative approaches can offer additional paths to relief from lingering complaints, as well as a stronger measure of control over your recovery. The techniques discussed below have been used successfully for PCS.

BODYWORK

This approach differs from conventional massage and its subtypes in that it focuses on neurological integration through body movement. There are two major types of bodywork, as follows.

- *The Feldenkrais method*, originally developed by Moshe Feldenkrais, is based on principles of physics, neurology, and physiology, and the conditions under which the nervous system learns best. Feldenkrais is recognized for the strategies it employs to improve posture, flexibility, coordination, chronic pain, and tension, along with neurological, developmental, and psychological problems. Many symptoms of PCS are reduced or eliminated through this method.

- *The Bowen Technique*, developed in 1950 by Tom Bowen, helps the body remember how to heal itself. The gentle yet powerful Bowen moves send neurological impulses to the brain, resulting in immediate responses of muscle relaxation and pain reduction. The moves create energy surges that, when sent to the nervous system, remind the body to regain normal movement in joints, muscles, and tendons. This helps relieve muscle spasms and inflammation.

ENERGY HEALING

This technique, also called biofields energy healing, involves the natural, subtle energy field (*qi*, pronounced *chee*) that surrounds and exists within a person. The International Society for the Study of Subtle Energies and Energy Medicine (ISSSEEM) was formed in 1989 to study the basic sciences and medical and therapeutic applications of subtle energies, including energetic and informational interactions resulting from self-regulation and other energy couplings of mind and body. It is known that energy pulses from the environment—for instance, low-level changes in magnetic, electric, electromagnetic, acoustic, and gravitational fields—often have a profound effect on both biology and psychology. In addition, it has been documented that people are capable of generating and controlling not-yet-measurable energies that seem to influence physiologic and psychical mechanisms. The following methods of energy healing are very effective for treating the symptoms of PCS and PTSD:

- *The Callahan Techniques*, now called Thought Field Therapy (TFT), were developed in the 1970s by Dr. Roger Callahan. Trained in both cognitive behavioral therapy and hypnosis, Dr. Callahan realized that when phobias or other symptoms shown by his patients were more severe or related to PTSD, the left brain and right brain became interconnected and "stuck" in the trauma, resulting in a wide array of problems. Using his knowledge of acupuncture meridians and their connections to specific emotions, Dr. Callahan developed techniques that employ a pattern of meridian points, eye movements, counting, and humming to reduce the impact of thoughts about the traumatic event on the body. This is highly effective against many symptoms of PCS and PTSD and started a wave of similar methods generally referred to as energy psychology.

- *Emotional Freedom Techniques* (EFT) were developed by Gary Craig, who was trained by Dr. Callahan. EFT is similar to TFT, but it uses a comprehensive acupoint tapping recipe rather than diagnosing treatment points in each person. EFT's results are often rapid and lasting in the treatment of depression, insomnia, and PTSD.

- *Energy medicine*, founded and developed by Donna Eden and Dr. David Feinstein, heals the body by activating its natural healing energies and by restoring energies that have become weak, disturbed, or out of balance. To accomplish this, energy medicine uses techniques from healing methods such as acupuncture, yoga, kinesiology, and Qi Gong. The various approaches in energy medicine work well against the symptoms of PCS and PTSD.

- *Energy psychology* is a term coined by Fred P. Gallo, Ph.D., who was trained by Dr. Callahan. Dr. Gallo's approach, sometimes referred to as Energy Diagnostic and Treatment Methods and/or NeuroSomatic Stimulation, is a combination of TFT that uses acupuncture points along with applied kinesiology using muscle testing to examine how a person's bodily energies are functioning. This approach also incorporates cognitive behavioral and mindfulness principles to balance the body's energy systems in relation to emotion, cognition, behavior, and health. Dr. Gallo's books *Energy Tapping* and *Energy Tapping for Trauma* offer excellent concepts and techniques for dealing with the symptoms of PCS and PTSD.

- *Kyusho* is an ancient form of Chinese self-defense and healing that involves the tapping of acupuncture points and is an excellent method of self-protection, especially after a concussion. Kyusho is effective in healing many symptoms of PCS and PTSD.

- *Reiki* is a form of energy healing that was developed in Japan in 1922. Reiki comes from two Japanese words: *rei*, which means "God's wisdom," and *ki*, which means "life-force energy." Thus, Reiki is actually spiritually guided life-force energy, similar to the laying on of hands to allow the life force to heal the body. In Reiki, the patient is passive and the practitioner active in the healing process. It is very effective for stress reduction and relaxation.

- *Polarity therapy* is based on the Eastern philosophy that everyone has an internal blueprint that controls everything from personal achievement to healing. The goal of this therapy is to identify blockages of internal energy and treat the resulting symptoms by placing you in better touch with your internal blueprint. Once back in balance, the body can better heal itself. A typical session lasts forty-five minutes to an hour, during which you lie on a polarity table while a practitioner uses Therapeutic Touch to increase your relaxation response and hasten healing. Polarity therapists should be certified by the American Polarity Therapy Association (APTA).

- *Qi Gong*, pronounced *Chee Gong*, was developed in China and, along with acupuncture, was for centuries the main form of healing of physical and psychological diseases and problems. Qi Gong is a system of exercises that incorporates physical postures, breathing techniques, and focused intentions to balance the energy in the body. It is used to improve health and has been known to help people alleviate pain and stress. The movements of Qi Gong reduce stress, build stamina, increase vitality, and enhance the immune system.

- *Therapeutic Touch* (TT) was developed by Dora Kunz and Dr. Dolores Krieger in 1979. TT is very similar to Qi Gong and Reiki. The method, first developed for use with cancer patients, involves a person remaining passive while the practitioner moves a hand over the body to detect and move the energy field. Research has shown that TT is useful in reducing pain, improving wound healing, aiding relaxation, and relieving symptoms of trauma associated with PCS and PTSD.

- *Quantum-Touch* is a method that focuses and amplifies life-force energy (*qi*, bioenergy, or *prana*) by combining various breathing and energy-awareness exercises. Quantum-Touch healers learn to increase and direct a person's life-force energy, facilitating the body's own healing process.

EYEQ

This software consists of a series of high-speed imaging exercises that use graphics and text to improve the brain's learning and processing abilities. EyeQ exercises promote concentration, focus, and memory much like physical exercise helps an athlete's performance. It is highly effective in recovering from a wide range of PCS symptoms, and it also improves performance afterward in the workplace, classroom, or sport/recreational activity. In fact, EyeQ is popular among athletes because it enhances peripheral vision and reaction time. In addition, it can improve reading speed and comprehension and increase the ability to process information quickly and efficiently.

FAITH HEALING

Faith healing is a way of improving health through spiritual means. Many people throughout the world have found vast relief from symptoms of PCS and PTSD through this alternative. Faith healing can include the laying on of hands, which is described in the Bible as the blessing of healing by a spiritual leader through actual touch or intent. Also included is prayer, an active solemn request to God or a deity. Research done in 1993 by psychologist Dr. Larry Dossey showed the effectiveness of prayer in healing many forms of illness, including the symptoms of PCS and PTSD.

HERBOLOGY

This practice combines age-old insight into healing with modern pharmacological research. An herbalist assesses your symptoms and treats them with herbal remedies tailored to your individual needs—for example, prescribing relaxing herbs for muscle tension or severe headaches. Herbal medicines originate from plant leaves, roots, and/or bark often boiled into soup or tea form. Today, many herbs are also prepared in tincture, powder, or pill form. No specific training is required of herbalists, though some states offer optional certification programs. It is recommended that you thoroughly check an herbalist's experience level before taking his or her advice.

HOMEOPATHY

This approach is based on the view that symptoms provide information about the body's attempts to heal itself. Homeopathic treatment involves the use of remedies made from naturally occurring substances that would cause particular symptoms if taken in large amounts, but that stimulate the curing of those same symptoms if taken in minute amounts in a highly diluted form. Before prescribing treatment, a homeopath evaluates symptoms according to their placement on certain mental, emotional, and physical planes. He or she will listen and observe as you speak in general about the influences in your life, and will be interested in the minute details of your symptoms. How you present this information is as significant to the practitioner as what you say. Upon evaluating your symptoms, a homeopath will prescribe a remedy or combination of remedies to stimulate your body's natural self-healing capacity.

Only three states—Arizona, Connecticut, and Nevada—have specific licensing boards for homeopathic physicians (DHts). Other states require homeopathic practitioners to have some form of certification or course work, though guidelines and requirements vary widely. It is wise, therefore, to inquire about credentials before working with a homeopath.

IRLEN METHOD

This method, developed by Helen Irlen, uses colored lenses to help with scotopic sensitivity syndrome, problems with the brain's ability to process visual information that involves light sensitivity. This symptom is one of the aftereffects of PCS, and the Irlen method is a highly effective treatment.

LIFE VESSEL/LIFE FORCE

This approach combines vibration energy, using sound and light frequencies, with Rife electrical therapy (see page 82). The patient lies in a box to receive simultaneous vibrations, sound, and light that creates a resonant frequency by which the body's autonomic nervous system comes into balance and is re-regulated. Treatment sessions vary, as different protocols are followed for specific symptoms of PCS.

NATUROPATHY

This method is based on the belief that the body has an innate healing ability. Naturopathic doctors, or N.D.s, teach their patients to use diet, exercise, lifestyle changes, and cutting-edge natural therapies to enhance their ability to ward off and combat disease. One approach, neurotransmitter/amino acid therapy, targets the neurotransmitters and neuromodulators discussed in Chapter 1, delivering specific amino acids that help combat various symptoms of PCS. The N.D. views the whole person rather than a specific symptom or disease and uses various forms of complementary and alternative methods of treatment, having been trained to work with other practitioners in those fields. N.D.s are trained in the art and science of natural health care at accredited medical colleges. Integrative partnerships between conventional M.D.s and licensed N.D.s are becoming more available.

LACE (LISTENING AND COMMUNICATION ENHANCEMENT)

LACE, an acronym for Listening and Communication Enhancement, was conceived by audiologists at the University of California at San Francisco. LACE includes interactive computerized aural rehabilitation programs that help people living with hearing loss increase listening skills by up to 45 percent. Since hearing is really done in the brain, and since a major symptom of PCS is difficulty with auditory processing, LACE develops skills and strategies for situations in which hearing is inadequate—just as physical therapy helps compensate for physical weakness or injury.

RIFE THERAPY

Rife is a form of electrical therapy in which specific electrical frequency protocols are used to relieve certain illnesses and the symptoms seen in PCS and PTSD. The Rife Machine was invented by Royal Raymond Rife in 1930.

SOLARIS HEALTH BLANKET

This device was based on Dr. Wilhelm Reich's research in the 1940s and re-emerged within the Russian space program when it was discovered that cosmonauts tended to recover from strenuous activity more quickly when they remained in their space suits longer. The Health Blanket contains reflective metallic material similar to that used in the lining of space suits and helps to activate and balance energy flow throughout the body. The blanket material acts as an electromagnetic mirror, reflecting the body's energy and optimizing adaptive reactions. It is highly effective in promoting recovery from PCS and PTSD.

VIBRATION THERAPY

Vibration therapy can take several forms. The following are vibration therapies that are beneficial in helping symptoms that can linger after a concussion:

- *Aromatherapy using essential oils.* Essential oils were the first medicines written about in Egypt and China, and the Bible contains 188 references to them. Aromatherapy is the practice of using natural oils extracted from flowers, bark, stems, leaves, roots, or other plant parts to enhance psychological and physical well-being. This approach works well against many of the symptoms of PCS and PTSD.

- *Bach Flower Remedies.* These remedies were developed in 1926 by Edward Bach, M.D., a physician, bacteriologist, and homeopath. His thirty-eight Bach Flower Remedies each include a specific flower essence that works in a way similar to homeopathic treatments. You can purchase Bach Flower Remedies over the counter to combat many symptoms of PCS and PTSD. However, for the best results, you may wish to visit a trained Bach Flower practitioner, who will develop a customized combination specifically for your symptoms. Such practitioners have more than two years of training and are registered with the Bach Centre as Bach Foundation Registered Practitioners. Some use the letters BFRP after their names.

CHOOSING A TREATMENT APPROACH

"What helped me? In 1994, I was told that I was permanently brain injured, and the only treatment offered was physical therapy and medication. I was never offered the wide variety of methods presented in this chapter, and in sheer desperation I started my own search for other approaches that could help me.

Because of my training as a neuropsychologist and health psychologist, I knew how important good nutrition was for the brain. Nutritional therapy was the first method I used, and I believe it made—and continues to make—an enormous difference in my symptoms. Since my accident in 1998, I've had additional concussions, as well as Lyme disease, which causes inflammation that also impacts the brain. To help with the PCS symptoms I've experienced, each of which is described in upcoming chapters, I have used most of the treatment methods described above and have found them to be very helpful. However, the fact that each person and each brain injury is unique keeps me from recommending any one method."

—D.R.S.

When considering your health care options, you should thoroughly research any and all treatments or approaches, whether conventional, complementary, or alternative. You need as much information as possible about procedures, costs, risk factors, and projected results in order to make informed choices. It is wise to consult with other people who have had concussions about their opinions and experiences. While no two people should expect the same recovery experience, it is a good idea to find out what is and is not working for friends and support-group contacts. Ask prospective practitioners about the possibility of contacting other patients or clients under their care to learn about their experiences. Additional information about people's experiences can be found through a local brain injury support group as well as online bulletin boards, newsgroups, chat rooms, or websites.

Finally, be prepared to be flexible. If you give an approach a fair trial without experiencing any improvement, or if you feel that a practitioner is either unsympathetic or underinformed about post concussion issues, you are justified in looking elsewhere for help.

FINDING THE RIGHT PRACTITIONER

Securing the services of the best practitioner or practitioners to treat your PCS symptoms can be quite difficult because of the number of options available and because initial evaluations and treatment are often done in a crisis situation over which you have no control. However, the selection of the right professional can have a significant impact on the length and speed of recovery from lingering symptoms.

Once you have received a tentative diagnosis of concussion and have decided upon an appropriate path toward recovery, the next step is to find someone in the chosen area who specializes in treating people with PCS and its unique symptoms. Doing so will guarantee a more refined diagnosis and, in many cases, more immediate relief from lingering discomfort or problems. The guidelines that follow can facilitate the decision-making process:

- Ask your primary health care provider (the family physician or other practitioner who sees to your routine health care needs) for advice and referrals. He or she can make recommendations based upon research into the treatment of concussion, your medical history, and, possibly, familiarity with the practitioner or practitioners you are considering. This advice can be invaluable.
- Make a point of seeking practitioners who have a thorough understanding of, and experience with, PCS and its symptoms. Always interview a prospective doctor or other practitioner to find out about his or her attitude toward, and experience with, the treatment of post concussion symptoms. (See "Assessing a Practitioner's Expertise with Concussion," page 85, for a list of suggested questions to ask.) When dealing with PCS, your health care providers' expertise can directly affect the outcome of treatment.

- Look for practitioners who are open to cooperating and coordinating treatments with professionals in other areas. This is particularly important if you are interested in pursuing complementary or alternative treatment approaches. Physicians are often skeptical about such things as herbology or acupuncture, or even chiropractic treatment or the use of nutritional supplements. Yet many of the most successful recoveries are the result of a team approach, in which a number of professionals cooperate out of concern for all aspects of the patient's health.

- Include key family members in the process of choosing a practitioner or practitioners. Be aware that brain trauma can interfere with your judgment and reasoning. It helps to have someone else, who can be objective, assist you with decision-making.

- Consider contacting me for a referral that can provide helpful details and direct you to many conventional and alternative treatments. (See my contact information on page 367.)

Assessing a Practitioner's Expertise with Concussion

Research into the lingering aftereffects of PCS is well documented, yet many doctors and other specialists lack expertise in diagnosing and treating the varied and sometimes elusive symptoms of this sort of injury. However, you are more likely to experience a complete recovery under the treatment of someone who has training and experience with concussion.

The following are some suggested questions to help you determine a prospective practitioner's level of expertise with PCS:

- *How many cases of PCS have you personally been involved with in the past three years?* If the practitioner lacks experience with PCS, look further.

- *What percentage of your practice is devoted to concussion patients?* Thirty percent or more is optimal. Less than 5 percent means that you should continue your search.

- *Have you attended any seminars or conferences during the past two years that involved concussion and specifically PCS?* Ideally, the answer should be yes. If it isn't, do not continue with this practitioner.

- *Have you written any articles on concussion in the past three years?* If the answer is yes, ask what types of articles. Publication does not signal good clinical experience.

- *Which resources do you refer to for information about PCS?* Take a look at any online resources that are mentioned. If a text or manual is cited, check the publication date. Developments in the field are ongoing, and your practitioner should be accessing the most current information.
- *Do you read or subscribe to* The Challenge *magazine, published by the Brain Injury Association;* Brain Injury Journal, *by published by the International Brain Injury Association;* The Perspectives Network *magazine, and/or any other periodicals about brain injury?* Routine reading of a TBI journal or magazine does not necessarily reflect a practitioner's competence, but it is desirable.

The greater a practitioner's interest in and recent experience with concussion, the better prepared he or she will be to assess your symptoms and prescribe and monitor your treatment.

As further study is done into the nature, range, and duration of PCS aftereffects, the medical community has become increasingly aware of the broad scope of this type of injury. Each concussion is unique. This makes both a tailor-made recovery approach and a diligent search for the right professional team imperative. In the chapters that follow, we will look in detail at many of the specific symptoms that are often seen in individuals with PCS, along with the types of treatment approaches that have been shown to be helpful for each one.

PART 2

PHYSICAL ASPECTS

PREFACE
SYMPTOMS OF POST CONCUSSION SYNDROME (PCS)

■

S PORTS AND RECREATIONAL INJURIES, ALONG WITH BLAST INJURIES, HAVE brought an awareness to the world of concussion (also known as *mild traumatic brain injury*, or mTBI) as well as its consequences, known as *post concussion syndrome* (PCS) or, in some parts of the world, post concussion disorder. Due to media attention and an increase in these types of injuries, the symptoms of PCS are recognized and understood to a greater degree than at the time *Coping with Mild Traumatic Brain Injury* was published.

Part 1 of this book included breakthrough research that characterizes the brain as dynamic rather than static, and amenable to healing rather than "once damaged, always damaged." With today's neuro-imaging, we know what happens when the brain is injured and understand how the injury relates to the wide variety of symptoms seen as part of PCS. Parts 2 through 4 cover the various symptoms of PCS. Physical symptoms are described in Part 2, while Part 3 covers the mental aspects of such an injury. In Part 4, information is given on the emotional aspect of PCS. Each of these sections includes real-life stories, a description of the nature of each problem, the reason it occurs, and how it can be identified and treated. These details will help you and your family to understand what you are experiencing and make informed choices about treatment of your symptoms.

INTRODUCTION

■

TERRIE HAD BEEN WORKING FOR FOUR MONTHS AT A TRANSITIONAL HOME FOR adults with traumatic brain injury in Maine. She learned a great deal about brain injuries, but then an auto accident taught her a great deal more.

On a rainy August morning, a squirrel ran in front of her car, which was traveling at about thirty miles per hour. Terrie hit the brakes, and her car hydroplaned and spun around three times before coming to rest against a rock wall. While the car was spinning, Terrie's body twisted and her ear struck the side window, but she was able to get out of the car afterward. When she did, onlookers noticed that she was swaying, and she complained of dizziness and neck pain.

Terrie lost consciousness on the way to the hospital. After undergoing X-rays and some observation, she was sent home—even though she could barely walk. In the weeks that followed, Terrie slept a lot and experienced headaches, hip pain, blurred vision, dizziness, fatigue, and numbness from her neck down into her arm. It felt as if someone were poking an ice pick into her left ear. The doctor never mentioned a brain injury, instead commenting that she looked fine. After Terrie spent two weeks on pain medication, the doctor extended her prescription and recommended that she go on disability.

Six weeks after her accident, Terrie met a doctor of osteopathic medicine (D.O.), who told her that her problems stemmed from *post concussion syndrome* (PCS). Despite this very telling diagnosis, Terrie was eventually fired from her job because she could no longer drive to work. She comments that people with concussion, also called *mild traumatic brain injury* (mTBI), are the true walking wounded—they look just as they did before, but have changed a great deal.

Because the various symptoms of PCS seem in such contradiction to an individual's outward appearance of well-being and good health, there is a need to understand and learn how to cope with the many limitations that can be imposed by this type of injury. Happily, there are several avenues through which this can be accomplished—among them education, conventional medical treatment, complementary and alternative approaches, and lifestyle modifications. Part 2 of this book covers specific physical symptoms and consequences of a concussion.

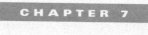
FATIGUE

G AIL WAS A 45-YEAR-OLD MARINE BIOLOGIST FROM OREGON WHEN SHE WAS broadsided while driving home from work and struck her head. Weeks after her accident, she struggled to live hour to hour, rather than day to day as in the past. Even going to the bathroom seemed like an ordeal.

Gail's fatigue is the biggest problem she faces as a result of her concussion, also called *mild traumatic brain injury* (mTBI). Because she is tired all the time, her possibilities for rehabilitation are limited. Gail has noticed that when she is tired, she doesn't cope well, sleep well, see well, or even speak properly. Gail's fatigue is worse during fine motor activities. In fact, writing a single check exhausts her more than scrubbing floors, because check writing calls for writing on lines, forming letters and numbers, knowing the date, and folding and inserting checks into stamped, addressed envelopes.

Gail wonders how to explain that she has a disability that does not affect her outward appearance but that keeps her from doing things she once was able to do. It is very difficult for her to convince people that her debilitating fatigue is a real consequence of her concussion.

When you have had an active day or a later-than-usual night, the sleepy, yawning feeling that follows is a signal that your body needs rest. The fatigue that so often accompanies a concussion is very different. Post concussion fatigue fogs your mind, saps your energy, deadens your limbs, and brings on an overwhelming need to sleep whenever and wherever the feeling strikes. The sleep you crave is often elusive and fragmented, however, and does little or nothing to relieve your bone-weariness and state of confusion.

Fatigue occurs three times as often among brain-injured people as it does among the uninjured population. Yet it is initially less noticeable than, say, balance problems or chronic headaches. As a result, it is frequently overlooked as an injury aftereffect. It is also easily misidentified. Post concussion fatigue is particularly easy to overlook during the initial recovery period, when you are likely to rest frequently as you nurse your visible injuries. However, once you attempt to resume your previous pace, your sleep-defying exhaustion quickly becomes apparent.

WHY FATIGUE CAN OCCUR AFTER A CONCUSSION

Much research has been done on both acute and chronic fatigue, but it remains unclear why people often have no reserve energy, or "second wind," after a brain injury. It is not known whether there is simply no energy left to use or whether the brain is unable to access it. There are some theories that this lack of reserve energy is due to failure of the *limbic input* to integrate with the motor functions affecting the *frontal cortical system*. Put more simply, the fight/flight area of the brain is overactive and is using up all of a person's energy and causing a disconnect in thinking processes. Regardless of the cause, we do know that once a person with a concussion uses up his or her energy, it takes longer to recharge than in the past—up to several days, in many cases.

You may feel extraordinarily tired if your concussion affects your ability to fall asleep or disrupts your customary sleep/wake cycle. This is a common complaint, because sleep patterns are fragile and can easily be affected by brain injury. A new awareness of the importance of restorative sleep has led to the inclusion of a chapter (Chapter 9) devoted to problems with sleeping in the aftermath of a concussion.

WHAT POST CONCUSSION FATIGUE IS LIKE

"Prior to my concussion, I maintained a very busy day. I would rise at 7:00 a.m., get my children off to school, go to the gym for two hours, have lunch, see five or six patients a day, and do supervision. After dinner, I would spend time with my family and end the night by writing progress notes on my patients until 12:00 a.m. Even at that hour, I had enough energy left to play my guitar and talk on the phone with friends.

After my concussion, I spent the first two months sleeping nineteen hours a day. When I was up, I felt very fatigued all the time. Even after several months, my energy was limited to the hours between 8:00 a.m. and noon. By 1:00 p.m., the fog started rolling in, making me feel inefficient or, at worst, spacey. By 3:00 p.m., my day was virtually over.

It took several years for the aforementioned fatigue to diminish. Eventually, I was able to resume my daily routine, until subsequent concussions caused consequences anew. However, there is always hope for recovery and living life again. At this writing, I am able to once again resume the lifestyle I had."

—D.R.S.

The fatigue that follows a concussion is lethargy in its most extreme form. It affects all aspects of your thinking, your physical abilities, and your emotional ability to cope with life. Many people with this type of fatigue first suspect a virus or a bad case of burnout, particularly if they fail to connect their exhaustion with other post concussion symptoms like headaches or neck pain. You may feel completely drained, as if you cannot make it through the day. Because fatigue affects your brain's ability to integrate information, your thoughts and responses may be as sluggish as your movements. You may sense that you have lost your mental stamina—that is, your power of concentration, your memory, and your sense of motivation. Your moods may also be affected, because frustrations mount—and your ability to deal with them diminishes—as your efficiency and productivity decline. Your ability to coordinate movements like walking and driving may be severely affected as well.

Like many people who have suffered a concussion, you may find yourself battling your exhaustion with frequent naps, caffeine, and lots of carbohydrates and sugary snacks. But these and other tactics, which provide an energy boost under normal circumstances, now fail to bring on that second wind. In fact, what you are eating is probably causing your symptoms to worsen, particularly if you are eating anything with sugar in it. The energy reserves that you normally depend on have suddenly vanished. Instead, you are likely to find that it takes several days to recover expended energy and that you have just a few "good" hours a day—usually in the morning. If you try to push your body beyond its new limitations, you may well experience something akin to circuit overload: an uncontrollable heaviness comes over you, as if you were being piled with lead weights; the need to lie down and rest is overwhelming; mental exhaustion leaves you confused, spacey, and faint; and the smallest frustrations make you feel emotionally wrung out. This opens the door to other emotional responses, such as grief over your lost or diminished abilities (this will be covered in detail in Chapter 27). Additional symptoms may follow, including insomnia, headaches, sexual dysfunction, depression, and/or irritability.

DIAGNOSING AND ASSESSING FATIGUE

It is easy to confuse post concussion fatigue with other conditions, including chronic fatigue syndrome, post traumatic stress disorder (PTSD), and various sleep disorders. Pervasive fatigue also shares symptoms with clinical depression, among them loss of appetite, insomnia, and chronic drowsiness. However, research has found no correlation between clinical depression and concussion-related fatigue, except in people who have had previous problems with depression.

Sometimes, the fatigue that follows a concussion is chronic, or ongoing. In other cases, it can strike in an acute form at unpredictable intervals. When you seek medical help, your doctor is likely to start by taking a thorough medical history. Because fatigue can be a symptom of so many different physical problems and since fatigue varies from person to person, a type of test called a subjective scale may be used to measure the effects of your fatigue. Examples of these scales include the Fatigue Severity Scale (FSS), the Visual Analog Scale for Fatigue (VAS-F), the Fatigue Impact Scale (FIS), the Barroso Fatigue Scale (BFS), the Barrow Neurological Institute (BNI) Fatigue Scale, and the Cause of Fatigue (COF) Questionnaire. The latter two, the BNI and the COF, were specifically designed for brain injury. While these scales are very helpful, it is important to note that the conclusion that exhaustion is due to a concussion may happen only through a process of elimination and careful evaluation.

TREATING POST CONCUSSION FATIGUE

The time-honored approach to treating fatigue is to isolate and eliminate the cause rather than focusing on the symptom. Of course, this can be extremely difficult to do when a concussion is the culprit, since the exact nature of this injury is so hard to pin down. Choosing an approach to treating concussion-related fatigue is further complicated by the fact that treatments for many other post concussion symptoms can induce tiredness on their own. Many medications, for instance, have the side effect of causing fatigue, and the physical toll taken by various therapies can easily compound your existing exhaustion. However, many people with a concussion have overcome, or at least reduced, bothersome levels of fatigue by trying one or more of the following conventional, complementary, and alternative approaches.

Conventional Approaches

Many doctors' plans for managing fatigue include a combination of medication and educating the patient about fatigue, the importance of regular exercise and restorative sleep, psychotherapy, lifestyle changes, and nutrition. Medications that are prescribed for fatigue include the following: psycho-stimulants, dopamine agonists, amantadine, modafinil, and selective serotonin reuptake inhibitors (SSRIs).

Your doctor may also recommend low-level regular exercise to be done at the time of day when you have the most vitality. Dietary modifications are another approach to treating fatigue, and your doctor is likely to recommend the avoidance of alcohol, caffeine, artificial sweeteners, and tobacco products, since these substances can play havoc with your stamina. High-energy foods that have undergone a minimum of processing are also likely to be helpful. These foods include fruits, vegetables, nuts, seeds, and protein-rich foods such as dried beans and fish (especially wild salmon, which contains lots of omega-3).

Complementary Approaches

Acupuncture, done by a licensed acupuncturist, can help combat fatigue. Long-term relief from chronic exhaustion has been reported after as few as six acupuncture treatments.

Recent studies have shown that biofeedback, neurofeedback, and light therapy can be effective against fatigue related to a concussion. There are also nutritional and dietary supplements such as bee pollen and vitamin B6 that are said to increase energy and combat fatigue. There is a wide variety of energy drinks on the market, including NingXia Red, which is a combination of various fruits. Most such energy drinks contain caffeine, however, and should be avoided or discussed with your doctor or dietician.

Alternative Approaches

Reiki, Qi Gong, and/or energy tapping are very helpful in re-energizing your body. In addition, there are numerous homeopathic remedies and herbal preparations that are advertised as energy boosters, among them the herbs ginkgo biloba and gotu kola, which are often recommended by medical doctors. Bach Flower Olive works to restore energy when you are physically and mentally exhausted.

Bear in mind, however, these over-the-counter products are designed for the general population, not as remedies for specific physical conditions and disorders. Moreover, each concussion is unique. It is therefore recommended that you consult with an appropriate and skilled practitioner before you use any over-the-counter herbal or homeopathic products. He or she can then recommend an alternative remedy or remedies especially suited to your individual symptoms and needs. If your physician is unable to help you with this or to provide an appropriate referral, organizations such as the Herb Research Foundation, the Bach Centre, or the National Center for Homeopathy may be able to help. For further information about these and other resources, you can reach me via the contact information on page 367.

PRACTICAL SUGGESTIONS

"I learned to cope with my fatigue by eating an anti-inflammatory/glycemic diet that keeps my brain sharp and my blood sugar level regulated during the day. When needed, I do take NingXia Red or Bach Flower Olive for extra energy. I have found that doing my writing or other thinking activities in the morning, when I have more energy, has helped. Then at midday when I feel fatigue, I try to exercise for the boost I need to see my patients later in the day."

—D.R.S.

As we have seen, post concussion fatigue has several different aspects. Each of them deserves attention during the treatment process. Sleep disruption may be the underlying cause of your exhaustion, and this is addressed in Chapter 9. Lost energy reserves may be the problem. Improper diet may be a contributor. Perhaps it is mental fatigue that troubles you the most. Or you may find yourself struggling with two or three of these problems. The following are a number of tried-and-true tactics to help combat each facet of fatigue. You may wish to experiment with a few of these suggestions, to see which ones best help you maintain control over this bothersome symptom:

- If your fatigue is overwhelming, try taking one midday nap to take the edge off your exhaustion. If your fatigue is extreme, this may help you sleep better at night.

- Take pain medication as prescribed, to minimize the possibility of interrupted sleep.
- To cope with physical fatigue, organize your daily activities according to a priority list. This way, by the time you become fatigued, your most important responsibilities will have been taken care of.
- Avoid getting overtired. This can set you back for days. Pace yourself, take frequent rest breaks, and solicit the help of others.
- Vary your activities to avoid monotony, but do not try to tackle more than one task or activity at a time.
- To combat intellectual and emotional fatigue, avoid excessive stimuli, such as sound and light. For instance, do your shopping by phone or online from home instead of subjecting yourself to crowded department stores. If you must go out shopping, do so when stores and roads are relatively quiet—say, at 10:00 a.m. or 2:00 p.m.
- Enlist your family's help in making your home a quiet place. Take a break from entertaining, turn down the telephone, and keep background noise to a minimum. Limit visitors to one or two at a time, and keep visits brief.
- Acknowledge your limited thinking capacity, and use it wisely. Schedule activities that require concentration for times when you are freshest. Research has shown that our thought processes tend to be clearer between 8:00 a.m. and noon, and again between 6:00 and 8:00 p.m. Conversely, the hours of least efficient mental function are in the area of 3:00 a.m. and between 1:00 and 3:00 p.m.
- Ration your mental energy carefully during a week that contains a big event.
- Use shortcuts. For instance, prepare a general grocery checklist on which you need only add or delete items. Ask a family member to draw simple maps of the places you need to go. Combat memory problems with a smartphone or pocket-sized digital recorder; do math problems with a calculator.
- Schedule limited, uninterrupted time for computer use and email.
- When planning your time, allow time-and-a-half for activities and take a short break every thirty to forty minutes.
- When scheduling activities, consider the components of the activity and schedule a break, rather than try to complete the task in one time period.
- Take periodic rest breaks. If you feel a wave of fatigue coming on, sit or lie down and relax.

The fatigue that follows a concussion strikes different people in different ways. That physically leaden feeling, that frustrating loss of focus, and the inability to get a decent night's sleep are all common aftereffects of brain trauma. These problems can occur individually or in any combination.

Recovery from post concussion fatigue, which typically takes six months to a year, usually begins with a slow, sporadic return of surplus energy. As with many symptoms, you will start to have good days—but you will have occasional relapses that are difficult to predict and are very frustrating when you are trying to make plans and live your life. Often, the reappearance of a mental second wind in the early evening will be the first sign that your fatigue is beginning to abate.

There is no simple cure for fatigue, but using appropriate medication; exercising; modifying your diet, surroundings, and activities; and rationing your stores of energy can bring relief and a welcome sense that you are regaining control of your life.

CHAPTER 8

HEADACHES

■

BARBARA WAS A PASSENGER IN A CAR THAT WAS STRUCK HEAD-ON BY ANOTHER vehicle. She was thrown forward into the windshield, then backward, and eventually out the car door. She spent weeks in the hospital because of her bodily injuries, but was also diagnosed as having a concussion, also called *mild traumatic brain injury* (mTBI).

Barbara suffered recurring mild headaches for many months after her accident. Ten years later, she began to experience agonizing head pain after exertion or an increase in her body temperature. Any activity that caused her to perspire also produced a massive throbbing in her head, along with projectile vomiting. The pain continued long after she cooled down from her exercise. Naturally, Barbara has long since given up most sports and aerobic activities.

Kelly, a forward on her school soccer team, is an aggressive player who is encouraged by her coach to "head" the ball, or use her head to redirect the ball while it's in the air. In the middle of a recent game, she was knocked to the ground and experienced a piercing pressure in her head. She was immediately sidelined and assessed for the ability to return to play. The trainer on hand kept her out of the game, and when the pressure and pain in her head increased, her family took her to the nearest emergency room, where she was diagnosed with a concussion. Kelly was advised by the ER staff to rest, stay home from school, take Aleve for headaches, and avoid physical activity for three weeks. No other suggestions were given at the time of discharge. During the prescribed recuperation period, Kelly's head throbbed daily, and she was unable to tolerate watching TV, reading, using the computer, or even texting her friends without a marked increase in her symptoms. Kelly was bored and slept a great deal, but while awake she discovered that keeping the shades drawn and the lights off in the room seemed to help, as did keeping background noise to a minimum. After three weeks, Kelly returned to school under the watchful eye of her parents and the athletic trainer. Because soccer season had ended, she was not given any post-injury testing to assess readiness to return to competition.

If you are bothered by headaches as a result of a concussion, you have plenty of company! Headaches, from the mildly uncomfortable to the simply agonizing, are among the most common physical complaints following trauma to the head or neck. In this chapter, we will look at the various types of post concussion headaches, their causes, and conventional, complementary, and alternative approaches to relieving headache pain. Also included are practical tips for minimizing or controlling headaches.

WHY HEADACHES CAN OCCUR AFTER A CONCUSSION

A single individual may experience headaches that range in intensity from mild to severe, and in quality from dull to sharp. The type of pain you experience depends on its point of origin. It can be experienced as a pounding, squeezing, tingling, or burning sensation; a touch-sensitive soreness; or a piercing jab that lasts anywhere from a second to several days.

Some headaches feel as though they originate deep within the skull; others seem to start externally and penetrate to the brain's very core. However, while it is the brain that perceives the discomfort of a headache, the brain itself is actually impervious to pain, because there are no nerve endings in the brain. What causes the experience of headache pain are pain sensors located in the arteries, nerves, and muscles of the head, as well as in the *meninges* (the thin membranes covering the brain), that have become distended, inflamed, or compressed.

TYPES OF HEADACHES THAT CAN FOLLOW A CONCUSSION

"During my recovery, I experienced two types of headaches. Days after my accident, an excruciating neuralgic headache appeared. It felt as if someone were putting a hot poker into my skull. This intense pain went away after two months of anti-inflammatory medication prescribed by my neurologist. The other type of headache presented itself as a varied collection of symptoms that included an aura of lights or a distortion of perception, followed by neurological symptoms of facial numbness, severe right-side weakness, slurred speech, and thinking problems. My neurologist thought that these problems stemmed from partial seizures and prescribed anticonvulsant

medication, which triggered numerous side effects, including dizziness. I was subsequently reevaluated by another doctor and diagnosed as suffering from post traumatic atypical migraines."

—D.R.S.

Medical researchers have identified more than a dozen different kinds of headaches. Of these, five are associated with concussion: tension, migraine, post traumatic, cluster, and analgesic-rebound. Each of these types of headaches has its own characteristics and causes.

It can be difficult to diagnose headaches precisely. After a concussion, a phenomenon known as *symptom overlap* can occur. This happens when two or even three pain sources have been activated by injury, and it means that you may experience more than one kind of headache at a time, or you may alternate between different types of head pain, depending on such factors as your activity level or the time of day. In addition, emotional stress, tension, or other physical pain can often increase headache pain.

Headaches come in many types and affect people differently. Even the dullest head pain can be incapacitating under certain circumstances. For the sake of clarity, we will look at each type of headache individually.

Tension Headache

If you suffer from tension headaches, you are already quite familiar with the two-sided sensation of squeezing or pressure that feels like a too-tight band around your head. The tightness continues for the duration of the headache, and may be accompanied by facial or back pain, particularly if you had a whiplash injury.

Tension headaches can be caused by worry, stress, poor posture, overwork, or inadequate ventilation. They often start late in the day, and they may prevent you from falling asleep. The pain may fluctuate from mild to moderate in intensity, but normal activity may not be affected. This is because physical activity does not generally aggravate tension headaches (in some cases, it may actually help).

Tension headaches are often described as either episodic or chronic. They are considered episodic if they occur fewer than fifteen times per month. Chronic tension headaches can persist for anywhere from fifteen days to six months at a time. These are often associated with depression—a common occurrence after a concussion.

Migraine Headache

Migraine headaches last from four to seventy-two hours and are experienced as an aching, pulsating, throbbing sensation at the forehead or temple. They may affect only one side of the head, or generalized areas of the skull. The physical effects may vary from one attack to the next or even within a single episode, and can include nausea and vomiting, muscle weakness, numbness, *phonophobia* (abnormal sensitivity to noise), *photophobia* (abnormal sensitivity to light), and *osmophobia* (abnormal sensitivity to smell). Migraines are typically intensified by physical activity and are often relieved by sleep.

Sometimes, migraines are preceded or accompanied by a set of sensory symptoms called an *aura*. An aura can include the perception of sudden brightness, jagged flashing lights, and/or blurred vision, and may also trigger problems with numbness, initiating movement, word-finding, speech, thinking and reasoning, disorientation, dizziness, and gastrointestinal symptoms. Most auras occur twenty to sixty minutes prior to the onset of headache pain and last for twenty minutes or less.

Migraines are classified according to the extent that sensory symptoms are involved. If head pain is the only symptom, the condition is called *common migraine* or *migraine without aura*. If the head pain is preceded or accompanied by sensory symptoms, it is called a *classic migraine* or *migraine with aura*.

It is also possible to have the sensory symptoms of migraine—the aura—without the head pain. *Migraine equivalent*, or *painless migraine*, is characterized by an aura without a headache. Symptoms can include mood changes, dizziness, blurred vision, unexpected fatigue, and stomach discomfort. Another painless type occasionally seen is the *atypical migraine*, or *complicated migraine*. In this condition, along with the various symptoms present in an aura, other neurological symptoms may also be present, such as slurred speech and one-sided muscle weakness. This type of migraine is difficult to diagnose correctly because its symptoms are similar to those seen in mild stroke and in certain types of seizures. The relatively uncommon *basilar artery migraine* (BAM) involves a very intense aura and physical symptoms originating from either the brain stem or both *occipital lobes* (see Chapter 1). Typical BAM auras involve vision problems in both eyes, dizziness, loss of muscle coordination, speech problems, ringing in the ears, and a decrease in one's level of consciousness.

All types of migraines can be initiated by certain triggers. Common migraine triggers include such ordinary things as coughing, bending over, emotional stress, physical activity, the menstrual cycle, odors, sounds, and irregular eating or sleeping habits. Certain foods or combinations of foods can also lead to migraines (see "Foods That Can Trigger or Worsen Headaches," below). Unusual fatigue, mood changes, bursts of energy, or excessive thirst or food cravings over a period of time can signal an impending migraine.

Post Traumatic Headache (PTH)

This type of headache is associated with head trauma and can arise months or even years after the original injury. A post traumatic headache (PTH) is not one specific type of headache, but rather can be a composite of a tension headache, atypical migraine, and neuralgic (nerve-related) head pain. In 2004, the International Headache Society developed criteria for placing post traumatic headaches into four categories: (1) acute post traumatic headache, (2) chronic post traumatic headache, (3) acute post whiplash headache, and (4) chronic post whiplash headache.

Most PTHs that follow a concussion stem from sudden injury to the vertebrae, muscles, ligaments, and tendons in the neck, or from an altered bite caused by damage to the teeth or injury to the *temporomandibular* (jaw) joint. Whichever of these is the case, the initial injury causes muscle spasms and inflamed, injured tissues, which in turn cause pain.

The pain occurs when the formation of scar tissue, usually at the site of head trauma, renders the nerve-cell fibers there unable to transmit information in the normal fashion. This disruption of impulses can cause the area of injury to become extremely sensitive, in a manner sometimes compared to that of the "funny bone" behind your elbow. The neuralgic component of this type of headache causes a burning or tingling sensation that radiates from the point of injury. The discomfort increases if any pressure is placed on the area, even pressure as light as a fingertip touch or a gentle hair combing. The pain can be continuous, but fortunately, most such headaches disappear within a year.

Foods That Can Trigger or Worsen Headaches

While not all headache sufferers are affected by what they eat, the consumption of certain foods can trigger headaches in some people. This is particularly true of people who suffer from migraines. Some of the most common headache-triggering foods and food ingredients include the following:

- Alcohol
- Avocados
- Bananas
- Beans (except green or wax)
- Cheeses (ripened types, such as Cheddar or Brie)
- Chicken liver
- Chocolate
- Cured meats (such as bacon, bologna, or ham)
- Fermented, pickled, or marinated foods
- Figs (canned)
- Monosodium glutamate (MSG)
- Nuts
- Onions
- Peanut butter
- Peas
- Pizza
- Sour cream
- Vinegar (except white)
- Yeast-raised breads and cakes
- Yogurt

If you are troubled by frequent headaches, you may be able to isolate a food culprit or two by eliminating all suspect items from your diet and seeing if your headaches improve. Then add back one food at a time to see which, if any, trigger headaches.

Cluster Headache

Cluster headaches are thought to be related to migraines. These severe headaches occur occasionally after a concussion, usually if injury to the back of the neck causes nerve damage and shooting pain or muscle spasms. A typical cluster headache appears suddenly and without warning, generally at a specific time of day, such as an hour or two after you fall asleep. The pain is an intense, steady, burning, penetrating sensation centered around or behind the eye and affecting only one side of the face. The involved eye may droop, tear, or become bloodshot; the cheek may be flushed; and the nostril on the affected side may be stuffy or runny. During an attack, symptoms may fluctuate from one side of the head to the other.

Cluster headache pain is quite severe and generally lasts from fifteen minutes to three hours. After that, discomfort may return in "clusters" of one to three headaches per day. Sometimes cluster headache episodes alternate with periods of remission, but in some 20 percent of cases, the pain is chronic—occurring daily for a year or more. These headaches can be triggered by cigarette smoking, alcohol consumption, extreme emotion, overwork, or even unaccustomed relaxation.

Analgesic-Rebound Headache

This type of headache is a reaction to withdrawal from prolonged or excessive use of analgesics or ergot derivatives, which are drugs prescribed for pain relief. The pain may be severe and generalized across the head. Ironically, it is often more intense than the headache for which the medication was taken in the first place. The head pain may be accompanied by restlessness, irritability, nausea, difficulty concentrating, and feelings of depression. Some sufferers have difficulty falling asleep or staying asleep, or may be awakened very early by new head pain. Analgesic-rebound headaches can occur daily for as long as the problem medication is used, and can continue for several weeks beyond that until the offending drug is completely out of your system.

DIAGNOSING AND ASSESSING HEADACHES

If you experience an acute PTH, it is important to go to an emergency room for evaluation to rule out a life-threatening condition, such as bleeding in your brain. A thorough history, physical, and neurological exam will be done, along with a computed tomography (CT) scan or magnetic resonance imaging (MRI), to assess the reason for the PTH. If there are causes for concern, from structural damage such as skeletal injuries or bleeding resulting from a sports collision, fall, or motor vehicle accident, immediate treatment will be given. You may need to stay at the hospital for observation. Otherwise, if there are no obvious causes for your headache, you will be sent home with instructions and prescribed medication.

For chronic headaches, a headache profile is one of the best ways to document your symptoms. This includes a pre-injury headache history (many people's pre-injury headaches were very different from those after the injury), a description of what the pain feels like, possible triggers, information about the pain's location and duration, and your thoughts on what seems to help. While headaches can have numerous symptoms and causes, and cover a broad spectrum of intensity, the acute symptoms are all treatable. Optimally, your head pain will subside completely once the right approach is found, but failing that, there are many ways to make any lingering discomfort quite manageable while you wait out the recovery process.

You will always have greater success nipping a headache in the bud than trying to end a full-blown episode. The key to doing this lies in correctly linking the headache's characteristics to its source, which in turn determines an initial course of pain relief. This is no easy task, however, since headaches can be difficult to identify and their causes hard to pin down. Also, people react to pain differently, often according to their background and upbringing. Experiments with biofeedback have shown that the same bodily sensation that is called "uncomfortable" by one person may be termed "intolerable" by another. In addition, headache symptoms sometimes mimic other problems, including eyestrain, temporomandibular (TM) disorder, sinus infection, and seizure disorder. Moreover, as mentioned earlier, a concussion can spawn more than one kind of headache, with symptom overlap that further complicates the issue.

It is therefore vital that you have professional input into your case, preferably with a treatment team that includes a neurologist who specializes in headaches. Depending on the location and circumstances of your injury, you may also benefit from the services of an orthopedist (a physician who specializes in disorders of the musculoskeletal system), a dentist, an ophthalmologist (eye doctor), an otolaryngologist (ear, nose, and throat doctor), a physical therapist, and/or a psychologist. Together, you will have the best chance of understanding and eliminating the conditions that trigger your headache pain.

TREATING CONCUSSION-RELATED HEADACHES

In general, headaches stop when the conditions that cause them are eliminated. Accomplishing this may be no small task when a concussion is involved, but there are a number of conventional, complementary, and alternative approaches that can act as preventive measures, and other treatments that offer temporary pain relief when a headache occurs.

Conventional Approaches

"Since my concussion, I suffer from occasional migraine headaches. After discovering that I had developed extreme sensitivity to prescription medication as a result of my concussion, I found taking the herb feverfew or the homeopathic remedy Natrum muriaticum, combined with electroencephalography (EEG) biofeedback, to be extremely effective for this type of pain. If I occasionally have a migraine without head pain, my neurologist suggests taking both acetaminophen and ibuprofen, and this seems to work. For general headaches, I take additional magnesium or use acupressure

on the headache point in the webbing between my thumb and index finger. Both give rapid relief."

—D.R.S.

Over-the-counter painkillers are the ideal starting place for anyone suffering from headaches, and they often bring relief to people with a concussion, many of whom find themselves newly responsive to low doses of medication. Well-known examples of these drugs include acetaminophen (Tylenol, Datril, and others), aspirin (Bayer, Bufferin, Ecotrin, and others), ibuprofen (Advil, Motrin, Nuprin, and others), ketoprofen (Actron and Orudis), and naproxen sodium (Aleve). There are also over-the-counter pain products that are combinations of aspirin and caffeine (Anacin) or acetaminophen and caffeine (Excedrin).

Each group of painkillers has specific advantages and particular side effects. The most appropriate way to select medication or a combination of medications is to weigh the different side effects and decide which are most endurable. Because your body can develop a tolerance to a single product, you can increase the effectiveness of over-the-counter drugs by varying the types you take—say, alternating between acetaminophen and ibuprofen. It is important to be cautious about doses, since analgesic-rebound headaches are a possibility with any pain medication.

Severe or persistent head pain may call for prescription medications. Many of these were initially developed for other maladies but can also be effective against headaches. For instance, certain drugs used for cardiovascular problems, particularly beta-blockers and calcium-channel blockers, reduce pain because they interfere with the transmission of nerve impulses in the circulatory and respiratory systems, thus keeping the blood vessels in the head from becoming constricted. Other types of drugs, including some antihistamines, anticonvulsants (anti-seizure medications), ergot derivatives, antidepressants, and even steroids can also block the pain of certain types of headaches by reducing inflammation, relaxing muscles, or disrupting nerve activity in key areas of the body. (See Table 8.1 for a list of medications commonly used to prevent and treat headaches related to concussion.)

Your choice of headache medication will depend on several factors: the nature of your concussion, the type and intensity of resulting pain, your medical history and the other medications you take, and the results you have experienced with other headache remedies. Your health care provider should tailor his or her

TABLE 8.1. DRUGS USED FOR HEADACHES

There are many different medications that have helped people who suffer from headaches following a concussion. Some of these are used to relieve headache pain; others are more useful as preventives. This table lists some of the types of drugs most commonly used for headaches, plus examples of each type. For each drug listed, the generic name is given first, followed by the brand name or names in parentheses.

TYPE OF DRUG	USE	EXAMPLES
Analgesics	General pain relief and headache prevention	Acetaminophen (Tylenol, Datril, and others) Aspirin (Bayer, Bufferin, Ecotrin, and others) Combinations (Anacin, Excedrin, Fiorinal, Medigesic, and others)
Anticonvulsants	Headache prevention; also used to control seizure activity	Carbamazepine (Tegretol) Gabapentin (Neurontin) Phenytoin (Dilantin) Topiramate (Topamax) Valproic acid (Depakene)
Antidepressants	Pain relief and headache prevention; also used for treatment of depression	Amitriptyline (Elavil, Endep) Doxepin (Adapin, Sinequan) Fluoxetine (Prozac) Nortriptyline (Aventyl, Pamelor) Phenelzine (Nardil)
Beta-blockers	Headache prevention; also used for treatment of high blood pressure and heart problems	Atenolol (Tenormin) Nadolol (Corgard) Propranolol (Inderal) Timolol (Blocadren)
Calcium-channel blockers	Headache prevention; also used for treatment of high blood pressure	Diltiazem (Cardizem) Nifedipine (Adalat, Procardia) Nimodipine (Nimotop) Verapamil (Calan, Isoptin)
Ergot derivatives	Pain relief and headache prevention, especially for migraine and cluster headaches	Dihydroergotamine (D.H.E. 45) Ergotamine (Ergostat) Ergotamine combinations (Bellergal-S [also contains phenobarbital, belladonna alkaloids], Cafergot [also contains caffeine]) Methylergonovine (Methergine) Methysergide (Sansert)
Narcotics	Treatment of intense, persistent pain	Meperidine (Demerol)/Oxycodone combinations (Percocet, Roxicet, Tylox [also contain acetaminophen], Percodan [also contains aspirin])
Nonsteroidal anti-inflammatories (NSAIDs)	General pain relief and headache prevention	Ibuprofen (Advil, Motrin, Nuprin, and others) Indomethacin (Indocin) Ketoprofen (Actron, Orudis) Naproxen (Naprosyn) Naproxen sodium (Aleve, Anaprox)

TYPE OF DRUG	USE	EXAMPLES
Steroids	Treatment of intense, persistent pain	Dexamethasone (Decadron, Hexadrol, and others)
		Prednisone (Deltasone, Sterapred, and others)
Tranquilizers	Treatment of intense, persistent pain	Chlorpromazine (Thorazine)
		Haloperidol (Haldol)
		Thiothixene (Navane)

recommendations to your particular circumstances and monitor your usage carefully. Diagnostic tests and a trial-and-error approach may be necessary to find the most effective medication for you.

Arnold Sadwin, M.D., pioneered two office treatments that bring quick relief to headache patients. The first, which stops an ongoing migraine within twenty minutes, is a scalp injection of 1 cc of Marcaine 0.5% in an insulin syringe with a short needle. It can be injected above the ear or over the occipital area, unilaterally or bilaterally, depending upon the severity of the pain. This injection, which has been 90 percent effective in hundreds of patients, can be taught to a responsible family member or friend and can be used several times a week if necessary. Another treatment pioneered by Dr. Sadwin is the administration of oxygen at eight liters for twenty minutes using a simple face mask. If this procedure is effective in twenty minutes, it can be prescribed for home use. The treatment can also be helpful in preventing the onset of migraine headaches when used for twenty minutes twice a day. Dr. Sadwin has noted a 75 percent success rate in over one hundred patients.

Not all drugs help all individuals. It may be necessary for your doctor to try several different prescriptions before finding the one that works best for you. It should be noted that sumatriptan (Imitrex), one of the newer drugs used to treat acute migraine episodes, is generally not recommended for people who have suffered a concussion.

In addition, like almost all medications, headache drugs have numerous potential side effects, ranging from upset stomach to blurred vision, and from dizziness to slowed heart rate. Some drugs can worsen preexisting health problems or have serious, even deadly, side effects if taken in improper doses. If you are taking medication for headaches, following your doctor's usage instructions carefully can mean the difference between pain relief and permanent problems.

Another approach that may be helpful for headaches is psychotherapy. Psychotherapy can help to pinpoint and alleviate depression, which can precede or accompany chronic headaches. Cognitive behavioral therapy (CBT) is an excellent method to help you cope with and understand the changes in your life and find ways of dealing with headaches. CBT is often combined with biofeedback and/or hypnosis. This type of therapy involves exploring the connection between cognition (thoughts), beliefs, feelings, behavior, and pain. A licensed psychologist who is board certified in behavioral or health psychology can provide these tools for coping with the lifestyle repercussions of long-term pain, along with strategies for managing stress and other conditions that contribute to headaches.

The hands-on techniques of physical therapy, including craniosacral therapy, massage, and stretching exercises, can be effective against headaches associated with muscle spasms and pain in the face and neck. Water therapy and ultrasound techniques are similarly helpful. Other methods that can control headache pain include aerobic exercise, such as brisk walking or swimming; maintaining consistent sleep patterns; and dietary monitoring to avoid trigger foods (see "Foods That Can Trigger or Worsen Headaches," page 105). If you smoke, quitting may help. For the most stubborn pain, headache clinics and pain clinics can teach additional methods of controlling your discomfort.

Complementary Approaches

Acupuncture helps control headache pain by stimulating the release of endorphins, body chemicals that act as natural pain relievers. After an initial evaluation, an acupuncturist inserts hairlike needles into specific points on your body. A session usually lasts thirty to fifty minutes. While improvement generally begins in twenty minutes, subsequent sessions are usually needed to control chronic headaches. A related type of treatment, acupressure, can be effective at the onset of headache pain. This involves pressing and then rotating the fingertips firmly against certain points on the body, such as the temples, the top of the head, the hollows in front of the jaw muscles, or below the bones at the base of the skull. The appropriate points depend on the nature and location of your headaches. It is best to consult with a licensed acupuncturist to determine your specific acupressure needs.

Behavioral medicine, a branch of psychotherapy that includes such techniques as biofeedback, hypnosis, and relaxation training, has been helpful for some people with post concussion symptoms. Extensive research has shown that biofeedback—specifically, hemoencephalography (HEG) neurofeedback done by a licensed clinical psychophysiologist—can be very effective against chronic headache pain. One downside of this type of treatment, however, is that the numerous sessions that may be required can become costly if not covered by insurance.

Hypnosis is similar to biofeedback in that it can help you learn to control bodily sensations. While biofeedback, neurofeedback, and light therapy use mechanical devices to do this, with hypnosis you learn to monitor your body through intense focusing, initially with the aid of a health psychologist and then on your own. Pain-control techniques for chronic headaches may involve visualizing a cold compress on your forehead or an on/off "pain switch" similar to a light switch. With instruction and a bit of practice, even children can become adept at this practice. However, the effective use of hypnosis does require concentration, which is often a problem after a concussion.

Developing a relaxation response is a good way to reduce stress, release tensed muscles, and combat hormonal changes that can result in headaches. Proficiency at yoga, meditation, visualization, and other relaxation techniques, such as those described in Herbert Benson's *The Relaxation Response*, can give you a natural defense against pain. The degree of relaxation needed to minimize pain varies from person to person and according to the specific type of headache.

The relaxation response is easy to practice. You need ten to twenty minutes of free time—perhaps before breakfast—and should arrange not to be disturbed. Find a place where you are comfortable, close your eyes, and relax your muscles. Breathe slowly in through your nose and out through your mouth while repeating and focusing on a word or phrase. When you finish, sit quietly for a minute or two—first with your eyes closed, then with them opened.

Chiropractic treatment, including myofascial therapy, has been shown to be effective in treating post traumatic, tension-type, and some migraine headaches. Chiropractic manipulation by a licensed chiropractor reduces abnormal motion and irritation to the neck muscles, nerves, and other tissues.

Alternative Approaches

While medication is likely to be an element in the treatment of concussion-related headaches, there is also much to be said for other approaches to pain relief. Nondrug treatments, which are far less risky than drug therapy, may reduce the frequency and intensity of your headaches. Even if a nondrug approach to headache pain is not completely effective by itself, it can often reduce your need for medication. It is advisable, therefore, to consider and experiment with other approaches to headache pain—under your doctor's supervision, of course.

You may also want to consider using homeopathic remedies and herbal preparations for headaches. Herbs such as arnica, feverfew, peppermint, skullcap, and white willow bark have long been used to relieve headache pain, and feverfew is in fact approved as a migraine treatment by many neurologists. Relaxing herbs such as chamomile may be helpful as well. Homeopathic remedies that may be recommended for headaches include *Bryonia*, *Ferrum phosphoricum*, *Gelsemium*, and *Natrum muriaticum*. There are also homeopathic combination remedies available for headaches. Combining a specific Bach Flower therapy, such as Agrimony for tension headache, with Elm may be helpful. To gain the best results, consult a Bach Flower practitioner. As with all homeopathic treatments, the appropriate remedy depends on the precise nature of the symptoms. Herbal and homeopathic remedies should be treated with the same respect as any other type of medicine. It is wise to consult a professional herbalist, homeopath, or Bach Flower practitioner who has experience in treating concussions to ensure that over-the-counter herbs and homeopathic remedies are right for you.

Reiki, polarity therapy, Qi Gong, Kyusho, and meditation are all effective methods for treating the various forms of PTH. Reiki, polarity therapy, Qi Gong, and Kyusho are passive approaches in which another party is doing something to you to relieve your symptoms, while meditation is an active method that depends on your ability to concentrate (often a problem after a concussion).

PRACTICAL SUGGESTIONS

Controlling headache discomfort can be a formidable task. A good place to start is with identifying and eliminating environmental factors that seem to bring on head pain. There isn't always a single headache trigger, of course, but you can cultivate habits to counteract factors that often lead to headaches. You can also take action to stop a developing headache before it takes hold. The following are practical suggestions that can help:

- Schedule time—even if just ten minutes a day—to learn how to relax. Find a pleasant location, wear loose clothing, and practice simple visualization or deep breathing.

- Document each headache episode. Each time a headache strikes, record the date, the time of day, foods eaten recently, your emotions and activity level around the time of the attack, and anything else that may be relevant. Then try to modify your environment to eliminate potential headache causes.

- Eliminate from your diet any foods that have been shown to trigger headaches. If you are not sure which foods may be involved, start by eliminating the most common offenders (see "Foods That Can Trigger or Worsen Headaches," page 105).

- Try not to deviate from your normal sleeping, exercise, and mealtime schedule.

- Try to determine whether certain activities—say, bending over, drinking alcohol, or squinting—seem to trigger headaches. Then avoid suspect activities as much as possible.

- Increase your level of aerobic fitness (but stick to low-impact exercises such as swimming or walking).

- Be aware that weather conditions, such as high humidity and the drop in barometric pressure that often precedes a summer storm, can contribute to migraines. It is advisable to monitor the weather as well as to experiment with controllable triggers.

- Avoid fluorescent lighting and computer use, if possible. Pulsating or flickering light causes stress on the eyes as well as mental strain.

- At the first sign of a tension headache, apply heat to your forehead and temples using warmed hands or a dampened facecloth. If heat brings no relief, try placing a cold gel pack or ice pack on your forehead or the top of your head.

- At the first sign of a migraine headache, change your surroundings for a relaxing setting. If possible, lie down and sleep.

- At the first sign of a neuralgic headache, lightly brush or comb your scalp. This may help to minimize head pain.

Often the success of a headache treatment strategy relies on recognizing and distinguishing migraine from tension headaches. Since there is no one medication that can treat both well, physicians often have to take a dual approach. A tension headache from TM disorder caused by head injury, for example, may trigger a migraine episode in a migraine-prone patient. The reverse is equally true. This duality often exists in a headache patient and is considered a pearl of wisdom not to be ignored by either the well-seasoned headache specialist or the patient.

There is no question that chronic headaches leave their mark on all aspects of your life. Remember that your concussion has made you somewhat fragile. It is acceptable—even advisable—to pamper yourself physically throughout the healing process and to make avoiding stress a new priority in your life. Patience, a positive attitude, your doctor's guidance, and the understanding of your family and friends are the tools that will best help you to minimize and cope with your discomfort.

CHAPTER 9

SLEEP DISTURBANCES

■

AS A YOUNG CHILD, TOMMY WAS EXTREMELY ACTIVE. HIS MOTHER REPORTS that he was always on the move, jumping off swings in midair and leaping to the ground. She also recalls numerous bumps and bruises from falling out of trees or off his bicycle. Tommy learned to ski at age 5, and he was active in every seasonal sport, be it skiing, ice hockey, soccer, baseball, or football.

Tommy's mother asserts that he was an excellent student and always slept well. However, after a football game when he was 17 years old, he began going to bed early and having trouble getting up for school. His mother noticed Tommy's increased need for sleep but at first attributed it to adolescence. When Tommy's grades began to fall, she became concerned and decided to take him to his primary care physician (PCP) to see what was going on.

Tommy had no medical history of head trauma or loss of consciousness, and there hadn't been an apparent knockout or episode of unconsciousness in his past. Yet subtle signs of memory loss about events were obvious to Tommy and his mother, such as when he had trouble recalling the details of his last football game. Only after extensive neurological testing and evaluation, along with a susceptibility weighted imaging (SWI) MRI, was Tommy diagnosed with *post concussion syndrome* (PCS), due to repeated hits to the head over time.

THE IMPORTANCE OF RESTORATIVE SLEEP

To appreciate the dramatic effect that sleep disturbance has on your brain and your health, it is important to understand both the stages of sleep as well as what is meant by restorative sleep—the completion of all five stages of sleep and the chemical changes that occur within a twenty-four-hour period that allow the brain and body systems to be repaired, heal, and grow. People follow a natural sequence of sleep called the *circadian rhythm*, which is the sleep/wake cycle within twenty-four hours. As the day wears on, we begin to desire rest and sleep. Melatonin, a naturally occurring hormone, helps regulate the sleep/wake cycle by lowering the body temperature and inducing drowsiness. Melatonin affects a small area, the *suprachiasmatic nucleus*, in the *hypothalamus*, or upper brain stem.

A concussion/*mild traumatic brain injury* (mTBI) changes the chemistry of sleep. First, melatonin is reported to be reduced in the presence of a concussion. Another hormone, orexin, sometimes called hypocretin, is responsible for arousal, wakefulness, and the stimulation of interest in food. Orexin is also reduced following head injury, and this decline causes a patient to experience excessive daytime sleepiness and poor quality of sleep. This condition, occurring after a concussion, is sometimes called *secondary narcolepsy*. Thus, a concussion not only can cause problems with going to sleep and staying asleep, but it also can cause daytime drowsiness.

STAGES OF SLEEP NECESSARY FOR RESTORATIVE SLEEP

There are two kinds of sleep: non-rapid eye movement (NREM) sleep and rapid eye movement (REM) sleep. NREM and REM sleep encompass five stages of sleep, all of which are necessary to achieve restorative sleep (Figure 9.1). Each stage is characterized by different brain wave activity and varying levels of neurotransmitters and neuromodulators (see Chapter 1):

Stage 1 (4 to 7 cycles per second). In Stage 1, your sleep is light and you can easily be awakened. Your body temperature and heart rate slow down, your muscles become more relaxed, and you may have some muscle jerking, called *hypnic myoclonia* or *myoclonic jerks*. You can hear sounds and are aware of your environment. This stage, which takes place as you are falling asleep, typically lasts for about five minutes. It is similar to the state you are in when relaxing on a summer day. Approximately 2 to 5 percent of our nightly sleep is spent in Stage 1 sleep.

Stage 2 (11 to 15 cycles per second). Stage 2 sleep involves brief bursts of rapid brain activity called sleep spindles. During this stage, eye movement is at its maximum, and your heart rate and breathing slow down. You spend approximately 50 percent of your nightly sleep in this stage.

Stage 3 (0.05 to 2.5 cycles per second). In this stage of sleep, your breathing, heart rate, and blood pressure are steady, slow, and regular. If you wake up during this phase, you will feel groggy and confused. Stage 3 makes up 4 to 6 percent of total nightly sleep time.

Stage 4 (0.05 to 1 cycle per second). Also known as deep sleep, this stage takes the brain off-line from the body, and it is difficult to awaken the sleeper. There is no eye movement or other activity. Repair and growth of cells occurs, along with regeneration of tissue and nerves, and a boosting of the hormone and immune systems. Stage 4 sleep is similar to roadwork, with most repairs being done when there is the least amount of traffic and lanes can be closed to more efficiently complete the job. If Stage 4 sleep is disrupted, brain regeneration and neuroplasticity is impeded. Deep sleep makes up 12 to 15 percent of total sleep time and is essential for a healthy brain and body.

Stage 5, REM sleep. You do dream in other stages of sleep, but during REM sleep your dreams are more lucid and vivid. During this phase, which lasts five to thirty minutes, your body temperature and heart rate increase, while the body becomes dead weight. Your skeletal muscles are paralyzed, and you are unable to move. There is rapid eye movement and irregular electroencephalogram (EEG) waves, including heightened gamma wave activity (see Chapter 1). Some of the greatest creative discoveries were conceived while dreaming, and medication, alcohol, drugs, and emotional trauma can either produce or suppress dreams during REM sleep. When deprived of this phase of sleep, a person becomes moody and irritable. During restorative sleep, a person goes in and out of REM sleep every ninety minutes. Typically, a person spends about 25 percent of a night's sleep in REM sleep and the rest of the time in NREM.

All five stages of sleep are critical to enjoying restorative sleep to repair the brain, achieve brain wave regulation, and make needed connections throughout the brain. Disturbances in sleep can cause problems with memory and thinking, mood issues such as depression and anxiety, chronic fatigue, and chronic pain. The chart that follows illustrates the effect of different stages of sleep on the brain's neurotransmitters and neuromodulators.

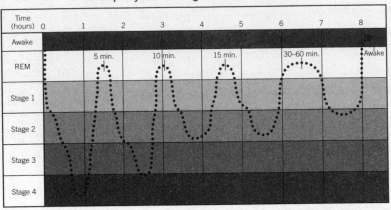

Figure 9.1.

WHY SLEEP PROBLEMS CAN OCCUR AFTER A CONCUSSION

A concussion causes dysregulation within the brain, resulting in sleep disturbance. You may feel extraordinarily tired if your concussion affects your ability to
fall asleep or disrupts your customary sleep/wake cycle. This is a common complaint after a concussion, because sleep patterns are fragile and can easily be
affected by injury to the brain. You may notice that in the first four to six weeks
following injury, pain and other symptoms may play havoc with two key facets of
sleep: sleep initiation, or the ability to fall asleep, and sleep maintenance, the ability to stay asleep. Often, people with a concussion awaken several times each
night for no apparent reason. Their sleep patterns may appear inverted, because
they sleep more during the day and less at night.

Sleep problems may stem from *intrinsic sleep disturbances* such as pain, problems with sleep apnea, or narcolepsy that was present before the injury but has
been worsened by brain trauma. Or you may experience *extrinsic sleep disturbances*,
which are environmental disruptions of sleep patterns due to noise, temperature
fluctuations, or other stimuli that you would have been able to ignore in the past.

TYPES OF SLEEP DISTURBANCES THAT
CAN FOLLOW A CONCUSSION

There are four types of sleep disturbances that can follow a concussion. The first,
insomnia, is the inability to fall asleep or remain asleep. It is the most common

THE EFFECT OF NEUROTRANSMITTERS AND NEUROMODULATORS ON SLEEP/WAKE CYCLES			
NEUROTRANSMITTER/NEUROMODULATOR	LEVELS PRESENT DURING SLEEP/WAKE STATE		
	Wakefulness	Deep Sleep	REM Sleep
Acetylcholine	High	Low to none	High
Serotonin	High	Low	None
Norepinephrine	High	Low	None
Histamine	High	Low	None
Orexin	High	Low	Low
GABA	Low	Medium	High

TABLE 9.1. *Neurotransmitters and neuromodulators in sleep.*

sleep problem among the world's population and has increased with the fast pace of today's lifestyle. Insomnia often occurs immediately following a concussion and, if not treated, may continue for years. *Hypersomnia* is the inability to become fully awake or the need for excessive quantities of sleep. This is a very common symptom after a concussion, as in my own case, when I would sleep for nineteen hours a day. *Sleep/wake cycle disturbance*, or *circadian rhythm disturbance*, is an interference with one's inner clock that regulates periods of sleep and wakefulness. This condition may predate a concussion but be worsened by the injury, or it may be caused by the injury itself. Finally, *parasomnias* are a type of motor problem that includes night terrors, nightmares, periodic leg kicking, or the twitching of restless legs syndrome.

WHAT CONCUSSION-RELATED SLEEP PROBLEMS ARE LIKE

"Prior to my concussion, I slept soundly for six hours a night and had great dreams. I never woke up during that time and always awakened alert and refreshed. After my concussion, I would sleep for nineteen hours and wake up groggy and disoriented. It would take me almost an hour to get focused. With the use of neurofeedback, cranial electrotherapy stimulation (CES), and changes to my diet, my sleep cycle once again provided restorative sleep—until I had a subsequent concussion. Each new concussion threw my sleep cycle off again, but I am now able to go to bed at 1:00 a.m. and wake up refreshed at 8:00 a.m. My mother, who had three concussions, used to be up all night and sleep all day. After I introduced her to audio-visual entrainment (AVE) and CES, however, she was able to re-regulate her brain and resume a normal sleep schedule."

—D.R.S.

DIAGNOSING AND ASSESSING SLEEP DISTURBANCES

It is easy to confuse concussion-related sleep problems with other conditions such as depression, chronic fatigue, chronic pain, post traumatic stress disorder (PTSD), and certain sleep disorders. Disturbances in sleep also share symptoms with clinical depression—loss of appetite, insomnia, and chronic drowsiness.

An evaluation of sleep disturbances after a concussion should include the following:

- A detailed history of sleep patterns prior to injury
- A current sleep log
- The type of work and shift the patient was doing prior to injury
- An account of alcohol, substance, and medication use
- A history of physical injuries and chronic pain
- A list of current medications and stimulants
- A history of psychiatric and/or mental health issues
- The duration and description of current problems

In addition, there are sleep centers that can perform in-depth sleep studies that include the use of a polysomnogram (PSG). This is the standard tool for measuring sleep disturbances, and it incorporates the assessment of breathing, respiratory muscle effort, muscle tone, REM sleep, and the four stages of NREM sleep. However, this procedure may be costly if not covered by your health insurance provider. Also used are the multiple sleep latency test, the EEG, the electrooculogram (EOG), and the electromyograph (EMG). In addition, there is actigraphy, which uses a small wristwatch to measure muscle movement during sleep.

TREATING POST CONCUSSION SLEEP DISTURBANCES

Treating sleep disturbances encountered after a concussion is vital to recovery. Your physical, mental, and emotional health is based on restorative sleep, plus sound nutrition and reduction of stress. The following are conventional, complementary, and alternative approaches to helping you with sleep disturbances.

Conventional Approaches

There are two conventional medical avenues to the treatment of sleep disturbances. The first is behavioral and/or environmental intervention, which includes the following:

- Stable wake and sleep times. It is important to go to bed and wake up at the same time each day.
- Reduction of or avoidance of caffeine and alcohol
- Elimination of tobacco
- Eating a higher protein diet while eliminating sugar, artificial sweeteners, and processed foods
- Phototherapy, or the careful use of and exposure to light
- Environmental controls such as turning off lights and minimizing background noises
- Regular exercise (however, do not work out within four hours of your bedtime)
- Limiting time in bed by not watching TV in the bedroom
- Napping, or not napping. Recent research shows that a ninety-minute nap during the day promotes restorative sleep at night. It is recommended that you discuss this with your doctor.
- Selection of the proper bed, pillow, and mattress for the promotion of restorative sleep
- Psychotherapy; specifically, cognitive behavioral therapy (CBT), to learn new cognitive approaches to sleeping and daily living, and/or trauma therapy, to minimize the effects of PTSD

The second conventional approach to correcting sleep disturbances is pharmacological treatment. The following substances can help if taken on a limited, short-term basis and under your doctor's supervision:

- Melatonin is a naturally occurring compound found in animals, plants, and microbes. Taking 8 mg at bedtime helps improve total sleep.
- Gamma-aminobutyric acid (GABA; see Chapter 1) is a neurotransmitter that is helpful in promoting sleep.
- Trazodone (Desyrel) and some other low-dose antidepressants may help sleep problems, though their side effects may worsen such symptoms as daytime fatigue and memory difficulties.
- Zolpidem (Ambien), zaleplon (Sonata), and eszopiclone (Lunesta) are nonbenzodiazepines used to treat transient insomnia.
- Acetylcholinesterase inhibitors such as Aricept (Donepezil), Razadyne (Galantamine), and Exelon (Rivastigmine) are wake-promoting agents that increase vigilance while increasing verbal and visuospatial memory.

Complementary Approaches

Acupuncture and self-controlled energo neuro adaptive regulation (SCENAR; see Chapter 6) are very effective at correcting many aspects of sleep disturbance. Neurofeedback is an extremely helpful non-pharmacological approach to treating post concussion sleep problems. The drawback is that many insurance companies do not cover neurofeedback; thus, the thirty-plus sessions over the course of several years can be very costly.

Cranial electrotherapy stimulation (CES) uses a medical device approved by the Food and Drug Administration for insomnia. The blinking glasses of personal Roshi (pRoshi) help the brain to regulate itself, whether you wear them or have them blinking against the wall during the night. The Quantumwave Laser has a specific setting for sleep, while the Q1000 can be used with acupuncture points to improve sleep. Hyperbaric oxygen therapy (HBOT) has also been found to be helpful. (This is different from the continuous positive airway pressure [CPAP] or automatic positive airway pressure [APAP] used to manage sleep apnea.)

Alternative Approaches

Reiki and Qi Gong are very effective ways to treat sleep disturbances after a concussion. Bach Flower Rescue Remedy Sleep may also help. A Bach Flower practitioner can assess whether other remedies, such as Star of Bethlehem, are appropriate for you. Aromatherapy with lavender or chamomile oil is often used to promote sleep, as are a variety of homeopathic remedies and herbal preparations, such as valerian root. It is important to consult with a naturopath or homeopathic practitioner with a background in working with post concussion patients before using any alternative products.

Over-the-counter sleep products are designed for the general population, not as remedies for specific physical conditions or disorders. Before purchasing an over-the-counter product, please consult with your doctor. Remember that each post concussion sleep disturbance is as unique as the person who was injured. An experienced professional can give you the best information about remedies especially suited to your symptoms and needs.

PRACTICAL SUGGESTIONS

You may wish to experiment with a few of the following suggestions to see which ones best help you maintain control over post concussion sleep disturbances:

- Adjust your bedtime according to how you feel in the morning. If you are tired, go to bed thirty minutes earlier. If you awaken too soon, go to bed a half hour later. Make it a point to get up at the same time every morning.
- Avoid sleeping pills if possible.
- Avoid watching TV right before bedtime.
- Limit your intake of fluids after 8:00 p.m. to avoid having your sleep disturbed by a full bladder.
- Avoid catnaps. Brief snatches of sleep can play havoc with your body's ability to get a full night's rest.
- Listen to relaxing music or relaxation programs as you attempt to fall asleep.
- Take two to three hours to unwind from your day before trying to fall asleep.
- Consider meditation or prayer before bedtime.
- Take pain medication as prescribed to minimize the possibility of interrupted sleep.
- Avoid getting overtired, as this can set you back for days. Pace yourself, take frequent rest breaks, and solicit the help of others.
- Keep your bedroom cool.
- Reserve your bed for sleeping rather than for reading, texting, computer use, or watching television.
- Once you wake up after continuous sleep, do not try to "snooze." Instead, get up.
- Use relaxation techniques to calm worries and minimize excessive thinking before bedtime.
- Avoid foods that cause heartburn or *gastroesophageal reflux disease* (GERD).
- Avoid expectations and thinking about your ability to sleep, and avoid worrying about sleeping. Both of these can directly affect the ability to sleep.

Post concussion sleep disturbances affect people in different ways. The effects of this symptom dramatically influence your ongoing recovery and all aspects of your life. The placebo effect is a powerful sleep inducer, just as the nocebo effect is a powerful disrupter—in other words, your expectations have a lot to do with the effectiveness of any technique or substance that you try. This is true for both concussive and noninjured individuals.

Recovery from post concussion sleep disturbances typically takes six months to a year. Following the suggestions in this chapter will allow and promote restorative sleep. The internal and external stressors in your life won't be eliminated, but you will be better able to cope and function as you move toward wellness once again.

CHAPTER 10

DIZZINESS AND IMBALANCE

∎

NEW YORKER CAROL IS THE SURVIVOR OF TWO CONCUSSIONS, ALSO CALLED *mild traumatic brain injuries* (mTBI)—the second one eight years after the first, and both from skiing accidents. It was the second injury that really affected her. Someone skied into her at the bottom of a slope, striking her head, injuring her back, and knocking her jaw out of place. It took the ski patrol over forty-five minutes to come to Carol's aid, and when she was transported to the hospital, the emergency-room physician made several poor judgments. Carol said that every time she moved, the room spun as if she were on a carnival ride. The doctor dismissed this, saying that it was just a result of lying down for too long.

Carol was a program research specialist with the New York State Department of Health and an adjunct instructor at a community college. She continued to teach after the second accident, but her dizziness kept her from driving and caused her to feel that the room was spinning whenever she turned from the chalkboard to look out into the lecture hall.

Although a neurologist told Carol that she was "as normal as normal could be," her longtime family physician saw the change in her and helped her to seek the treatment she needed. She is now seeing a neuropsychologist and a psychiatrist to help her put her life back together. Her classroom dizziness has stopped and Carol can drive again. However, she still experiences occasional lightheadedness when she gets up too quickly—a feeling that she, rather than the room, is spinning.

At one time or another, virtually everyone—concussion survivor or not—experiences the unsettling sensation of dizziness. The room seems to spin, your vision dims momentarily, and you become aware of a slightly nauseated feeling. Dizziness can be related to several conditions, among them low blood sugar, extreme hunger, and low blood pressure.

WHY DIZZINESS AND IMBALANCE CAN OCCUR AFTER A CONCUSSION

Dizziness is a common complaint after TBI, and there are a number of reasons for the symptom. Double vision, injury to brain stem centers that monitor balance, or damage to certain areas of your *cerebellum* can trigger lightheadedness or a feeling of imbalance. Blood pressure fluctuations, caused by disruption of the nerve impulses that govern your heart rate or by trauma to the part of the brain that regulates blood flow, can also make you feel faint or unsteady. Extended use of a cervical collar, a supportive device for the neck that is often recommended after a whiplash injury, can lead to compression of nerves leading into the back of the head and, in turn, increased lightheadedness. Vertigo is usually caused by injury to an inner-ear structure called the semicircular canal.

WHAT POST CONCUSSION DIZZINESS AND IMBALANCE ARE LIKE

"After my concussion, I had problems with feeling lightheaded, unbalanced, and unsteady. In one situation, I was on a small rowboat for an hour and couldn't regain a feeling of steadiness for more than three hours after returning to land. Many of my medications increased these feelings, especially the products taken to combat high blood pressure and seizures."

—D.R.S.

There is a difference between dizziness—feeling lightheaded and unsteady—and the sensation called vertigo. If the dizziness you experience is true vertigo, you will feel that the room is spinning around you whenever your head or body moves into certain positions, particularly if the change in position is rapid. Research shows that 15 to 78 percent of people with a concussion experience vertigo as a consequence of their injuries.

If your dizziness stems from lightheadedness or an unbalanced feeling, you will not feel that your surroundings are spinning, but as if *you* are spinning. You may need to hold on to a chair or tabletop because your sense of where you are in the room seems so fleeting. The feeling of not having your "sea legs" may be constantly with you. You may find yourself avoiding unnecessary movement so that you won't trigger yet another unpleasant wave of disequilibrium—particularly in the morning hours, when unsteadiness is usually at its peak.

DIAGNOSING AND ASSESSING DIZZINESS AND IMBALANCE

To distinguish between post concussion vertigo and lightheadedness that may be caused by another problem, your doctor should take a medical history and check your blood pressure in a sitting or standing position. If your blood pressure is normal and your symptoms may be from true vertigo, your primary care physician (PCP) will likely refer you to one or more of the following specialists: an otolaryngologist (ear, nose, and throat doctor), an ophthalmologist (eye doctor), a neurologist, an audiologist, and/or an endocrinologist. These specialists can determine whether your dizziness symptoms stem from inner-ear, vision, central nervous system (CNS), or endocrine system disorders via a variety of tests too numerous to list.

Evaluating inner-ear function is important for distinguishing between true vertigo and other types of balance problems, which in turn is essential to formulating an appropriate treatment plan. Two important tests that may be done by a neuro-otolaryngologist to evaluate your vestibular system (the balance system in your inner ear) are the *caloric test* and the *rotary chair test*. In the caloric test, your inner ear is alternately cooled and heated by irrigation with water at controlled temperatures, while your eye movements are monitored by means of an instrument called an electronystagmograph. Because the body normally responds to such temperature stimulation with characteristic movements of the eyeball, this test can diagnose problems in the vestibular system. In the rotary chair test, your eye movements are measured as you focus on a fixed object while sitting in a slowly turning chair.

TREATING POST CONCUSSION DIZZINESS AND IMBALANCE

Fortunately, dizziness or vertigo that results from a concussion usually subsides within six to eight weeks. However, those long days of discomfort can seem interminable, particularly if the dizziness makes you feel nauseated or you are struggling to deal with other aftereffects of your injury. There are a number of approaches you can try to minimize your episodes of dizziness—or better still, to bring the entire malady to a quicker end. These can be used either by themselves or in conjunction with other approaches.

Conventional Approaches

Occasionally, vertigo can be so severe that it renders you unable to function. If this happens, an over-the-counter motion sickness product, such as dimenhydrinate (Dramamine) or cyclizine (Marezine), or a prescription medication for dizziness and nausea, such as meclizine (Antivert; also available in nonprescription strength as Bonine), can bring relief. Vertigo can sometimes be minimized through the use of sedatives such as diazepam (Valium). Another helpful approach is physical therapy with a practitioner who specializes in balance and spatial-orientation problems, though you may be asked to discontinue your vertigo medications during your sessions, since they can suppress necessary information needed by your therapist. Not every therapist is trained to treat dizziness and imbalance from a concussion. However, the right person can teach you exercises that temporarily overload the vestibular system. Overloading challenges the vestibular system to adapt to multiple atypical movements. For example, you may be asked to sit or lie atop a large ball and move your arms or legs in specific patterns. A similar type of approach is used by figure skaters, who practice spinning and twirling until they can perform such moves without dizziness. There is also a unique treatment for *benign positional vertigo* (BPV) that involves rotating the head very gently to remove loosened calcium crystals from the semicircular canal in the inner ear.

Complementary Approaches

Acupressure can help an attack of dizziness to abate. When dizziness strikes, try applying steady, firm pressure to your temples and to your jaw joints, directly in front of your ears, for several minutes or until dizziness subsides. *Auricular*, or outer ear, acupuncture has also been shown to be helpful in relieving dizziness, as well as in heading off future episodes. Biofeedback and neurofeedback are very effective at helping regulate the motor area of the brain. Chiropractic treatment may also help. Interactive Metronome (see Chapter 6) is designed specifically for problems with balance and motor issues.

Alternative Approaches

There are several herbs and homeopathic remedies that can combat dizziness problems. However, since dizziness that is related to concussion may be only one of your symptoms, you should consult with a qualified herbalist or homeopath about what is best for you rather than experimenting on your own with over-the-counter preparations. The Herb Research Foundation and/or the National Center for Homeopathy can be of assistance in locating an experienced practitioner in your area. Please contact me via the information listed on page 367 for information and assistance.

Reiki and Qi Gong are also effective against dizziness and imbalance, as are various methods used in energy medicine. Self-help books can provide insight, but it is wise to find an experienced practitioner who can work with your specific symptoms.

PRACTICAL SUGGESTIONS

"I've learned to cope with attacks of dizziness by casually leaning on a wall or gently touching a desk. When walking, I look for a straight-line focal point, like the grout line between floor tiles."

—JULIA

While it is always a good idea to seek professional assistance with a symptom as problematic as dizziness and imbalance, you can do a lot at home and at work to keep attacks at bay, or at least to lessen their severity. Here are a number of ideas:

- At the first sign of dizziness, stop moving and sit or lie down. In most instances, this helps the sensation to pass within a few minutes.
- Roll out of bed slowly in the morning rather than quickly sitting upright.
- Modify your activities and environment so that you either avoid or bombard your system with dizziness triggers. For example, sit and stand up slowly, so as not to set off the motion receptors in your inner ear, or try the opposite—repeating these movements in rapid succession until the accompanying spinning sensation stops.
- Note whether your dizziness is worse at certain times of day, when you are hungry, or if you spend time amid warm temperatures, bright sunlight, or noise. If it is, take steps to avoid these conditions.
- Try sleeping without a pillow so that your neck and upper spine remain perfectly straight and your head is not pushed forward while you sleep. A folded hand towel or piece of fabric tucked under or behind the neck can increase

your comfort in this position. Special cervical pillows, available in many drugstores, also offer gentle support for the neck.

- Use occasional support, such as a cervical collar—under a doctor's supervision, of course—if you have suffered a neck or whiplash injury. Doing so temporarily can take pressure off crucial nerves in the area. A soft cervical collar may also be used by a physical therapist who is trained in the *canalithic repositioning procedure*, a specific method of dealing with postural dizziness. You may be required to keep the soft collar on for twenty-four hours following this treatment for vertigo.

- Be aware that drugs such as oral contraceptives and blood pressure medications can cause dizziness as a side effect. In fact, some medication-sensitive individuals may even get dizzy after taking aspirin. Bear in mind that your concussion may have made you more sensitive than normal to medication. Be sure to confer with your doctor before taking any drug product.

- Avoid alcohol, cigarettes, and recreational drugs, since these substances promote dizziness.

- Limit your use of salt, which can cause fluid retention and increased vertigo. Also, stay well hydrated.

Dizziness is one of the more vague symptoms of *post concussion syndrome* (PCS) because it can be triggered by several different conditions. Happily, though, it is likely to be one of your shorter-lived complaints. While you wait for the unpleasant sensation to subside, it is worthwhile to experiment with different methods of making yourself more comfortable. With time, patience, and the right techniques, your dizziness and imbalance problems should soon be a thing of the past.

CHAPTER 11

VISION AND LIGHT SENSITIVITY PROBLEMS

■

ATRICIA SUFFERED A CONCUSSION, ALSO KNOWN AS *MILD TRAUMATIC BRAIN injury* (mTBI), when her car was struck head-on at thirty-seven miles per hour by a truck that failed to yield the right of way. In the early stages of her recovery, Patricia often saw double images and had problems moving her eyes across the page when reading. She also had difficulty watching moving objects and tolerating bright and fluorescent lights. Patricia found herself squinting when using the computer or the touch screen on her phone, and she was unable to watch television for any length of time.

These problems have improved over time, but Patricia still has days when she is extra-sensitive to visual stimulation. Busy, brightly lit places such as shopping malls, for instance, are often overwhelming to her. To cope with this sensitivity, Patricia sometimes plays games—for instance, telling herself that this is one of those days when she has to keep her eyes from wandering to nonessential sights.

While you might not immediately connect an injury to your neck or a blow to the back of your head with the onset of vision problems, the fact is that a great many people who have suffered a concussion experience trouble with their eyes. Dry eyes, a gritty sensation in the eyes, intermittent double vision (*diplopia*), and blurred vision are the most common complaints, but a wide range of other maladies, including partial vision loss, tracking difficulties (problems focusing on moving objects), seeing things in your visual field, and photophobia (abnormal sensitivity to light) can also occur.

As with other post concussion symptoms, the extent and duration of vision problems depend on the force, type, and location of brain trauma. In some cases, a complete return to normal vision may be unlikely; however, many people with a concussion experience significant if not complete improvement over the long term. Regardless of your prognosis, it is important to understand the nature of the vision problems brought on by a concussion.

WHY VISION PROBLEMS CAN OCCUR AFTER A CONCUSSION

Vision is a complex process that involves not only the eyes but also the brain. Light enters the eye and is focused by the lens and projected onto the retina, where an image of whatever the eye is looking at is formed. This image is then transmitted by means of the optic nerve to the *occipital lobe*, located at the back of the brain. This part of the brain houses the visual pathways that receive nerve impulses from the retina. It also controls your visual fields and your understanding of what you see. The process of seeing is made even more complex by the fact that, because of the way light enters the eye, the image that forms on the retina is reversed: images of things on the right form on the left side of the retina, and vice versa. This image reversal is itself compensated for—the image is re-reversed—by the way in which nerve impulses from the retina travel to the brain. Images from the right side of the retina go to the right side of the brain, and those from the left side of the retina go to the left side of the brain (remember that the right side of the brain controls the left side of the body, and vice versa).

The eye and the optic nerve therefore constitute an intricate instrument that is vulnerable to a number of different injuries. Sometimes the eyeball itself sustains a direct blow during a concussion. When this happens, the force of impact can bend, compress, twist, tear, or jolt the lens, the retina, and/or the optic nerve, all of which are critical to seeing correctly. In other instances, an impact injury to the base of the skull or the back of the neck may damage delicate tissues in the brain stem that regulate eye coordination and movement.

If a force or blow happens to strike the protruding back center part of the head, the impact may be

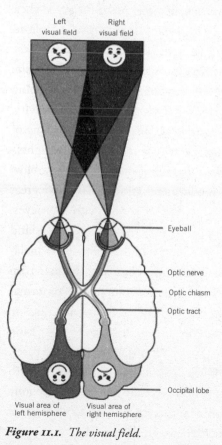

Figure 11.1. The visual field.

absorbed by one or both of the occipital lobes. An injury to the crown area (the top of the head) can affect the *parietal lobe*, which governs spatial awareness and such higher-level visual skills as reading. Wherever the location, bruising, bleeding, swelling, or nerve damage from a concussion can create havoc within your visual system.

It is important to pin down the source of any vision problems that occur after a concussion. Identifying the culprit helps you to understand your symptoms, know what to expect in terms of recovery, and make decisions about the best course of treatment.

TYPES OF VISION PROBLEMS THAT CAN FOLLOW A CONCUSSION

"I had trouble with double vision after my concussion; however, this problem was eventually found to be a side effect of medication. Over time, I also experienced blurred, weaker vision in my right eye—the side that was injured. Since this difficulty seems to be worsened by stress and fatigue, I do what I can to avoid these conditions. Of course, these fluctuations make prescribing and wearing corrective lenses a real problem. On occasion, I'm affected by unexpected light sensitivity, particularly from fluorescent lighting, though it has never been determined whether this problem is related to an injury in my eye or to brain injury. Once in a while, I'm also bothered by floaters.

In my concussion from the collision with the snowplow, one of my eyes was dilated. A physician friend thought I had a brain tumor. I had recently been diagnosed with a meningioma (a benign brain tumor) and feared that this symptom might signify yet another tumor. To my relief, an investigation revealed that my eye dilation was part of a traumatic atypical migraine."

—D.R.S.

Doctors who work with concussion patients treat a number of different visual problems, one or more of which may match your own post-injury symptoms. The characteristics of the most common eyesight-related complaints are described in this section.

Blurred Vision

Blurred vision—seeing objects out of focus—after a concussion can result from damage to the cornea, the clear, dome-shaped transparent membrane that covers the front of the eyeball; to the lens, which focuses light on the retina that processes the light image; or to the optic nerve, which transmits visual messages to the brain.

Even if only one eye has been damaged, everything you see will appear blurry. Some cases of blurred vision improve on their own and some can be improved with treatment—for example, *vitreous detachment*, in which the clear gelatin that holds the round shape of the eye is separated from the retina, forming a pocket—but if the blurriness is a result of retinal detachment or optic-nerve damage, you may be left with some permanent degree of blurred vision.

Cortical Blindness

Occasionally, a concussion involves such severe trauma to both occipital lobes that an intense blurring condition called cortical blindness can result. At best, you may be able to decipher a newspaper headline or other large print; at worst, this malady allows you to see nothing at all; the eye will be normal in appearance to an examining physician, but damage has occurred to the specialized cells of the occipital cortex (the area responsible for processing the visual signals received from the eye), rendering optic pathways unable to connect to the injured area of the brain. Some people eventually regain most of their original sight capacity, though a year or two often passes before it can be determined how much of your sight will return. There are some people who do not realize that they have damaged their visual cortex, because they claim they can still see people. This clinical phenomenon, called Anton's syndrome, has been described mostly in cases of stroke but has also been seen following head injury.

Double Vision

Under normal conditions, your eye movements are synchronized so that you see the images reflected on both retinas as a single picture. If the movements of your eyes are affected by nerve damage, however, you may see each retinal image separately—that is, you may see two distinct images instead of one. This phenomenon is called *diplopia*, or double vision.

Double vision makes resuming everyday activities quite difficult and can contribute to headaches, fatigue, and dizziness problems. Double vision may disappear on its own within a period of six weeks or so. Many eye doctors prefer not to prescribe new corrective lenses during the first three or four months following the onset of double vision after a concussion, because there are many instances where vision and focus improve gradually, thereby rendering a new prescription ineffective until stability of focus and fusion of images reoccur. However, the condition may linger for a year or more, or even be permanent, depending on the severity of nerve damage. Even so, it is possible to improve or correct residual vision through the use of prisms or corrective muscle surgery so the patient can see as normally as possible.

Floaters

Floaters—sometimes called *vitreous floaters*—cause moving spots to appear in your field of vision. Occasionally, tiny bits of chemicals (usually proteins) or solid matter develop in the vitreous fluid, the clear, protective gel-like substance that fills most of the space in the back half of the eyeball, between the lens and the retina. As these objects move, they reflect light onto the retina. You perceive these reflections as floating spots before your eyes.

Floaters are very common and can occur under ordinary circumstances. Usually, they cause no harm and do not signify a serious problem. When they occur after a concussion, it is often because the injurious blow causes minute hemorrhages within the eye, which result in the formation of numerous small, free-floating solid objects within the vitreous fluid. However, floaters can also be a sign of a serious retinal problem such as a detachment or tear. If you are experiencing floaters, it is important to be examined by an eye care professional to determine if the floaters are benign or of a more serious nature.

Optic Atrophy

If there is significant trauma to the optic nerve during a concussion, the nerve is unlikely to heal. It may then begin to atrophy, or waste away. Once this happens, the optic nerve can no longer transmit impulses from the retina to the brain, resulting in blurred vision and significant, if not complete, vision loss in the affected eye. This permanent loss of vision in one eye in turn hampers your perception of depth and distance.

Sympathetic Ophthalmia

This condition is triggered by direct trauma to the eye and is believed to result from the spillage of ocular proteins from retinal pigment cells. These proteins come into contact with immune cells that, once activated, begin to damage the contents of the eye. If the process is not corrected quickly, it can ultimately involve the opposite eye. Prevention of further damage from this condition requires professional attention within ten days and often requires surgery to either remove the contents of the eye or remove the eye completely, with the aim of stopping the threat of spreading.

Photophobia

Sometimes an injury to the visual system results in an unusual sensitivity to light. This condition can manifest itself as anything from seeing an annoying intermittent glare to a crippling intolerance for any sort of light—even through closed eyelids. Light sensitivity can be short-lived or chronic, depending upon the type and severity of injury.

Tracking Problems

Tracking is the ability to follow and maintain your focus on a moving object with both eyes. Tracking problems may result from an injury to the brain stem or the *cerebellum*. A concussion in the area of the brain stem sometimes causes *nystagmus*, or rapid oscillations of the eyeball that interfere with smooth, coordinated eye movement when looking to the right, left, up, or down. Slowed eye movement due to a concussion can also cause tracking problems and can hamper your ability to read or process visual images.

Visual Agnosia

In rare cases, a person who is experiencing *post concussion syndrome* (PCS) will see an image but be completely unable to attach meaning to it. For instance, you might be handed an apple, but it would remain a meaningless object until you put your senses of touch, smell, and taste to work to help you identify it. This phenomenon, called *visual agnosia*, can occur during recovery from cortical blindness due to injury to specific areas within the occipital lobes. In its various forms, it can cause spatial confusion; an inability to read, write, draw, or follow a map; or an inability to recognize familiar faces. Visual agnosia is distinct from cortical blindness or Anton's syndrome in the sense that visual agnosia causes difficulty interpreting visual signals, while in cortical blindness, there is no signal to process. In Anton's syndrome, there also is no signal to process, but the person doesn't recognize this and continues to behave as if he or she can see despite not observing, and, as a result, bumping into, objects in his or her path.

Visual Overstimulation

People with PCS often find themselves visually overstimulated in the months after injury—they cannot tolerate changing light patterns and/or the sight of movement, clutter, or detail. This condition is tied to trauma to one or more areas of the brain responsible for processing images. It may range from intermittent to long-term, and from mildly inconvenient to completely incapacitating. It is important for a person recovering from a concussion to avoid excessive visual stimulation as well as other forms of sensory stimuli.

Visual Field Changes

The visual field is the full extent of your sight capacity when your eyes are looking straight ahead, including your central and side, or peripheral, vision. Sometimes a concussion causes a loss of vision in one area of your visual field. For example, you may clearly see the center of what you are focusing on, but have a blurred or completely missing area to the left or right, depending on the area of the brain that was injured. In some cases, side vision can disappear completely. Left- or right-side vision loss is generally caused by injury to the visual pathways behind the eyes; central visual field problems result from injury to one eye or to both of the occipital lobes; and upper or lower visual field problems stem from damage to the optic nerve. With an occipital cortex lesion, the central field of vision can be damaged while the peripheral vision field is preserved.

DIAGNOSING AND ASSESSING VISION PROBLEMS

Whether mild or severe, temporary or permanent, visual problems that result from a concussion are sure to interfere with many aspects of daily living. If you experience problems with your eyesight in the weeks after your injury, it is a good idea to obtain a thorough evaluation by an ophthalmologist—a medical doctor who specializes in diagnosing and treating eye disorders. This examination will determine the scope and nature of your condition, rule out the possibility of further visual deterioration, and ascertain whether treatment is possible. Computerized visual fields, such as computer campimetry, along with other forms of visual mapping, such as Goldman perimetry, may be done in a special dark room in which small, lighted targets are presented and you are given a push button to press when you see the light. Based on your diagnosis, your ophthalmologist can also direct you to additional sources of information and support.

TREATING POST CONCUSSION VISION PROBLEMS

There is often no treatment other than time for vision problems resulting from a concussion. Patience may therefore be your doctor's first prescription. Fortunately, some eyesight difficulties eventually diminish or disappear on their own. This is particularly true of problems that arise from injury to the brain, such as cortical blindness, tracking problems, visual agnosia, and visual field problems. However, it may take some time. For example, recovery from cortical blindness is slow, with vision gradually improving over a two-year period. Similarly, visual field problems often fade, but it may take as long as a year or two before there is noticeable improvement. With visual agnosia, it is impossible to predict how long healing may take or even what the chances of recovery are.

Any recovery from damage to the optic nerve usually occurs within six months following the injury. After that time, improvement is unlikely. Your ophthalmologist should tell you at what point you should cease to expect any further improvement in your condition. In addition to an ophthalmologist, there are eye care professionals (mainly optometrists) who specialize in pinpointing and rehabilitating the visual consequences of TBI.

Of course, many eye problems do respond well to medical, surgical, and alternative approaches. Arming yourself with information about available treatments can help you understand and participate in the healing or coping process, as the case may be. A number of commonly recommended treatments are described below.

Conventional Approaches

Appropriate treatment, if any, for a PCS-related vision symptom depends on the nature of the problem. If blurred vision results from damage to the cornea, antibiotics such as ofloxacin (Ocuflox) and/or anti-inflammatory medications such as prednisolone (Pred Forte) can promote healing. If not, a corneal transplant may be needed to restore your sight.

Prescription eyeglasses are helpful for lens problems, but severe damage may require cataract surgery. An eye patch is often used to help eliminate troublesome double images. If double vision persists for a year or more, surgery on the eye muscles may be done to reposition the eye. Nystagmus is difficult to treat, and time may be the best healer.

In addition to prescribing specific treatments, an ophthalmologist can advise you on ways to compensate for visual deficits. If you experience blurriness in your left visual field, for instance, the doctor may suggest that you hold printed matter to the right of your nose when reading to avoid experiencing a blind spot (an area that does not register visual information), or that you turn your head to move your stronger right vision into your left-side blind spot. If you are light sensitive or suffering from visual overstimulation, your doctor will likely discuss with you ways to avoid painful and distressing visual stimuli. There are no corrective measures for floaters, but most people with floaters eventually become used to them, especially once they settle below the line of sight.

Complementary Approaches

Acupuncture by a qualified licensed acupuncturist may be effective against visual problems such as nystagmus, photophobia, and blurred vision. Neurofeedback can also be helpful in this area. In addition, Interactive Metronome (see Chapter 6) can help with balance and visual field problems.

Alternative Approaches

EyeQ is specifically designed to help with tracking and reading problems, while the Irlen method uses various colored lenses to help with symptoms of visual disturbances, specifically double vision. Various visual problems have been helped by herbal preparations such as bai shao, bilberry, and eyebright. Homeopathics such as *Bryonia album*, *Gelsemium*, and *Causticum* are also commonly prescribed. As always, what is best for you depends on your specific needs and symptoms. If you are considering such remedies, it is important to consult an herbalist or homeopathic practitioner who can help you, rather than self-prescribing or experimenting with over-the-counter products. If your primary care physician (PCP) is unable to help you, or to supply a referral to a qualified herbalist or homeopath, the Herb Research Foundation and/or the National Center for Homeopathy may be able to help. For further information, please call or email me via the contact information listed on page 367.

PRACTICAL SUGGESTIONS

While you wait out the weeks or months necessary to determine the extent of your recovery from PCS-related vision problems, it pays to do what you can to make yourself comfortable, safe, and better able to cope with day-to-day life. You may find some of the following techniques quite helpful:

- If you have problems with depth perception, use extreme caution when going up or down stairs and curbs. If a handrail is available, use it. Also be cautious when crossing streets—it may be difficult to tell exactly how much space there is between you and oncoming traffic, or how fast that traffic is approaching.

- Before getting behind the wheel again, have your driving skills assessed to make sure it is safe for you to do so. Tests of this type are available through most rehabilitation hospitals.

- If reading is a problem, find large-print books and newspapers (or use a magnifier), and use a ruler or blank index card to help you keep your place when reading a printed page. Or make use of audio recordings of books, magazines, and newspapers from your local public library, or computer programs. Many e-readers also allow you to adjust the size of the text so you can make it as large as you need to see it comfortably.

- For computer work, most Windows and Apple products have the ability to read text aloud. Also, online software such as Natural Reader, a free download from www.naturalreaders.com, can read aloud what is written. Read:OutLoud, a text reader that's part of the Solo 6 Literacy Suite by Don Johnston Assistive Technology, can be similarly helpful. Text Assist, a text reader by Creative Labs, is found on Creative's Sound Blaster sound cards. You can reach me via the contact information on page 367 for further information about this.

- If you find you have developed light sensitivity, cater to this condition. Use dark glasses, keep blinds or shades lowered, and avoid brightly lit places.

- Avoid becoming visually overstimulated. Choose calm surroundings over chaotic places such as shopping malls and crowded parties. Try to sleep during car trips.

- Seek the support of friends and family. Help them understand the exact nature of your visual problems, delegate responsibilities that cause you great difficulty, and ask for their assistance with environmental and scheduling modifications.

- If you find yourself in a fragile emotional state due to worry and frustration over eyesight problems, ask your ophthalmologist or PCP about a referral for mental health assistance.

If your vision remains impaired over the long term as a result of your concussion, you may qualify for special services such as job retraining, visual aids, a guide dog, and/or assistance with reorganizing your home and work space. In most states, your ophthalmologist can register you for consideration for these benefits. Fortunately, though, in most cases vision slowly but surely improves after a concussion. Time, patience, medical advice, and concessions made with your specific visual problem in mind will combine to make the recovery period much easier.

CHAPTER 12

HEARING AND NOISE PROBLEMS

■

ETER, A 35-YEAR-OLD SHEET-METAL WORKER FROM SOUTH DAKOTA, WAS ON the job when a tool fell a distance of some six feet and struck him on the top of the head. He immediately began hearing a ringing sound in both ears that wouldn't stop. The sound seemed even louder when Peter left the construction area for quieter surroundings. Peter consulted his family physician, who found no marked hearing loss or visible middle-ear damage. The doctor identified the ringing sound as a neurological consequence of being hit on the head and said that it would improve in time. Over a year later, however, Peter was still grappling with the constant ringing sound, most noticeably at night. A neurologist suggested biofeedback, which provided a measure of relief, but Peter now realizes that he may well have to learn to live with the ever-present ringing in his ears.

While Peter's hearing problem occurred after being struck in the head, the same symptoms were experienced by Josh, a high school ice hockey player, and Pat, a second lieutenant stationed in Iraq, following sports and blast injuries. Josh collided with another player while skating after the puck in a game, while Pat was riding in a Humvee when an improvised explosive device (IED) detonated just outside the vehicle. All three people are now living with hearing and noise problems.

Most people tend to associate hearing problems with old age or with damage from middle-ear infections in childhood. As many people with a concussion, also called *mild traumatic brain injury* (mTBI), can attest, however, a force or blow to certain areas of the head also can cause changes in one's ability to hear, as well as problems with noise.

WHY HEARING PROBLEMS CAN OCCUR AFTER A CONCUSSION

In a healthy, normal ear, sound waves cause vibrations of the eardrum, which are then transmitted to the middle ear, and, in turn, to a fluid-filled structure called the *cochlea*, located in the inner ear. In the cochlea, vibrations are changed into electrical impulses that are transmitted to the brain by the auditory, or acoustic, nerves (although certain vibrations, such as those caused by one's own speech, are conducted to the inner ear directly through the skull). The brain interprets these electrical impulses as sound.

Most hearing problems are the result of either *conductive failure* (a mechanical problem in the middle ear that keeps vibrations from reaching the cochlea) or *sensorineural failure* (damage to the inner ear that prevents sound impulses from being relayed to the brain). Typically, these conditions occur as a result of middle-ear fluid entrapment, wax buildup, exposure to noise, and age-related nerve degeneration. However, it is not unusual for a number of hearing problems to arise suddenly after a concussion.

In some instances, brain trauma is centered in areas of the *parietal* or *temporal lobes* that are linked to ear-related functions like balance and spatial awareness or the interpretation of sounds. Usually, however, post concussion hearing problems are the result of damage to the middle or inner ear. For instance, an eardrum may rupture. Or there may be swelling around the *eustachian tube* (a drainage tube that connects the ear to the throat) or bleeding into the middle ear, either of which can cause sound-blocking fluid buildup behind the eardrum. Or tiny, sensitive bones in the middle ear may be destroyed, which also hampers sound transmission. If the cochlea or the surrounding nerves bear the force of impact, all hearing in the affected ear may be lost, or you may become unable to interpret auditory messages.

It is important and reassuring to realize that many concussion-related hearing difficulties are temporary and treatable. Learning as much as you can about your particular problem can help you take the right steps toward recovery.

TYPES OF HEARING PROBLEMS THAT CAN FOLLOW A CONCUSSION

Trauma to the head or neck can result in a variety of difficulties that either reduce or interfere with your ability to hear, process, or tolerate sounds from your environment. The problems most commonly encountered after a concussion are described below.

Hearing Loss

Hearing loss, or hearing impairment, is a reduction in the ability to hear certain sounds due to nerve damage or a malfunction in the conduction of sound waves in the ear. Low-volume and high-pitched tones are the hardest sounds to hear; rapid or monotone dialogue also is difficult to understand. Hearing loss can rule out comfortable use of the telephone and make everyday interactions quite stressful. In conversation and circumstances in which there is competing noise, you may find yourself having to watch the speaker for clues as to what is being said.

Hearing loss may be temporary or permanent, depending on the cause of the impairment. Fortunately, most types are treatable.

Ménière's Syndrome

This condition, which can occur with or without a concussion, is characterized by one-sided low-frequency hearing loss with a sensation of fullness in the same ear, ringing or buzzing noises in the ear, and severe, even violent, attacks of vertigo (for a detailed discussion of vertigo, see Chapter 10). The amount of hearing loss may fluctuate, and the attacks of vertigo may vary in frequency. When the condition is in full swing, it can effectively render you immobile. While it is known that Ménière's syndrome stems from fluid buildup in the inner ear, there is a great deal of debate as to the underlying cause of this condition. Some treatments that may be suggested include diuretics (medications that alleviate fluid retention), limitation of movement, and, sometimes, surgery to release fluid from the middle ear. At present Ménière's syndrome is incurable, but various symptoms, such as vertigo and ringing in the ear, are treatable.

Noise Sensitivity

In many cases of inner-ear injury, the body attempts to compensate for loss of function. This can result in extreme sensitivity to loud sounds or noises of a certain pitch. In other cases, a concussion leads to sound-selection problems that render a person unable to discriminate between certain sounds or filter out background noise. Either condition poses a challenge to such everyday activities as conversing in a moving car or following the dialogue in a television program. Further compounding the problem is the fact that noise sensitivity often occurs in conjunction with tinnitus and hearing loss.

Sound Agnosia

In rare cases a condition called *sound agnosia*, or the inability to comprehend everyday sounds, may occur during recovery from a concussion. This malady is the result of injury to the temporal-parietal area of the brain's right hemisphere (see Chapter 1), and it leaves you able to participate in conversation but unable to identify or locate the source of such ordinary sounds as a ringing doorbell or barking dog. In some cases, there is complete loss of hearing in one ear. Naturally, sound agnosia poses a significant handicap to everyday functioning.

Tinnitus

Like Peter, in the story at the start of this chapter, many people with concussions are troubled by *tinnitus*, or the perception of sounds in the ear that are unrelated to any actual external sound. Ringing and buzzing noises are common. Some people hear fluctuating high-pitched tones like those from the uppermost keys on a pipe organ. Still others hear roaring or hissing noises. The problem is often worse at night or in very quiet surroundings. Needless to say, it can be extremely annoying and, consequently, stressful. Post concussion tinnitus may be temporary or lifelong.

DIAGNOSING AND ASSESSING HEARING PROBLEMS

If you experience a hearing problem after a concussion, it is essential that you be evaluated by an otolaryngologist, or ear, nose, and throat (ENT) specialist. Your primary care physician (PCP) should be able to refer you to a qualified professional, whose evaluation should include your family and medical histories, a review of the circumstances of your injury, an examination of your ears, and an audiogram, or hearing assessment, by an audiologist. Many ENT specialists have audiologists on staff. The results will enable the otolaryngologist to establish a diagnosis, prescribe corrective treatment, and suggest techniques to provide relief. He or she can also furnish educational materials and information about support organizations that deal with your particular problem. Because long-term hearing problems can affect speech and language—particularly in children—a referral to a speech/language pathologist may also be in order.

TREATING POST CONCUSSION HEARING PROBLEMS

The nature and severity of a hearing problem are usually good predictors of its curability. Happily, many hearing problems are correctable through a number of approaches. Others respond to a lesser extent to various treatments and practices. What follows is a look at the most successful approaches to resolving hearing problems.

Conventional Approaches

Your doctor will no doubt inform you that many types of hearing problems respond to available medical treatments. For instance, if hearing loss results from damage to the eardrum or inner-ear bones, surgical repair may be in order. Antibiotics, decongestants, antiemetics (medication for motion sickness), and changes in one's intake of sodium, tobacco, alcohol, and caffeine are often effective at reducing middle-ear fluid buildup that interferes with hearing, as occurs in Ménière's syndrome. In some cases, corrective surgical procedures to drain middle-ear fluid may help to decrease pressure on the vestibular system (the balance system in your inner ear).

Sound agnosia resulting from a concussion usually resolves itself over time. Tinnitus can be difficult to treat because the exact source of the problem is often impossible to pinpoint. In addition, this problem is often accompanied by hearing loss, and corrective measures for that problem can make tinnitus worse. Antidepressant medication may be used to relieve the emotional stress related to this annoying symptom. If you suffer from tinnitus, it is important to have your doctor assess *all* of the medications you are taking, since dozens of drugs—particularly those containing alcohol—are known to aggravate the condition. An adjustment to your prescription medications may bring significant relief. Hearing aids and tinnitus-masking devices can do a great deal to minimize the effects of long-term hearing problems as well. Niacin by prescription and over-the-counter no-flush niacin may also be helpful in reducing tinnitus.

Complementary Approaches

Certain complementary health practices have been shown to effect improvement in hearing problems such as noise sensitivity and vertigo. Acupressure and both traditional and *auricular* acupuncture can be particularly helpful. The appropriate type and frequency of treatment varies depending on individual needs and symptoms, so it is necessary to consult with a licensed acupuncturist to determine your specific needs.

Another complementary method for treating tinnitus is thermal biofeedback. This can help you learn to relax and tune out the annoying sound, while traditional neurofeedback can help you consciously alter the brain waves that perceive the sound. NeuroField, another form of neurofeedback described in Chapter 6, has been effective in many cases. In addition, hypnosis may be suggested to help you cope with tinnitus or the psychological effects of hearing impairment.

In many cases, the brain eventually becomes used to the constant noise of tinnitus, making the condition less annoying over time. LACE (Listening and Communication Enhancement), an interactive computerized aural rehabilitation program conceived by audiologists at the University of California at San Francisco, has been shown to help increase listening skills. Just as physical therapy can help rebuild muscles and adjust movements to compensate for physical weakness or injury, LACE will help you develop skills and strategies to deal with situations when your hearing is inadequate. We don't really hear in our ears; we hear in our brains. While hearing aids can help a person detect softer sounds, they don't necessarily provide good listening skills. So, whether you wear hearing aids, are just acquiring aids, or simply wish to improve your listening skills, LACE training can be very beneficial.

Alternative Approaches

There are no herbs or homeopathics to eliminate specific hearing-related symptoms such as tinnitus. However, based on your makeup, there may be remedies that can lessen your symptoms. It is best to consult with a qualified herbalist or homeopathic practitioner to see if help is available to you.

PRACTICAL SUGGESTIONS

As is often the case with post concussion symptoms, time can play an important role in correcting your hearing problems. While you follow your doctor's recommendations and wait out the recovery process, there are a number of steps you can take to help minimize the effects of hearing problems on your everyday life:

- Avoid nicotine, caffeine, alcohol, and recreational drugs. These substances have been shown to exacerbate tinnitus.

- Limit your use of salt, which can cause fluid retention and increased vertigo, and stay well hydrated.
- Stick to a regular sleep schedule to reduce stress and anxiety, both of which are tinnitus triggers.
- Sleep with a radio playing softly in the background, or run an electric fan or other source of "white noise" to minimize the effects of tinnitus. There are clock-sized noise-generating machines available that are designed specifically for this purpose.
- Call your telephone company's customer service number to inquire about special audio equipment that can make conversing by telephone easier.
- Ask your doctor about the advisability of a lip-reading course. Most rehabilitation facilities offer this type of training.
- Don't hesitate to inform people about sound-selection problems. Ask them to speak one at a time, or find a quiet place to hold conversations.
- Cater to your sound sensitivity by avoiding large-group functions and noisy places. If possible, do your shopping and other necessary errands when public places are least crowded—say, between 10:00 a.m. and noon. If that is not possible, ask a family member to do these chores for you while you are recovering.
- If you find yourself extremely anxious about your hearing problem, ask your doctor about sources of support and psychological help.

The effects of hearing problems on daily living are significant and undeniable. However, it is reassuring to know that many such disorders are cured by time and that others can be brought under control, if not completely corrected. If your concussion has left you with hearing difficulties, you can contribute a great deal to your recovery by seeking the expertise of a specialist, taking good physical care of yourself, being forthright about your impairment, and establishing home and work environments in which you can function most comfortably.

CHAPTER 13

MUSCULAR AND MOTOR PROBLEMS

■

B RIDGEPORT, CONNECTICUT, RESIDENTS HELEN AND MOE WERE AGES 79 AND 80 when they both suffered whiplash after their car was struck in the rear when stopped at a traffic light. When the police arrived, Helen complained of facial numbness and severe head pain, and Moe felt neck pain. They were immediately taken to a local hospital for testing. After a brief examination, it was suggested they have physical therapy for their neck spasms. Days later, Helen noticed severe headaches, writing problems, muscle weakness, unsteadiness, and poor coordination in addition to her facial pain and numbness. She was seen by a neurologist, who diagnosed a concussion, also known as *mild traumatic brain injury* (mTBI), and explained that her symptoms were related to her brain injury rather than the whiplash. She was put on Elavil to control her pain.

Nine months later, Moe completed his course of treatment for whiplash, fully recovered. Helen hasn't been as lucky. While physical therapy has eased her neck pain and headaches to some extent, she is still plagued by facial pain and numbness, fatigue, dizziness, continual muscle weakness, poor coordination, unsteadiness, and difficulty writing.

These symptoms were also present for Ted, who sustained a concussion while playing football. A fellow player used a face-mask tackle, pulling aggressively on the face mask of Ted's helmet. This type of tackle is illegal in American football, as it causes a player's head to snap around and can result in a *rotation injury* to the head. Ted was luckier than Moe and Helen, because he was immediately evaluated by an athletic trainer and treated by a sports medicine doctor, both of whom had experience dealing with concussions. When they noted signs of a concussion, Ted was told to immediately restrict his activities and rest in a quiet, darkened room while his brain healed. Ted felt better within a week, but he was not permitted to return to practice until he passed a concussion test administered by the athletic trainer and team physician.

The majority of concussions are the result of auto accidents, recreational activities, sports injuries, falls, physical assaults, and blast injuries in combat. In these types of traumas, both the brain and surrounding muscles are affected. The results can interfere with your ability to work, sit, drive, climb stairs, tie your shoes, and do many of the other intricate tasks that most of us do each day without thinking. Muscular injuries from any type of direct trauma are painful and may be slow to heal, but movement problems and chronic central nervous system (CNS) pain from *diffuse brain injury* may linger even longer or, in some instances, become permanent (see Chapter 15).

WHY MUSCULAR AND MOTOR PROBLEMS CAN OCCUR AFTER A CONCUSSION

"After my concussion, I had two major issues: hemiparesis, or muscle weakness on my entire right side, and a fine motor tremor in both of my hands, similar to an essential familial tremor. This meant that my hands shook all the time, more so when I felt anxious. As a musician and painter, this was a particular challenge. I used to do some fine fingerpicking on my guitar and have learned to compensate in this area. However, my hardest fine motor task is putting on eye makeup. Obviously, this is something male concussion patients can't relate to, but trust me, it is a huge issue. I learned to either have someone else apply my makeup or not use it."

—D.R.S.

Injury to the brain's motor areas, such as the *parietal lobe, cerebellum,* and *brain stem,* can directly affect your coordination, strength, balance, muscle tone, and posture. Numbness can be a result of injury to the sensory cortex in the front of the parietal lobe. A discussion of the different parts of the brain can be found in Chapter 1.

TYPES OF MUSCULAR AND MOTOR PROBLEMS THAT CAN FOLLOW A CONCUSSION

There are several types of muscular and motor problems that can occur as a result of a concussion. Like many effects of brain trauma, these can be intensified by fatigue and other factors. The most frequently cited complaints are described below.

Muscle Coordination

"As mentioned, I had tremendous difficulty with fine motor activities right after my accident. I had a moderate hand tremor and could no longer hold a pen or play my guitar. Several months later, feeling better, I promised my youngest son that I would perform for his class on the last day of school. A longtime guitarist, I never imagined I would have a problem. But to my great embarrassment, my right hand stopped responding in mid-performance."

—D.R.S.

Depending on the location and severity of your concussion, you may have slow, jerky, or uncontrolled movements. You may also encounter tremors—small, involuntary muscular movements that most often affect the head and hands. Even when you know exactly what you want to do—sign your name, thread a needle, or walk up stairs—and you can picture yourself doing it, step by step, in your mind, you may find yourself unable to make your body perform the needed motions. You may also have trouble trying to learn new motor skills, a problem caused by uncoordination or by difficulties with learning or memory. (A more detailed discussion of learning and memory problems will be found in Chapter 19.)

Loss of Muscle Strength

Loss of muscle strength can occur as a result of a concussion if the injured region of the brain is responsible for controlling muscular activity. *Hemiparesis* is the medical term for weakness and difficulty with movement affecting one side of the body. This is most likely to occur with injury that affects one side—the opposite side—of the brain. Paralysis of an entire side, called *hemiplegia*, may occur, although it is uncommon after a concussion. Muscle weakness can also occur due to injury to the muscles themselves or to the nerves that serve them, as a side effect of medications like carbamazepine (Atenonal, Tegretol), or as a result of sleep problems.

Perhaps the most common cause of muscle weakness after a concussion is simple disuse atrophy resulting from inactivity. While this problem is not painful, it can disrupt the range of your daily activities.

Loss of Muscle Tone

Brain injury can affect muscle tone, which is the tightness of the muscles when they are at rest. When muscle tone is normal, your body moves smoothly and easily. Injury to a CNS motor area can cause muscle tone to be too tight. You may experience muscle spasm, or tightening of a single muscle or muscle group, or *hypertonicity*, the tensing of all muscles, which causes your limbs and trunk to stiffen. Because muscle spasm is also the bodily response to pain, it can be difficult to determine whether the problem is from a brain injury or a muscle injury. There is a close relationship between spasticity and bladder function when there is brain or spinal cord injury. Nervous system connections to the bladder travel closely together with motor fibers that control the limbs, especially the lower extremities, which is why leg spasticity can be linked to spasticity of the bladder. When spasticity of the legs is severe, the legs can cross and "scissor," which can result in problems with personal hygiene.

Posture Problems

Brain injury can affect the muscles that control your head, neck, shoulders, and the rest of your body. If your neck muscles are in spasm from a brain or muscle injury, this can cause your body to go out of proper alignment, resulting in limited range of motion, muscle weakness, pain, and reduced muscle tone.

Both body movements and posture involve your bones, joints, and surrounding soft tissues—specifically, your muscles, tendons, and ligaments. If a joint between two bones is placed in a position that overstretches the surrounding soft tissues, injury occurs. This is true for all joints in your body, but has particular importance where the spine is concerned. In the spine, the soft tissues also support the soft discs that separate and cushion the vertebrae. Therefore, determining whether a posture problem is due to brain injury or direct bodily trauma is extremely difficult. Brain injury can affect the tone of the antigravity muscles in the trunk and limbs, producing flexion of the arms and legs. This may make it difficult to extend the arms, legs, and trunk against gravity since increased tone can diminish the cooperation between gravity and antigravity muscle effort.

Muscle Injuries

There are several muscular problems that can occur after a concussion. In these cases, the brain injury does not cause the injury to the muscles; rather, the same head trauma that results in brain injury also causes injury to the muscles and tendons near the impact area. Understanding the origin and nature of your particular complaint can help you understand your discomfort. The most frequently cited muscle injuries occurring in association with concussion are discussed below.

WHIPLASH

The impact of a blow to the head can cause whiplash, the stretching and tearing of the neck muscles, tendons, and ligaments because of hyperextension (excessive backward motion) or hyperflexion (excessive forward motion) of the cervical (upper) spine. This type of injury is most often a result of a motor vehicle accident or sports collision. Nerves may be pinched or damaged, and the neck muscles, tendons, and joint-stabilizing ligaments may be injured, resulting in acute or chronic pain. Muscle damage that leads to the formation of *adhesions* (bands of fibrous material that form unnatural attachments between tissues or structures in the body) between or within the muscles can prohibit free movement of the head and trigger painful spasms affecting the upper back, neck, face, and/or jaw muscles.

MYOFASCIAL DYSFUNCTION

This problem is an offshoot of whiplash that involves the muscles surrounding the neck, some of which continue up into the face. With this type of injury, the *fascia*, a cellophane-like membrane between the muscles, can become adhered to the muscle, resulting in restricted movement of the neck and facial muscles, and pain that radiates into the face, jaw muscles, cheek, arm, and/or hand.

FIBROMYALGIA

This muscle-pain syndrome—once known as *fibrositis, myofascial pain syndrome,* or *psychogenic rheumatism*—often develops following injuries to the neck and back. Localized or radiating pain may be traced to walnut-sized tender nodules, called "trigger points," within certain muscles. This condition often affects muscles of the neck, shoulder, buttocks, or anywhere along the spine. Pressure on a trigger point produces local tenderness as well as pain that radiates upward to the back of the head, or outward into the upper arm or thigh. The exact cause of these symptoms is unknown, but it is known that they can be aggravated by stress.

TEMPOROMANDIBULAR (TM) DISORDERS

This is another type of muscular problem associated with whiplash. *Temporomandibular* (TM) disorders, formerly called TMJ syndrome, include a variety of painful conditions of the TM (jaw) joint and muscles. Other complaints sometimes accompany the TM condition, including pain and a sensation of fullness in the ear, *tinnitus*, dizziness, and even hearing loss. The fact that these symptoms suggest problems within the ear can make it very difficult to identify TM disorders.

DIAGNOSING AND ASSESSING MUSCULAR AND MOTOR FUNCTION PROBLEMS

Most people who experience a concussion receive little or no professional evaluation of muscular or motor function immediately afterward. Treatment usually focuses on obvious physical injuries, if any—broken bones, cuts and bruises, and the like. If you can walk and talk normally, it is often assumed that all is well.

Later, if you go to your primary care physician (PCP) complaining of motor and/or muscular difficulties along with chronic pain, he or she may refer you to an orthopedist, physiatrist, or neurologist for evaluation and rehabilitation. These specialists may prescribe further diagnostic tests, such as a computed tomography (CT) scan or magnetic resonance imaging (MRI). (See Chapter 5.) If you have complaints involving an ear, you may also need to see an otolaryngologist (ear, nose, and throat doctor), who will do a structural assessment and hearing test. Other diagnostic tests commonly used to assess muscular and motor difficulties are described below.

Flexion/Extension X-Rays

This diagnostic test involves x-raying the neck or back during flexion, or bending forward, and extension, or bending backward. This can identify bone misalignment, such as two or more vertebrae out of normal position due to ligament or muscle damage. It can also identify muscle spasm, which can cause reversal of *lordosis*, the normal curvature of the spine.

Electromyography (EMG) and Nerve Conduction Velocity (NCV) Study

Electromyography (EMG) and the nerve conduction velocity (NCV) study are used to investigate where damage has occurred in nerves serving the various muscles in the body. EMG may be compared to testing the wiring in a wall of your house to investigate why the light switch is not working. It measures the electrical activity in the muscles to determine whether the nerves that serve the muscles in the injured part of the body are intact and the muscles are functioning normally. A thin insulated needle is inserted into the muscle, and measurements of electrical discharges are taken while the muscle is at rest and at work. EMG is usually done in the hand or foot, though other locations on the body are sometimes used.

The NCV study is similar to checking the speed with which electrical current travels from the power plant to the light switch. In this test, the speed and frequency of electrical impulses from your brain or spinal cord to the injured muscles are measured. A nerve is mildly shocked at one location and the response is measured at another location. Slower-than-normal conduction of nerve impulses can indicate nerve damage.

Both of these tests are often experienced as being uncomfortable, even painful. However, the doctors who administer them are aware of this.

Myelography

In this test, radio-opaque dye is injected into the spinal canal and X-rays are taken that show the dye as a white substance outlining the disc and nerve roots. This is done to pinpoint disc or nerve damage and scar tissue. Myelography is more effective at finding lesions than either the CT scan or MRI. However, because it is invasive, it is used less often.

Physical Capacity Evaluation

This consists of a series of timed tests to evaluate your balance, muscle tone, muscle strength, coordination, and flexibility. You may be asked to carry a box around a room, balance on a platform, or pick up small items. Your grip strength is measured by a small device that you squeeze with either hand. A physical capacity evaluation is usually done by a physical therapist or at a rehabilitation hospital.

Thermography

This test involves taking an infrared photograph of the surface of the body using a camera with heat-sensitive film. Thermography detects temperature differences in different parts of the body. These may be caused by injuries to nerves or blood vessels at the site of pain.

EVEN WITH modern diagnostic testing, it can sometimes be difficult to differentiate between brain injury that causes specific muscle, tendon, and ligament problems and direct injury to those same areas—particularly if chronic pain is involved. Your doctor will try to distinguish among the different tissue injuries, movement problems, and types of chronic pain, and prescribe appropriate treatment based on his or her assessment.

Fibromyalgia in particular is difficult to pin down, because the disorder leaves no neurological or orthopedic indicators on standard diagnostic tests. Some physicians will diagnose fibromyalgia if they can induce pain by applying pressure at several specific trigger points in various muscles throughout the body. Identifying TM disorders is another challenge, because the physical and ear examinations that are usually done in response to a patient's complaints typically yield only negative results. Myofascial dysfunction also can be difficult to diagnose because its symptoms can mimic (or coexist with) those of other disorders, including herniated disc, joint syndromes, and displaced vertebrae.

TREATING POST CONCUSSION MUSCLE AND MOTOR PROBLEMS

Depending on your physical makeup and the force of your injury, you may recover within a few weeks without treatment or suffer longer-term complications as a result of brain injury or nerve damage. In either case, recovery may be interrupted by setbacks and is rarely uniform.

Conventional Approaches

Various types of rehabilitative work can help to overcome motor difficulties, as well as chronic pain. Physical therapy techniques help with balance, motor coordination, muscle movement, tone, spasm, and strength. This type of therapy is also helpful in treating general inflammation and myofascial pain. For more extensive rehabilitation, you might need to see a physiatrist, a medical doctor who specializes in physical medicine and rehabilitation. Craniosacral methods, as explained in Chapter 6, are very effective in working with *post concussion syndrome* (PCS) muscle problems. Various types of massage therapy, such as Repetitive Usage Injury Therapy (RUIT), structural massage, and integrative massage, are also very helpful.

If there is any form of paralysis present, a possible treatment is the Taub method. Developed by Dr. Edward Taub, it is a revolutionary and extremely successful approach to physical therapy. His method uses the concept of restrictive therapy, which means restraining the limbs that work so that the body/brain is forced to reconnect to the paralyzed limbs.

Specialized treatment such as biofeedback can be obtained through rehabilitation hospital programs for people with a concussion. Biofeedback can be extremely helpful in many situations. Thermal and EMG biofeedback can increase muscle responsiveness and coordination, as well as help to control discomfort. Neurofeedback can help to normalize electrical activity in the motor areas of the brain, enhancing motor reflexes. However, all of these techniques can present a challenge for people with concentration or attention-span difficulties.

There are various types of indirect physical therapy treatments designed to heal and strengthen muscles and improve balance, coordination, and flexibility. One of these, the Burdenko method, involves dynamic water- and land-based movement exercises. The water portion is done in a vertical position using flotation devices to help you achieve natural traction, allowing gravity to gently separate the vertebrae. The land exercises are an extension of these therapeutic movements. For help finding a qualified Burdenko therapist in your area, feel free to get in touch with me via the contact information listed on page 367.

Another form of indirect physical therapy, the Feldenkrais method, is a series of subtle exercises designed to retrain your body's movement patterns for pain control and more efficient motor function. A practitioner teaches you alternative ways of moving to replace faulty patterns that may aggravate your injury. Again, you can contact me for help finding a qualified Feldenkrais therapist in your area.

Therapeutic horseback riding also helps to enhance balance, coordination, and physical stability.

Movement and dance therapy are forms of dynamic therapy that force the brain to adapt to injury by learning to use different parts than before to facilitate motor movement. This helps the brain to form new nerve connections to replace those impaired by injury. Music and dance therapy incorporate multiple movements and sensory input, and are available through many colleges, special education services, and dance studios.

If you need to overcome small motor impairments, or learn new techniques for dispatching troublesome tasks at home and at work, occupational therapy may be recommended. As an alternative, you may choose to undergo cognitive retraining, which involves learning new ways of accomplishing tasks that have become problematic. Or you may choose vocational therapy to learn skills that will prepare you to seek a different type of employment.

Complementary Approaches

Acupuncture helps the energy system to release the spastic muscles. Chiropractic adjustments can help to realign vertebrae in the neck, thus improving blood flow and nerve-impulse supply to problem muscles. This approach also allows for freer movement and more space between the joints. Many chiropractors also do myofascial release methods that are very helpful. In addition, light therapy can be effective at helping release muscle spasms.

Alternative Approaches

Polarity therapy, which maximizes the flow of internal energy and encourages the body to heal itself, may be effective against muscle and movement problems. Some people believe that reorganizing the body's energy structure, internal flow, and communication mechanisms can help improve balance and coordination.

PRACTICAL SUGGESTIONS

"Three years after my accident, I was still struggling with stability, balance, and walking. While in Switzerland, I discovered a telescoping walking stick that collapses to twelve inches in length and extends to almost four feet, and has straps and hand grips. In light of my balance problem, the Swiss shopkeeper advised me to use two sticks. Walking in the woods with only my hiking sticks for support gave me a wonderful feeling of freedom!"

—D.R.S.

"What works for me is a pen with a fat barrel, such as the Sheaffer Big Red, and a Mead fiber-tipped pen."

—BARBARA

"I still have difficulty remembering motor movements in my rehab program. I've found that when I feel a movement and sense it through a rhythmic beat, I can perform it immediately and remember it even days later."

—D.R.S.

Muscular and motor difficulties can wreak havoc with almost every activity on your daily agenda. While the prognosis for recovery is often quite good, the healing process can take time. In the meantime, there are steps you can take to make your life easier and more comfortable:

- If self-care tasks prove difficult during the early phase of your recovery, consider hiring a home health aide.

- Shop with an eye toward making home and personal care tasks easier. Look for items with Velcro closures or large handles, for example. I can assist you with finding a wide array of items designed specifically for people with muscular and motor problems. Simply call or email me via the contact information on page 367. A rehabilitation hospital can also help you.

- If fine motor problems make writing difficult, try using a clipboard and a felt-tipped or wide-barreled pen to make this task easier. Also consider using a slip-on pencil grip and number-three pencils, which have harder lead than customary pencils. If writing by hand is temporarily out of the question, use a computer instead.

- Join a local support group or communicate online with people affected by symptoms similar to yours. Through such contacts you can gain valuable advice, as well as emotional and psychological support, from others who have "been there." The wisdom and encouragement of others in your situation can be extremely helpful.

- Remember that a cycle of muscle deconditioning and weakness begins after only a few days of bed rest. Avoid what may become months of reconditioning therapy by engaging in whatever light activity you can manage.

- Avoid tension and stress, which place more strain on joints and muscles and may cause additional discomfort.

- Try hot or cold packs to help loosen or numb muscles in the affected area. Warm baths or showers can also be very effective.

- Add a regimen of stretching to your daily routine. This will help improve range of motion and flexibility.

- Practice yoga. These gentle exercises promote flexibility, strength, concentration, posture, breathing, balance, and relaxation.

- Improve your neck muscle strength if you are an athlete or participate in contact recreational sports.

- Use a mouth guard during contact sports or recreational pursuits. The majority of sports-related concussions are related to injury from hits to the jaw.
- Wear a helmet if you are riding a horse, skateboarding, skating, skiing, or using a bicycle or motorcycle.
- Make use of protective headgear designed for your sport, even if it isn't mandated that participants do so.

When muscle and motor problems follow a concussion, they are certainly an added challenge. However, working to find the best treatment for your particular symptoms and experimenting with strategies to help you cope with everyday life can go a long way toward making you feel better and more in control.

CHAPTER 14

SENSORY AND METABOLIC DISTURBANCES

∎

SINCE EXPERIENCING A CONCUSSION, ALSO CALLED *MILD TRAUMATIC BRAIN injury* (mTBI), Gail, whose story opens Chapter 7, has experienced a variety of sensory and other problems that were not immediately attributed to her injury. For example, certain foods now taste different to Gail, and some cause actual discomfort when eaten. In addition, because she is extremely sensitive to touch, an ordinary act such as opening a jar causes Gail to overreact and jerk her hand back. Cooking—which Gail refers to as a sensory-intensive operation—is a problem. She has to think carefully about every step of the process, to avoid feeling overloaded by smells, sights, and sounds.

No matter what the activity, Gail is fatigued by too much sensory stimulation, which in her case triggers episodes of double vision and a constant sensation of being cold. She also complains of having a metallic taste in her mouth, and she has gained twenty pounds since her accident. Her doctor attributes the last two problems to her medication.

Have you been annoyed by weight gain or by appetite, skin, or sensory problems since your concussion? Complaints of this type are common among people with *post concussion syndrome* (PCS). By themselves, these miscellaneous symptoms may not seem severe or constant enough to send sufferers to a doctor. And when medical attention *is* sought, sensory and metabolic difficulties are generally viewed as separate from post concussion symptoms. As a result, problems of this nature often go undiagnosed.

The fact is that sensory and metabolic symptoms do occur, either as a direct result of injury to the brain or nearby areas or as a side effect of medication prescribed for other post concussion symptoms.

WHY SENSORY AND METABOLIC PROBLEMS CAN OCCUR AFTER A CONCUSSION

Doctors and researchers do not fully understand the connection between TBI and sensory and metabolic difficulties. However, it is known that even tiny *contusions* (bruising) in the sensory areas of the brain, which are localized in the *parietal*, *occipital*, and *temporal lobes* (see Chapter 1) can trigger complaints of this nature. Your concussion may have damaged nerves that facilitate the sense of taste or smell, or affected your *pituitary gland's* hormonal control of weight and appetite. Injury to the spinal column or nerve receptors in the skin can alter your sense of touch.

TYPES OF SENSORY AND METABOLIC PROBLEMS THAT CAN FOLLOW A CONCUSSION

Sensory and metabolic symptoms vary in type and degree, depending on the nature of your concussion. Some of the most commonly reported problem areas are described below.

Altered Sense of Smell

"I was walking to my mailbox one day when I slipped on some ice. I fell backward without catching myself and hit the right rear of my head on the cement driveway. My next memory is of twelve hours later, when I found myself in a Sioux City hospital. When I was served breakfast and lunch the following day, I blamed the food's tastelessness on institutional cooking. I was discharged from the hospital with a diagnosis of mild traumatic brain injury and the recommendation that I see a neurologist within two weeks.

At the two-week appointment, my neurologist realized that I had lost my sense of smell along with most of my sense of taste. He told me not to worry, for this was a common problem, and my sense of smell would probably return within six weeks. Two weeks after that, I developed a nauseating phantom smell that was very worrisome. Car exhaust and hair sprays in particular triggered a strong, unpleasant odor.

In the ensuing years, my ability to smell and taste has slowly improved. However, the phantom odor still intrudes off and on, making my life frustrating and difficult. As it happens, cooking had always been a major part of my life—in fact, before my injury, I had twice been a finalist in the Pillsbury Bake-Off. I have had to learn many new coping skills in order to continue entering cooking contests and catering luncheons. Fortunately, my efforts still receive positive reviews."

—DARLENE

Your ability to smell allows you to detect and identify odors. A concussion can result in *hyposmia* (a partial loss of the capacity to smell) or in *anosmia* (a complete loss of the sense of smell). Another complaint, *dysosmia*, is a change or changes in the sense of smell that cause you to perceive a phantom smell that can be either pleasant, neutral, or, more commonly, distinctly unpleasant. However slight they may be, changes in your ability to smell can be difficult to adjust to.

The sense of smell is probably the least appreciated of all the senses. It affects our lives in many ways, not the least of which is our ability to appreciate the flavor of food. Your sense of smell also acts as a signal, alerting you to the presence of such things as gas leaks, spoiled food, and smoke. Dysosmia, or phantom smells, can distract and disgust, while some odors can actually trigger a migraine headache. Research in aromatherapy has shown that our moods, metabolism, and ability to become sexually aroused are all affected by the sense of smell. Clearly, problems in this area can have far-reaching and dramatic effects. An olfactory loss of some type, whether partial or complete, can be seen in about 20 percent of individuals after a concussion.

Loss of the Sense of Taste

Under normal circumstances, your tongue can distinguish four basic tastes: sweet, sour, salty, and bitter. However, a disruption along the nerve pathways from the taste buds to the brain can prevent taste messages from being interpreted properly. The result is *hypogeusia*, or decreased ability to taste, while the ability to distinguish food texture, temperature, and spiciness remains intact. Frequently, when a person cannot appreciate the flavor of food, he or she is actually experiencing flavor loss caused by hyposmia or anosmia. Most people with PCS do retain the ability to detect the irritating properties of certain substances— the burn of chili peppers or the tingle of alcohol, for example. In the case of loss of smell as a result of a concussion, there is often also a change in taste reported due to the close relationship that exists between the two senses. The question for the treating doctor becomes, does the patient have loss of taste because there is true loss of smell and taste still works? Or is it true loss of taste? Or is it both? In most cases after a concussion, it is a patient's olfactory (smell) system that is impaired rather than the gustatory (taste) system.

Changes Involving the Skin

Your skin is your body's largest organ and may undergo changes in sensitivity after a concussion. Occasional or localized numbness can occur. And, although it is less common, you may experience a heightened sensitivity to touch, sometimes to the point that the feeling of anything—even clothing—touching your skin is unbearable. You may also experience occasional skin rashes or the chronic itching and superficial inflammation of *atopic dermatitis*, a skin disorder that involves scaly and itchy patches. Both skin rashes and atopic dermatitis are unexplained but not uncommon results of trauma to the brain.

Appetite and Weight Changes

A decrease in appetite may appear immediately after a concussion, but this is more common with moderate or severe brain injuries. More characteristic of a concussion is an increase in appetite. Injury to your short-term memory and/or the *hypothalamus* (the portion of the brain that controls hunger) can play havoc with your appetite, making you feel hungry even when you have just eaten. Also, if you are having problems with short-term memory, you may not *remember* that you have eaten.

Inflammation in the brain due to a concussion can trigger the release of cortisol, which then triggers the storage of fat to protect the body. A concussion can also alter your body's metabolism of food, so that you may find that your appetite has increased. Or you may find that you are gaining weight even though your eating habits remain the same, because you are now burning calories more slowly. Weight gain can also occur as a side effect of anticonvulsants or other medications, such as antidepressants or sleep aids. Another factor in weight gain is an overall decrease in activity level as a result of chronic fatigue—a major problem after a concussion.

Bladder and Bowel Control Problems

Bladder-control problems (incontinence) and bowel problems, such as diarrhea or constipation, are embarrassing but not uncommon after a concussion. Brain injury may cause confused messages to be sent to or from the muscles in the bladder and/or the bowel. Incontinence may lead to bladder infections. Constipation may also be caused by inactivity during the period after your injury or occur as a side effect of medications.

DIAGNOSING AND ASSESSING SENSORY AND METABOLIC PROBLEMS

If your concussion leaves you with symptoms such as those previously described, it is important to tell your neurologist about them. To determine the exact nature of your problem, he or she should do a thorough evaluation, including family and medical histories, a review of the circumstances of your injury, and an examination of the affected area. Additional specialists may be called upon, including an otolaryngologist (an ear, nose, and throat specialist), a dermatologist, an allergist, or a gastroenterologist.

A comprehensive measure of sensory deficits is best done through an established chemosensory clinic. An institution such as the Taste and Smell Clinic at the University of Connecticut Health Center can provide a multidisciplinary approach to these problems, to determine whether your sensory deficits are neurological in origin. Please contact me via the information on page 367 for further details.

Once a diagnosis has been made, your doctor or doctors can prescribe corrective treatment, suggest techniques to provide relief, and furnish educational and support materials.

TREATING POST CONCUSSION SENSORY AND METABOLIC PROBLEMS

"Although I was on a one-thousand-calorie, twelve-grams-of-fat-a-day diet prescribed by the head of nutrition at a major Boston hospital, I gained over twenty pounds after my concussion. It was clear that metabolic changes caused by my brain injury, together with side effects of my seizure medication, could override even the healthiest diet. I found going from a well-toned size eight to an out-of-shape size fourteen to be really discouraging. I felt as if I was living in a "fat suit." I eventually decided to focus on the fact that I'm lucky to be alive—even as I was determined to get into the best possible shape for my circumstances by maintaining healthful eating habits and working out as much as my body would permit."

—D.R.S.

The precise nature and the severity of your symptoms may be good predictors of their curability. Many sensory and metabolic problems reverse themselves over time. Others can be expected to respond to treatment. What follows is a look at the most successful approaches.

Conventional Approaches

Between 5 and 30 percent of people with PCS lose or face alterations in their sense of smell, sense of taste, or ability to detect common chemicals. However, there are treatments that can help. If the decreased sensory ability is from brain swelling or injury to the nerves for taste or smell, this can be treated with steroids. Examination of a person with smell and taste problems following a concussion requires evaluations by a neurologist and an otolaryngologist. For use in the doctor's office, a scratch-and-sniff test has been developed, along with an alcohol sniff test. In the emergency room, it is important to evaluate the severity of the injury causing the complaint by checking computed tomography (CT) scans of the brain for evidence of skull fracture and looking for evidence of leaking spinal fluid from the nose or ear. In certain instances, surgery will be required.

If tests indicate that your problem is neurologically based, time will generally be the best healer. There are some medications, such as valproic acid (Depakene), and experimental surgical procedures available to treat distorted or phantom smells. Drug treatment for loss of the sense of taste is under research.

In general, skin sensitivity is difficult to treat. You can try treating the various symptoms of skin sensitivity with a minor analgesic like acetaminophen (Tylenol, Datril, and others) to reduce pain, an antihistamine such as diphenhydramine (Benadryl) to relieve itching, or aloe vera gel to reduce a dry, uncomfortable feeling.

Treatment for problems with appetite or weight changes caused by a concussion is geared toward the symptoms rather than the cause or injury. Typical approaches may include appetite suppressants and weight-control programs such as Weight Watchers, Jenny Craig, and Diet Workshop. Your neurologist may also recommend consulting a nutritionist, who can assist you in revising your diet.

Bodily changes can be very upsetting from an emotional point of view. Cognitive behavioral therapy (CBT) can help you cope with weight gain or loss and the sense of having lost control. In some situations, antidepressants may be needed.

Bowel problems can often be helped by increasing water or fluid intake, exercising, and using an over-the-counter stool softener. Incontinence is best treated by a urologist, who may recommend specialized muscle exercises called Kegels (see page 186). There are medications available to help with bladder retraining, but the side effects, such as light sensitivity, can worsen other post concussion symptoms.

Complementary Approaches

Both traditional and *auricular* acupuncture have been found to be effective against various sensory and metabolic complaints. Acupressure may also be helpful for bladder control. To determine which treatment to use, it is best to consult with a licensed acupuncturist. Neurofeedback can sometimes help by changing your perception of sensation and helping with the neurological "disconnect" in the brain. Also, light therapy and self-controlled energo neuro adaptive regulation (SCENAR) are very effective at improving perception of smell and perception of sensation (see Chapter 6).

Alternative Approaches

There are a number of herbal and homeopathic remedies that may bring some relief. For bladder problems, the herbs sang piao xiao, fu shen, couch grass, or buchu, or the homeopathic *Nux vomica*, may be helpful. Wu yao is an excellent herb for bowel problems. The homeopathics *Aconitum napellus* or *Natrum muriaticum* may be appropriate for problems with the sense of smell. *Plumbum metallicum*, another homeopathic remedy, may be used for skin sensitivity. Before using these or any other alternative remedies, it is best to have a thorough medical evaluation and then to consult with an experienced herbalist or homeopath who has experience in treating people with brain injuries. He or she will be able to prescribe remedies according to your individual needs and symptoms.

PRACTICAL SUGGESTIONS

"When I found myself bothered by skin sensitivity and hot flashes, my doctors first suggested that I stop the medication I was taking at the time. This helped to some degree, but my skin was still more sensitive than usual. My dermatologist suggested experimenting with different detergents and body and facial soaps, and I kept trying different products until I found ones that worked for me."

—D.R.S.

As with many symptoms associated with PCS, it helps—indeed, it can be necessary—to be inventive and willing to explore alternatives that bring relief. The following suggestions may prove helpful for sensory and metabolic problems:

- Don't assume that your complaint is too minor to mention, or that nothing can be done. Bring sensory and other problems to your doctor's attention.
- Indulge your particular sensitivity. If you are prone to sensory overload, ask for help rather than placing yourself in situations that are physically uncomfortable.
- Experiment with different foods and methods of preparation to determine which tastes or smells are absent or bothersome. Plan meals and snacks around your findings.
- Seek expert help for skin or weight problems. Mainstream corrective measures such as moisturizers or fad diets may not work for you.
- Make sure to have functioning smoke and gas detectors in your home if you're experiencing difficulty with your sense of smell.
- Be exceptionally careful with the preparation of foods and beverages. Refrigerated foods should be date-labeled and stored at appropriate temperatures, and discarded if they look or feel suspicious. When in doubt, have a friend or family member check perishables for spoilage.
- To enhance your enjoyment of food, add texture, contrasting temperatures, and spices. For example, try spicy chips and taco sauce, or ice cream with crunchy nuts and hot syrup.

Bear in mind that you, your concussion, and your symptoms are completely unique. Listen to your body, and be aware that it may be necessary to experiment in order to find techniques that are effective against sensory and metabolic symptoms. Also, keep in mind that even if they are relatively minor, long-term problems of any sort can exact an emotional toll that may impede your recovery. Don't hesitate to ask for medical and family support when you need it.

CHAPTER 15

CHRONIC PAIN/POST TRAUMATIC PAIN (PTP)

■

BOTH HELEN AND TED, WHOSE STORIES APPEARED IN CHAPTER 13, DID RECOVER from their muscular injuries; however, both continued to suffer from chronic pain. In Helen's case, she continued to experience scalp and tooth pain, while Ted felt as if he was walking on crushed glass. He reported that whenever he took a step, he felt like he was getting an electrical jolt throughout his body. Due to his chronic pain, he was unable to resume playing football during the next two seasons.

Karl, who served in the military and sustained a blast injury, reported that one of the most difficult parts of his life since is dealing with the chronic pain in his body.

Muscular and emotional injuries from any type of direct trauma can be painful and slow to heal, but movement problems, emotional trauma, and chronic central nervous system (CNS) pain from diffuse brain injury, rotation injury, and blast injury may linger even longer. In some instances, these conditions may become permanent.

WHY CHRONIC AND POST TRAUMATIC PAIN (PTP) PROBLEMS CAN OCCUR AFTER A CONCUSSION

"For over six years, I had chronic neck and shoulder pain from my auto accident, especially from the seat belt—a very common muscular injury. Numerous tests, including nerve conduction velocity, were done to pinpoint the source of my pain. Eventually, I was diagnosed with CNS pain that was causing muscle spasms in my neck and shoulder. Various treatments proved unsuccessful until I discovered EMG biofeedback (see Chapter 6). This technique helped stop my muscle spasms and increased my mobility. But it was not until I used neurofeedback, which actually changed my pain perception, that my CNS pain stopped completely."

—D.R.S.

Pain, as defined by the International Association for the Study of Pain, is "an unpleasant sensory and emotional experience associated with actual or potential tissue damage, or described in terms of such damage." Pain is neither good nor bad; rather, it is a warning signal that something is wrong. This signal helps you to react and respond. The perception of pain is a complex operation that involves an intricate network of connections to and from the spinal cord and brain, which collectively make up the CNS. The location of the brain's pain centers and the fine points of pain perception remain under research, but it is known that the CNS allows you to sense pain when something is not right with your body. Acute pain is an early warning signal. Its psychological component is anxiety, which helps you to react quickly to the threat. For example, acute pain tells you to react to the heat of fire so that you can move away to avoid getting burned.

In a typical muscle or soft-tissue injury, the brain perceives that the area has been injured and sends a message to the muscle to respond by tightening, or spasming. This in turn causes the sensation of pain to be sent back to the brain, completing what is called the pain/spasm cycle. In addition, the actual injury causes the body to react and repair through an inflammation response.

Chronic pain is long lasting, often having a life of its own. Its psychological component is depression; thus, chronic pain and depression often go hand in hand. Chronic pain is also called post traumatic pain (PTP), since the source of the depression and pain has often happened at a much earlier time.

PAIN ASSESSMENT

Pain can be extremely difficult to assess, because it is personal and unique to the person experiencing it. Therefore, both subjective methods (what a person feels) and objective methods (diagnostic assessments) of scientific measurements are used in the assessment of pain.

How Your Pain Feels to You

"For over a month following my concussion, I thought worms were crawling over my head. Thankfully, my neurologist explained that this was a symptom of nerve pain."

—D.R.S.

The mnemonic device "COLDER" helps in assessing what your pain feels like. The letters stand for *Character* (whether the pain is stabbing, pinching, burning, etc.), *Onset, Location, Duration, Exacerbation* (what makes the pain worse), and *Relief* (what makes the pain better). In addition, the frequency and severity of the pain are also assessed.

In questioning the character of your pain, your doctor may ask you to rate it from 0 to 10, with 0 meaning no pain and 10 meaning the most pain. He or she may also ask you to rate the pain's sensation, with 0 being dull pain and 10 being very sharp pain. Thus, a 10–10 would indicate the highest level of extremely sharp pain. The book *Conquering Chronic Pain after Injury*, by Doctors William Simon, George Ehrlich, and Arnold Sadwin, contains the following descriptions of the sensation of pain:

- *Hyperesthesia.* An increased sensitivity to stimuli, such as pain felt when stroking, brushing, or lightly touching the skin
- *Dysesthesia.* An abnormal sensation, such as a feeling of hot and cold, ants crawling, or water dripping
- *Paresthesia.* A tingling sensation
- *Hypesthesia.* A decrease in normal sensation
- *Anesthesia.* A loss of sensation

A history is also taken to see if the type of pain being experienced existed prior to the concussion, also known as *mild traumatic brain injury* (mTBI). If so, the concussion may have caused the preexisting pain to increase. A review of medical records is needed to pinpoint what caused the pain before and what methods were helpful in its relief.

Diagnosis and Assessment

There are a vast number of clinical tests done to assess chronic pain. There is electrophysiological testing, such as the nerve conduction velocity (NCV) study, which is used to investigate where damage has occurred in nerves supplying the various muscles in the body (see Chapter 13). Also, there are imaging tests to look for structural damage, along with psychological pain assessments, such as the Vanderbilt Pain Management Inventory, Cognitive Coping Strategy Inventory, and the Multidimensional Pain Inventory, to name a few. Each of the test methods provides information to help the clinician make a proper diagnosis and provide the most suitable treatment to help you manage and cope with your chronic pain.

TREATING POST TRAUMATIC PAIN

Since PTP can affect you emotionally (see Chapter 23 on PTSD), psychologically, physically, and spiritually, successful treatment requires a complex program. Depending on your physical makeup and the force of your injury, you may recover within a few weeks without treatment, or you may suffer longer-term complications as a result of brain injury or nerve damage. In either case, recovery is often interrupted by setbacks and is rarely uniform.

Conventional Approaches

Traditionally, there have been four conventional methods of treating chronic pain: surgical intervention (such as on a bulging disc), medication, physical therapy, and psychotherapy.

Physical therapy is helpful in treating general inflammation and *myofascial pain*, or pain in the covering of the muscle. Muscles normally move smoothly next to each other; however, an injury can cause the myofascia to become stuck together, causing pain. Craniosacral therapy, a specific form of physical therapy, is very effective against chronic pain, as is the Burdenko method of dynamic water- and land-based movement exercises (see Chapter 13). In addition, cognitive behavioral therapy (CBT), a form of psychotherapy, can help ward off depression, manage stress, and find the emotional tools for coping with long-term pain.

Over-the-counter and prescribed medication for chronic pain can be extremely helpful. However, after a concussion, you should bear in mind that you may be newly sensitive to even low doses of over-the-counter products. Additionally, side effects—a fact of life with any medication—can play havoc with your recovery, so be sure to start with minimal doses and follow your doctor's instructions carefully.

Minor aches and pains are best treated with aspirin and/or nonsteroidal anti-inflammatory drugs (NSAIDs) such as ibuprofen (Advil, Motrin, Nuprin, and others) and naproxen sodium (Aleve). These products block the production of body chemicals called *prostaglandins*, which play an important role in the pain, heat, and swelling that occur with tissue damage. Prescription-strength NSAIDs are available for people who do not respond to over-the-counter drugs. Topical ointments that include aloe or capsaicin are also helpful.

Prescription medications used by pain sufferers also include diazepam (Valium), a muscle relaxant, and amitriptyline (Elavil, Endep), an antidepressant that when taken at bedtime can be useful for sleep and pain management. It is still unclear how and why these medications work to reduce pain; however, they are often found to be very effective. Corticosteroid injections may be used for treatment of joint pain, particularly in the hands, ankles, feet, hips, or knees.

Narcotics, which block the transmission of pain messages to and from the brain and spinal cord, are an option for extremely severe, persistent pain. If you require more powerful pain medication, such as the narcotic meperidine (Demerol), you may be able to reduce the amount you need by supplementing the prescription drug with over-the-counter medication, such as aspirin, acetaminophen (Tylenol and others), ibuprofen, and/or naproxen sodium. By alternating different products, you are more likely to feel relief with lower doses of medications. Keeping your use of powerful prescription medications to a minimum has several benefits. First, it helps prevent your body from building up a tolerance to the drug that would make you require progressively stronger doses for pain relief. Second, it helps minimize side effects. In addition, taking an over-the-counter product in conjunction with a prescribed pain medication—with your doctor's guidance and approval, of course—can sometimes enhance the prescription drug's effectiveness. Furthermore, your symptoms can be complicated by the rebound phenomenon, in which increasing the dose of pain medication actually causes more pain as the medication begins to wear off. Occasionally, anticonvulsants are prescribed for severe piercing, stabbing pain. A form of continuous administration called epidural therapy involves injecting narcotics directly into the membrane around the spinal cord. This helps to avoid numerous side effects associated with these drugs.

There are several non-pharmacological pain-control options, two of which are medical devices approved by the Food and Drug Administration. Transcutaneous electrical nerve stimulation (TENS) involves the wearing of a small battery-powered generator that transmits electrical impulses to underlying nerves. This electrical activity can block pain signals traveling to the brain and may also stimulate the body's production of natural pain-control substances. Cranial electrotherapy stimulation (CES) is similar to TENS, but the electrodes are attached to the ears and the electrical impulse is sent directly to the brain's pain center to decrease the sensation of pain. Implantable spinal cord stimulators with adjustable settings may also be used with the strongest types of pain. These are implanted by pain specialists or neurosurgeons and are effective in controlling severe pain that does not respond well to oral medications.

TABLE 15.1. MEDICATIONS USED FOR PAIN MANAGEMENT

CATEGORY	
Antidepressants	Amitriptyline (Elavil)
	Desipramine (Norpramin)
	Nortriptyline (Pamelor, Aventyl)
	Fluoxetine (Prozac, Sarafem)
	Paroxetine (Paxil, Paxil CR, Pexeva)
	Duloxetine (Cymbalta)
Analgesics	Acetaminophen (Tylenol)
	Tramadol (ConZip, Rybix ODT, Ryzolt, Ultram, Ultram ER)
Steroids	Prednisone (Deltasone, Liquid Pred)
	Dexamethasone (Decadron, Dexasone, Diodex, Hexadrol, Maxidex, DexPak)
Anticonvulsants	Carbamazepine (Tegretol, Tegretol XR, Equetro, Carbatrol)
	Valproic acid (Depakote, Depakote ER, Depakene, Depacon, Stavzor)
	Phenytoin (Dilantin)
	Clonazepam (Klonopin)
	Gabapentin (Neurontin)
	Levetiracetam (Keppra, Keppra XR)
	Lamotrigine (Lamictal)
	Oxcarbazepine (Trileptal)
	Pregabalin (Lyrica)
Local anesthetics	Lidocaine
	Mexiletine
	Flecainide
Topical anesthetics	Capsaicin
	Lidocaine patch
	Compounded neuralgic preparations containing ketamine, bupivacaine, diclofenac, gabapentin, topiramate, orphenadrine, doxepin, and others in various formulations

These traditional methods remain very effective; however, there are now integrative approaches available that are very helpful. These approaches are often found in clinics that specialize in PTP.

One integrative approach is through nutrition. The first step in dealing with chronic pain is to change what you eat, because a traumatic injury, regardless of cause, produces inflammation in your body and brain. To reduce this inflammation, it is important to follow a diet high in omega-3, including foods such as wild salmon, sardines, chia seeds, flaxseed, cherries, broccoli, and avocado, while eliminating cane sugar, artificial sweeteners, and corn syrup. The spice turmeric also helps with inflammation. A licensed dietitian or nutritionist with training in brain injury can help design an anti-inflammatory diet specifically for you. An over-the-counter medication called Wobenzym N, which is designed for healthy inflammation and joint support, and gamma-aminobutyric acid (GABA), a neurotransmitter, help soreness and tenderness. Both of these products are recommended by many physicians worldwide.

Complementary Approaches

Acupuncture has been found to work well at controlling chronic pain. Hypnosis and relaxation training are effective as well; however, you may have to wait to try this method if you are having problems with concentration or your attention span. The supplement S-adenosylmethionine (SAMe), a synthetic form of a compound formed in the body from the essential amino acid methionine and the energy-producing compound adenosine triphosphate, is helpful for depression and pain management.

Bioenergetics therapy, developed by Dr. Alexander Lowen, is a body-oriented approach to psychotherapy that is effective for chronic pain. Thought Field Therapy (TFT), energy psychology, and energy medicine (see Chapter 6) are all helpful as well. Biofeedback can be very useful in pain management, as can heart rate variability (HRV) training methods. Electromyography (EMG) biofeedback and neurofeedback can help to normalize electrical activity in the motor areas of the brain, enhancing motor reflexes and changing the perception of pain. Self-controlled energo neuro adaptive regulation (SCENAR) and use of the Photonic Stimulator for light therapy have been used by NASA for pain management aboard the space shuttle.

Alternative Approaches

Polarity therapy, which maximizes the flow of internal energy and encourages the body to heal, may be effective against muscle pain and movement problems. Some people believe that reorganizing the body's energy structure, internal flow, and communication mechanisms can help improve balance and coordination. Therapeutic Touch (TT), Reiki, Quantum-Touch, and Qi Gong can be very useful in pain management. Watsu, a form of bodywork that combines water, shiatsu massage, and yoga, may be helpful as well.

Ayurvedic medicine is a Hindu system of traditional medicine that relies on plants and minerals and includes various treatments for pain management. Ayurvedic practitioners can be found in most major cities. In addition, there are Buddhist and Chinese herbalists who offer many effective remedies for pain.

Aromatherapy, using the Young Living Essential Oils blends Relieve It and PanAway, can be useful in pain management. Bach Flower Rescue Remedy, along with Star of Bethlehem, Cherry Plum, Sweet Chestnut, and White Chestnut may be effective as well. To gain the best results using Bach Flower products, it is best to contact a Bach Flower practitioner to have a formula designed just for you. A supplement used in Europe to help with bodily inflammation is avocado-soybean unsaponifiables (ASU). Other products that help combat inflammation are borage oil and evening primrose, both taken orally, as well as Topricin, a homeopathic topical ointment. Both herbal and homeopathic preparations are available for pain relief. Herbal remedies sometimes recommended for pain include white willow bark, bai shao, and ye jaio teng. Among homeopathics, *Arnica* is recommended to relieve muscle soreness, while *Natrum sulphuricum*, *Bungaris*, and *Carbo vegetabilis* help with muscle, headache, and generalized pain. Traumeel, an over-the-counter homeopathic, is specifically designed for pain and inflammation. As always, it is best to consult with an herbalist or homeopathic practitioner who knows your history and needs before trying an over-the-counter herbal or homeopathic remedy.

PRACTICAL SUGGESTIONS

"What has really helped with my chronic pain over the years was changing my diet to an anti-inflammatory one, exercise using the Burdenko method (which I lovingly call "Igoretics" after its founder, Dr. Igor Burdenko), and stress reduction, which was not so easy (however, the breathing methods and little monitor of emWave did help, along with EMG biofeedback and neurofeedback). When needed, I did take a small dose of Valium, Neurontin, or the homeopathic Traumeel. Also, I used the topical ointment Topricin. Along with this, I used monthly acupuncture and chiropractic myofascial release or structural massage as needed. Also, I worked with a homeopath and nutrition educator, along with taking Wobenzym N, Alka-V, and GABA. Lastly, I found a pillow that really helps with pain at MyPillow.com. The bottom line is that I have a life again! I'm back at work, spending time with my friends and family, and enjoying life—not just enduring it."

—D.R.S.

The prognosis for recovery from post concussion symptoms is often quite good, but the healing process can take time. In the meantime, there are steps you can take to make your life more comfortable:

- Take your over-the-counter or prescription medication before you feel pain.
- Change to an anti-inflammatory diet.
- Exercise. Water therapy, yoga, and T'ai Chi are gentle exercises that are helpful for both body and mind.
- Rest often, and pace yourself.
- Get restorative sleep (see Chapter 9).
- Try hot or cold packs to loosen or numb muscles in the affected area. Warm baths or showers can also be helpful.

The pain that follows a concussion can indeed be difficult to live with. However, a positive attitude is one of the keys to a faster recovery. Chances are good that the weeks and months after injury will be much easier to bear if you refuse to be victimized by discomfort. Instead, retake control of your life by working with your health care provider and searching for your own creative solutions to chronic pain.

CHAPTER 16

SEXUAL PROBLEMS

■

B EVERLEY, A SUCCESSFUL REAL ESTATE BROKER AND NATIONALLY RATED GYM- nastics judge, had been happily married for thirty-two years. Prior to her brain injury, she often initiated lovemaking with her husband, whether by preparing a candlelit dinner, wearing an alluring nightgown, or just engaging in provocative play. After her concussion, also called *mild traumatic brain injury (mTBI)*, she felt as if sexuality did not exist. Sex never entered her mind, she never felt aroused, and the idea of initiating sexual intimacy was completely foreign to her. It took almost two years before Beverley began to make overtures toward lovemaking, and even then, it took a very conscious effort.

You may have found your sexual side to be curiously absent in the time since your concussion. Or perhaps the opposite is true—since your injury, you may have found yourself consumed with thoughts of sex and the desire for intimate physical contact. In either case, you may be relieved to know that this is no mere coincidence. While sexual issues are rarely granted the attention paid to other post concussion symptoms, there is a sound basis for these problems.

WHY SEXUAL PROBLEMS CAN OCCUR AFTER A CONCUSSION

Contrary to popular belief, the state of sexual arousal has its roots in the brain, not in the sex organs or erogenous zones. Just as your brain signals the need for nourishment or sleep, it also determines when—and if—you become sexually aroused. Specifically, the desire for sex is regulated by the *hypothalamus*, as well as the brain stem and surrounding structures (see Chapter 1).

"My accident took place in March, and I thought that by November, my life would be like it used to be—including a normal sex life. I had a healthy, active sexual response prior to my concussion, but for eight months after, my sex life with my then-husband

came to a halt. I had no desire and was sexually numb and unresponsive. Extremely concerned, I asked my neurologist about this. His response was, "This can happen with a TBI. The problem you're experiencing might also be caused by your medication." I wanted to scream. No one had ever told me that this could happen because of a brain injury!"

—D.R.S.

A normal, active sexual relationship has interrelated physical, mental, and psychological components. Understandably, a problem with even one facet can have a significant effect on the quality of the relationship as a whole. If, six months after your concussion, you are still having sexual problems that are unrelated to medication, assume that the problems are a direct result of brain trauma. If you had sexual problems prior to your injury, your symptoms may intensify.

If your concussion is localized in this area, your brain may be unable to properly receive, interpret, or relay information transmitted by other parts of the body. Thus, what seems like a sudden loss of sex drive is actually a neurological malfunction that blocks pleasurable images, thoughts, and sensations. Less commonly, a force or blow to the brain's *frontal lobe* causes sudden problems in the ability to reason, make judgments, and conduct yourself in a socially appropriate manner. One result of such an injury can be a sharp, even problematic, increase in sexual desire and activity.

Sexual difficulties can also stem from concentration problems. (Problems with concentration will be discussed in detail in Chapter 18.) The extent to which you can relax and enjoy physical contact is directly related to your capacity to screen out distractions. Loss of the ability to focus in this manner can make it difficult, if not impossible, to become and remain aroused. Chronic pain, sleep deprivation, and emotional upheaval—also common occurrences after a concussion—can have similar effects on sexual desire. In addition, prescription medications that are used to treat post-injury headaches, seizures, and other symptoms may dull sexual response by interfering with nervous system signals that accompany arousal. Most antidepressants are similarly troublesome in that they alter brain chemicals, including those that determine desire, sensation, and climax time. Pain medications may also alter and decrease sexual interest.

TYPES OF SEXUAL PROBLEMS THAT CAN FOLLOW A CONCUSSION

Loss of Desire

Whether it is your concussion or subsequent medication that has interrupted the transmission of pleasure signals, affected your ability to concentrate, or triggered pain, worry, or sleeplessness, you are likely to experience diminished sex drive. In light of the strain of your injury and the energy you are devoting to recovery, sex may start seeming unimportant or just like more trouble than it's worth.

Altered Sensation

If the brain's pleasure center fails to interpret incoming nerve impulses properly, sexual contact can fail to have its customary arousing effect. Instead, normally erogenous areas of the body may seem deadened and disconnected from the arousal process. In other cases, the breasts, genitals, and other sexual areas may become unbearably sensitive, so that sexual touch feels annoying or uncomfortable.

Physiological Problems

In the absence of brain signals of arousal—or in spite of them, where certain medications are concerned—physiological changes that normally precede intercourse may fail to occur in the usual fashion. For men, this can mean an inability to achieve or sustain an erection due to diminished blood flow to the penis. A woman may be unable to lubricate or to relax the vaginal muscles. Many different medications, some of which are often prescribed for post concussion symptoms, can interfere with normal sexual functioning. In addition, anyone who has suffered a concussion may be rendered more sensitive to medications in general, whether taken for post concussion problems or not, even if these drugs previously caused no adverse effects. Table 16.1 gives examples of medications often prescribed for people with a concussion that can cause sexual dysfunction as a side effect.

Intensified Sexual Desire (Hypersexuality)

While a significantly heightened sex drive is usually associated with moderate and severe brain injuries, this condition occasionally occurs as a result of a concussion. In some cases, this intensified drive is manageable. In other instances, it can become overwhelming and compel an individual to make inappropriate

TABLE 16.1. DRUGS THAT CAN CAUSE SEXUAL DYSFUNCTION

MEDICATION	POSSIBLE SEXUAL EFFECTS
Antianxiety Agents	
Diazepam (Valium)	Reduced sexual desire, impotence, inhibited orgasm, inhibited ejaculation
Lorazepam (Ativan)	Loss of desire
Anticonvulsants	
Carbamazepine (Atenonal, Tegretol)	Impotence
Ethosuximide (Zarontin)	Increased sexual desire
Phenytoin (Dilantin)	Reduced sexual desire; impotence; persistent, painful erections
Primidone (Mysoline)	Reduced sexual desire, impotence
Antidepressants	
Amitriptyline (Elavil, Endep)	Loss of desire, impotence, inhibited ejaculation
Doxepin (Adapin, Sinequan)	Reduced sexual desire, inhibited ejaculation
Fluoxetine (Prozac)	Reduced sexual desire, inhibited orgasm, inhibited ejaculation, loss of penile sensation
Nortriptyline (Aventyl, Pamelor)	Reduced sexual desire, impotence
Phenelzine (Nardil)	Impotence; inhibited orgasm; inhibited ejaculation; persistent, painful erections
Sertraline (Zoloft)	Sexual dysfunction
Beta-Blockers	
Atenolol (Tenormin)	Impotence
Labetalol (Normodyne, Trandate)	Reduced sexual desire; impotence; inhibited ejaculation; persistent, painful erections
Metoprolol (Lopressor)	Impotence
Propranolol (Inderal)	Loss of desire, impotence
Timolol (Blocadren)	Reduced sexual desire, impotence
Calcium-Channel Blockers	
Nifedipine (Adalat, Procardia)	Persistent, painful erections
Verapamil (Calan, Isoptin, Verelan)	Impotence
Pain Medication/Anti-inflammatories	
Indomethacin (Indocin)	Reduced sexual desire, impotence
Naproxen (Naprosyn)	Impotence, inhibited ejaculation
Naproxen sodium (Aleve, Anaprox)	Impotence, inhibited ejaculation
Tranquilizers	
Chlorpromazine (Thorazine)	Reduced sexual desire, impotence, inhibited ejaculation
Haloperidol (Haldol)	Impotence, pain upon ejaculation
Thiothixene (Navane)	Impotence; persistent, painful erections; spontaneous ejaculation

MEDICATION	POSSIBLE SEXUAL EFFECTS
Miscellaneous	
Acetazolamide (Diamox)	Loss of desire, impotence
Baclofen (Lioresal)	Impotence, inhibited ejaculation
Dextroamphetamine (Dexedrine)	Impotence, inhibited orgasm, inhibited ejaculation

jokes, comments, and physical advances, or to engage in public exhibitionism (the act of exposing one's body parts—specifically the genitals or buttocks) and other overtly sexual behavior.

Narcotic Pain Medications

The use of opioid narcotics for the treatment of chronic pain is generally avoided in cases of TBI due to their potential for causing impairments in thinking. Another important side effect is a decrease in the sex drive. Medications such as oxycodone (Oxycontin, Percocet, and Roxicodone) can interfere with testosterone, an important hormone that determines your sex drive. These drugs can affect the metabolism of testosterone, and in men, decrease its production. They do this by affecting the hypothalamus through the inhibition of luteinizing hormone (LH), a pituitary hormone important to the making of testosterone. This problem is not well known among treating doctors and goes under-recognized.

Chemotherapy Drugs

If you sustain a concussion and are on a chemotherapy regimen, it is important to know that, because of your concussion, your medication can trigger hypoactive sexual drive disorder—a very stubborn loss of a woman's sexual desire. In men, chemotherapy drugs used to treat prostate and testicular cancer may also suppress testosterone production, leading to loss of libido.

Anti-HIV Drugs

If you are taking anti-HIV medication, a concussion can affect the way your medication is processed by your body. After a concussion, lower testosterone levels have been reported in advanced HIV patients receiving antiviral medicine. Also important is that the virus itself may damage the nerve endings of the sexual organs, leading to problematic sexual arousal. Administering testosterone supplements has been helpful to these patients.

Relationship Problems

Changes in desire or drive can trigger other problems in your relationship with your sexual partner. For example, if a concussion causes you to lose interest in sex, it is not unusual to fear that your partner will take offense or lose patience and seek sex elsewhere. A diminished sex drive can also lead you to withhold affection, become less communicative, and otherwise avoid situations and behavior that might lead to intimate physical contact. Anxiety over your ability to perform or to enjoy sexual activity can compound sexual problems by adding an element of stress. A sudden increase in the sexual demands of one partner can cause stress in a relationship as well.

Unfortunately, we often do not see sexual problems as serious enough to need attention until they have lasted long enough to cause emotional or marital problems—in fact, it is usually these secondary problems that cause people to seek professional help.

DIAGNOSING AND ASSESSING SEXUAL PROBLEMS

If you are troubled by changes in your sex drive or ability, it is important to volunteer the information promptly and candidly when your primary health care provider asks the customary question "How are you doing?" Understandably, most doctors rely on their patients to advise them of less-than-obvious symptoms and complaints. Since sex is a more personal topic than, say, dizziness or memory problems, few medical professionals probe this aspect of their patients' post concussion symptoms. Some may be reluctant to address the issue even if it is raised by the patient. In addition, many doctors feel that warning people with a concussion about the possibility of sexual problems may cause unnecessary worry and anxiety—not all people are affected by this problem, and those who are may be affected for only a relatively short time. However, if you do experience sexual problems and they are not addressed, your physical and emotional symptoms can escalate.

When discussing sexual problems with your doctor, it is important to emphasize the way in which your current situation represents a change from the past. After all, the definition of "normal" sexual desire and performance varies greatly from individual to individual and from couple to couple. The fact that your sexual responsiveness differs from what it was before the injury is what is most important. You should also consider your other post concussion symptoms— insomnia or inattentiveness, for instance—and raise the possibility of a link between these symptoms (and medications you may take for them) and your newfound sexual difficulties.

Your primary care physician (PCP) will probably suggest an examination by a gynecologist or urologist to rule out physical dysfunction unrelated to your brain injury. Also, since a concussion can affect and disrupt your hormones (see Chapter 1), it is important to be evaluated by an endocrinologist who has an understanding of brain injury. As part of your assessment, you may also be referred to a mental health professional for emotional support and further consideration of your problem.

TREATING POST CONCUSSION SEXUAL PROBLEMS

Of all post concussion symptoms, sexual problems can be among the hardest to cope with. This is because it is often harder to obtain support from your partner, who is directly affected by the situation. Also, it can be difficult to discuss this topic with family and friends. Knowing this, you may be tempted to wait out your difficulties or let them go unattended while you focus on other aspects of recovery. However, it is critical to your state of mind—and quite possibly to your relationship with your partner—that you obtain the help you need to get your sexual side back on track. A number of approaches to resolving sexual problems are presented below. Additional information and support can be obtained by contacting me via the information on page 367.

Conventional Approaches

If your sexual problems are medication related, time will not improve things. Discuss with your doctor the possibility of switching medications or modifying dosages to reverse, or at least minimize, sexual side effects. Prescription medications such as Viagra and Cialis are effective at increasing sexual desire and performance in both males and females. Specific hormone treatments are also very helpful. It is important to consult with an endocrinologist before taking any over-the-counter remedy.

Psychotherapy, including cognitive behavioral therapy (CBT) and behavioral sex therapy by a physician-recommended specialist, can provide insight into sexual difficulties and often reignite—or, if necessary, temper—your libido.

Couples counseling can also be extremely helpful for promoting mutual understanding of your problem and reducing tension between you and your partner. If your problem involves inappropriate sexual remarks or behavior, the professionals at either a rehabilitation facility or, if you are a veteran, a VA hospital can refer you to a specialist with experience in sexual disorders stemming from brain injury.

For women, if arousal is a problem, you might consider the use of an artificial lubricant such as K-Y jelly and/or do Kegel exercises to tone the vaginal muscles. Both of these measures can make sexual stimulation and intercourse more pleasurable. Kegel exercises consist of tightening and squeezing the vagina and rectum by drawing the muscles inward and upward, holding this position for five to ten seconds, then relaxing. This can be done virtually anywhere, at any time. You should try to do at least thirty repetitions a day. For males for whom erectile problems or loss of sensations appear to be permanent, a urologist may recommend one of a number of approaches to reverse impotence (usually medication, a penile implant, or a vacuum device). For women, surgery to expose the clitoris or tighten the pubococcygeus muscle, in which are located the nerve endings responsible for sensation in the outer section of the vagina, may be an option.

Complementary Approaches

Hypnosis and relaxation methods—such as biofeedback (including heart rate variability, or HRV, training) and neurofeedback—are very effective at increasing sexual desire. Acupuncture can also be helpful.

Alternative Approaches

Reiki, Qi Gong, and the use of Therapeutic Touch (TT) (see Chapter 6) are effective at increasing sexual response. Certain herbal remedies, when used appropriately, can bolster libido or counteract the effects of medication on drive and performance. Damiana, suo yang, yin yang huo, ba ji tian, green oats, and wild yam, for instance, have long been considered to enhance sexuality when taken in balanced herbal preparations. Ginkgo biloba may be helpful in reversing medication-related impotence and loss of desire. It is best to consult with a qualified herbalist who has training and experience in treating people with head injuries and sexual dysfunction. Similarly, a homeopathic physician may be able to recommend appropriate remedies, as well as dietary changes and other natural measures that can produce positive results. Homeopathic remedies often recommended for sexual problems include *Sepia, Silica, Natrum muriaticum*, and *Kali phosphoricum*.

PRACTICAL SUGGESTIONS

While it is crucial to seek professional help for sexual and other difficulties triggered by your concussion, there are helpful measures that you can try on your own. The first and most important thing is to be forthright with your partner about the existence and nature of the changes in your sexual side. You may wish to consider and discuss the following suggestions:

- Try various methods of relaxation before engaging in sex, including a warm bath, massage, meditation, or deep-breathing exercises. Maintain your state of relaxation by allowing sufficient time for leisurely paced sexual activity.
- Do what you can to block out distracting stimuli during sex. Lock the door, darken the room, warm the sheets with an electric blanket, and shut out noise with music or the drone of an electric fan.
- Consider props to increase arousal. The use of candles, body oil, soothing music, erotic apparel, and visual aids such as books or films can help you stay focused during sex.
- Do not use a mechanical device for stimulation. While these may work at first, the brain will become sensitized to the device's speed and sensation and will therefore be less responsive to your partner's natural rhythm and speed.
- Consult the *Physicians' Desk Reference (PDR)*, found in the reference section of most public libraries, for information about potential adverse reactions to any drugs you take, including such "ordinary" drugs as antihistamines, diuretics, and cholesterol medication. If "changed libido" or "genitourinary complaints" are listed as a possibility, ask your doctor whether you might stop the medication or switch to a different drug. *Do not*, however, discontinue any prescribed medication without consulting your physician.

Above all, it is important not to minimize your sexual difficulties, and it is equally important not to blame yourself for them. Remember that in more than half of all cases, these problems have a physical cause, and that in fully 25 percent of such cases, sexual problems are directly related to medication.

While time may be the best healer for many post concussion problems, treatment is widely available for most types of sexual dysfunction. You will be best able to cope with sexual changes that are concussion-related if you communicate with and muster the support of your partner, and then arm yourself with knowledge about aspects of your injury that might be contributing to your problem. Having done that, you can continue consulting and working with appropriate professionals until you find the help you need.

CHAPTER 17

POST TRAUMATIC SEIZURES (PTS)

■

B EVERLEY WAS ON HER WAY HOME FROM A GYMNASTICS MEET WHEN SHE LOST control of her car. The car fishtailed, accelerated, flew over a snowbank, and landed sideways. Beverley suffered a concussion, also called *mild traumatic brain injury* (mTBI), and spent two weeks in an acute-care hospital before being sent to a rehabilitation hospital for ten weeks. She was discharged from there with the assurance that her various problems would go away with time.

Twelve months later, Beverley had a seizure. Within twenty-four hours, she had two more. Her diagnosis at the time was either a stroke in the left brain or a seizure with paralysis. Her neurologist put her on Tegretol, an anticonvulsant (anti-seizure) medication. Unlike many people who have seizures, Beverley experiences no auras, peculiar smells, or other signs warning of an oncoming seizure. As a result, her medication level must be kept high so that she can continue to drive. Unfortunately, the medication severely limits both her creative expression and her sex drive.

There is neither rhyme nor reason for Beverley's seizures. Sometimes she loses the thread of conversation at one point and picks it up at another. Other times, she has no lapse of memory but simply falls to the floor. Usually, she has no recollection of what happens during her seizures and is confused and disoriented when she comes to. Beverley suspects that she experienced seizure activity in the weeks before her second hospitalization but never knew what was happening. Only when her seizures occurred in the presence of a professional trained in treating brain injury was the problem identified and treated. For that, Beverley considers herself lucky.

Seizures are not as rare as you might think. Sometimes called *ictal events*, they involve a sudden, temporary, unusual discharge of electrical impulses in one focal area of the brain (this applies only to partial seizures, since generalized seizures do not necessarily start in one focal area) that may quickly spread, or diffuse, causing uncontrolled stimulation of nerves and muscles. Seizures can result in abnormal or arrested movement, alteration of consciousness, disorders of sensation or perception, and behavior disturbances. *Convulsion* refers to the involuntary muscle or body movement that can occur during a seizure. People can develop seizures due to birth defects, metabolic or circulatory disorders, brain tumors, or brain injury. Often, the cause of seizures is unknown.

The term *post traumatic seizures* (PTS) refers to seizure activity after a TBI. Seizures that occur within minutes of brain trauma are called *concussion convulsions*. Recurrent seizures are termed *epilepsy*, a condition that affects up to 1 percent of the general population. Epilepsy that results from injury is called *post traumatic epilepsy* (PTE). This diagnosis is given when there are two or more unprovoked seizures that occur after a brain injury. PTE is more common in teenagers and young adults, especially as a result of auto accidents, sports collisions, and blast injuries.

Simple partial seizures are seizures beginning in one part of the brain when there is no alteration of consciousness, while in *complex partial seizures* there is such a change. *Status epilepticus* are seizures that do not stop by themselves or occur so frequently that consciousness is not restored between seizure events. In general, seizures are not thought to cause brain damage by themselves unless they last for a long time—a circumstance that is extremely rare following a concussion. However, inherent in seizure disorder is a loss of control that is particularly dismaying to people with *post concussion syndrome* (PCS), many of whom are already wrestling with other aftereffects of brain trauma that may make them feel they have lost control of their lives.

WHY SEIZURES CAN OCCUR AFTER A CONCUSSION

Seizures, one of the most serious consequences of brain trauma, are most often associated with moderate and severe brain injury. However, they do sometimes occur after a concussion as well. Neurologists are not entirely sure what causes the irregular discharge of energy that produces seizures in such cases, but some speculate that trauma excites nerve cells (neurons) within the brain, causing them to go out of rhythm. Seizures, then, are the body's efforts to correct this irregularity. Another theory is that the misfiring of electrical signals after a concussion stems from bleeding from broken blood vessels or capillaries or the shearing of nerves within the brain that forms scars from which a seizure focus evolves.

In some cases, this unusual discharge of energy, visible on an electroencephalogram (EEG), takes place across almost all of the brain, causing a *generalized seizure* to take place. Other times, irregular impulses are limited to one section of the brain, resulting in what is termed a *partial seizure.* There are also *unilateral seizures*, which affect only one side of the brain (and, therefore, the body), and *unclassified seizures*, another type of partial seizure, for which no specific location can be pinpointed but which are characterized by unusual discharge. There is still another type, called *psychogenic nonepileptic seizures*, where no abnormal EEG activity or other clinical evidence of a seizure can be detected, yet the person presents in thought, mood, and behavior similar to a person with seizure activity. This type of seizure is related to underlying psychiatric or psychological disorders and is often confused with various emotional and mental disorders (see Chapters 23–27). In most instances, a given individual will have only one type of seizure problem, yet it is possible to have both partial and generalized seizures.

Seizures often originate in the *temporal lobes* (see Chapter 1). This part of the brain is particularly vulnerable to seizure-causing damage because the structures within it require high levels of oxygen, and it is anatomically more susceptible to impact. In fact, complex partial seizures so often originate in this area of the brain that you may hear them referred to as *temporal lobe seizures.* Less frequently, seizure activity may also involve the *frontal, occipital,* or *parietal lobes.*

Depending on where your seizure is located, you may experience a variety of symptoms, including sensory, motor, emotional, mental, and cognitive changes. A partial seizure in the temporal lobe can cause a feeling of fear, forced thought or actions such as aggression, a dreamy state, a feeling of disconnection from people around you, and the impression that you are having a mystical or religious experience. If you are having seizure activity, it is important to tell your neurologist of these experiences.

If you experience seizures as a result of a concussion, there are often contributing circumstances. For example, a family history of seizures may give you a propensity for this type of irregular electrical activity, enabling even a mild jolt to your brain to act as a trigger. Or you may have suffered meningitis or seizures in childhood, or had a previous brain injury. Overuse of drugs or alcohol can also be a factor in the development of seizures. Research shows that the risk of seizures continues for many years after a concussion and increases significantly if a seizure occurs shortly after the injury.

Certain physical, external, and internal events can act as seizure triggers—that is, they can cause irregular impulses to begin. Physical triggers can include medications, alcohol, and illness, as well as certain light or sound patterns. There are also external triggers that stem from situations in the home, work, or school environment, and internal triggers that can ignite the same chain of events from within. A list of common seizure triggers appears in Table 17.1.

TYPES OF SEIZURES THAT CAN FOLLOW A CONCUSSION

The symptoms that accompany PTS differ from person to person, depending on the pattern and spread of the irregular electrical discharge in the brain.

Generalized Tonic-Clonic Seizures (GTCS)

Generalized tonic-clonic seizures (GTCS) are generalized seizures, once referred to as *grand mal* ("great illness") seizures, that cause you to lose consciousness and shake and twitch uncontrollably. Your muscles convulse for up to several minutes, after which movement subsides and you awaken with no memory of the incident. You are likely to feel dazed, confused, and sleepy, but in most cases can resume your previous activities after resting.

Simple Partial Seizures (SPS)

Simple partial seizures (SPS) take place without impairment of consciousness. Partial seizures can involve autonomic symptoms, such as fluctuations in your heart rate or blood pressure; sensory symptoms, such as hearing or seeing things that are not present; or motor symptoms—most often a sudden, jerky movement of one part of your body.

Complex Partial Seizures (CPS)

Complex partial seizures (CPS) take place when an extra discharge of electrical energy in the brain propels electrical impulses to certain parts of the brain but without involving the entire organ. A complex partial seizure may cause symptoms such as numbness or muscle weakness. You usually experience an alteration of consciousness, sometimes associated with motor or sensory symptoms. Your level of awareness decreases, but you do not lose consciousness. Additional symptoms can include sensations such as butterflies in the stomach, changes in heart rhythm, and tingling in the face or arms.

TABLE 17.1. POSSIBLE SEIZURE TRIGGERS

TYPE OF TRIGGER	EXAMPLES
Physical	Holding your breath
	Hyperventilating
	Illness, fever, injury, or pain
	Insufficient sleep
	Missed medications
	Menstruation
	Over- or underexertion
	Overuse of alcohol or stimulants
	Poor nutrition or skipped meals
	Specific light, sound, or touch patterns (flashing lights, for example)
	Withdrawal from alcohol or drugs
External	Arguments
	Criticism
	Death of a loved one
	Failure
	Overwork
	School, job, marital, or financial pressures
	Threatened loss of relationship
	Threatened loss of job
Internal	Agitation
	Anger
	Anxiety
	Boredom
	Depression
	Excitement
	Fear
	Feelings of inadequacy
	Grief
	Tension
	Worry

Auras

An aura precedes a seizure and is actually the beginning of the seizure itself. An electrical discharge is already happening. *Aura* is a lay term for a simple partial seizure before it spreads to become complex or generalized. Auras may be experienced in many different ways—as changed thinking, reasoning, perception, sensation, or body movement. You may have a feeling of *déjà vu*, a recurrent daydream, or a rush of paranoia. Occasionally, involuntary muscle movement is also involved. The type of aura you experience depends on the area of the brain

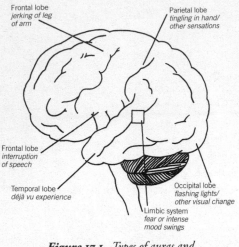

Frontal lobe
*jerking of leg
of arm*

Parietal lobe
*tingling in hand/
other sensations*

Frontal lobe
*interruption
of speech*

Temporal lobe
déjà vu experience

Occipital lobe
*flashing lights/
other visual change*

Limbic system
*fear or intense
mood swings*

Figure 17.1. *Types of auras and
their origins in the brain.*

from which the seizure originates
(see Figure 17.1.)

Interictal Behavior Syndrome

After a seizure, you are likely to feel
disoriented and fatigued. You may
feel spacey and confused, but this is
usually temporary and disappears
after a period of rest. This is called
postictal (or sometimes *interictal*)
behavior. However, current research
has questioned whether this behavior is truly an aftermath of a seizure
or if it stems from some other cause.

DIAGNOSING AND ASSESSING PTS

Since many of the symptoms of migraine headaches mimic those of seizure activity, it can be difficult to distinguish between the two maladies. However, it is
important to determine the true cause of your symptoms, from a legal as well as
a medical standpoint. In some states, your right to drive a car may depend on the
diagnosis. In addition, some of the manifestations of seizure activity can be
symptoms of more than one kind of ictal event. While you might expect symptoms to overlap in this way, considering the complex neurological problems
involved, this can make it difficult to categorize seizures.

If you suspect that you might be experiencing seizures as a result of your
concussion, it is imperative that you ask your primary care physician (PCP) for a
referral to a neurologist who specializes in epilepsy. This specialist will ask you for
an in-depth medical history and give you a thorough neurological examination.
He or she will probably perform an EEG to determine the focal point, nature,
and frequency of any irregular electrical impulses within your brain. Your symptoms will also be considered. The neurologist may suggest additional diagnostic
testing, such as magnetic resonance imaging (MRI) or a computed tomography
(CT) scan, to determine whether there is any structural damage to the brain (see
Chapter 5 for an explanation of these diagnostic procedures).

TREATING PTS

It is important to realize that while seizures can usually be suppressed, they cannot be cured. However, you can gain a sense of control over this disorder by determining whether certain events or circumstances tend to set off your seizure activity. You may find it helpful to keep a record of your surroundings, activities, experiences, and moods over a number of days. Also make a note of all food, drink, and medications you consume. Then record the approximate times of any suspected seizures. Share all of this data with your specialist.

The approach taken toward seizure management is usually based on whether part or all of your brain is involved. Typical courses of treatment are described below.

Conventional Approaches

"After my accident, I experienced intermittent facial numbness, motor problems, and postictal behavior. Despite the fact that I had never had an abnormal EEG, based on my symptoms, my neurologist felt that I was having partial seizures involving the temporal lobe, cerebellum, and reticular formation system. I was placed on Tegretol, an anticonvulsant medication, and had a toxic reaction that caused me to become highly agitated and see four of everything. The dosage was lowered and these symptoms went away, but months later, I began noticing muscle weakness. I was taken off Tegretol and started on Depakote, another anticonvulsant. On this medication, I gained twenty pounds, felt spacey all the time, and had periods of imbalance, slurred speech, and lightheadedness. Eventually, I was weaned from anticonvulsant medication and showed marked improvement in memory, balance, and endurance."

—D.R.S.

Anticonvulsant medication is the primary treatment for seizures. Of course, your biological makeup and concussion are unique, and these medications can cause side effects such as sleepiness, stomach upset, anxiety, and fluctuations in heart rate. Therefore, your medication and dosage must be tailored to meet your individual needs. The goal is to inhibit seizures with the fewest possible side effects, and without compounding other post concussion aftereffects. While multiple medications are sometimes necessary, the use of a single medication at the lowest possible dosage is the method of choice. A trial-and-error approach is often necessary to find the right medication and dosage, so it is important that your neurologist be available for consultation about any problems you encounter.

Generalized seizures are often treated with phenytoin (Dilantin) and phenobarbital, along with valproic acid (Depakote); partial seizures with lamotrigine (Lamictal), oxcarbazepine (Trileptal), and carbamazepine (Carbatrol, Tegretol). (For a more complete list of anticonvulsant medications, see list on page 197.) It is not fully understood how these medications work, but it is known that they somehow inhibit the excessive electrical discharges that are responsible for seizures. The prescribed amount and frequency of medication depend on such factors as your weight, your age, other drugs taken regularly, and your sensitivity to drugs in general.

If you must take anticonvulsant medication, you should become familiar with such terms as *drug level* (sometimes also called *serum level*), which refers to the amount of medication in the liquid portion of your blood at any one time. It is also important to understand about a drug's *half-life*, which is the amount of time it takes for half of a dosage of a drug to be metabolized—that is, to become inactivated—within your body. A drug's half-life can vary widely from person to person; therefore, calculating the speed at which your body inactivates a particular drug is critical to determining the appropriate dosage, and is also important when mixing or discontinuing medications. If too much medication accumulates within your body, you may experience signs of toxicity, with symptoms that can include breathing or visual problems, anxiety, tremors, skin rashes, impaired memory, and heart rhythm problems. You may also be allergic to a particular medication and suffer symptoms ranging from skin rash to arthritis to cardiac arrest. In addition, if you must take an anticonvulsant, you should always remember the following points:

- Be aware that over-the-counter medications can interfere with the action of anticonvulsant drugs. Consult your doctor before using any nonprescription product.
- Never discontinue a medication on your own. Doing so can sometimes trigger potentially damaging seizures. If you have problems and complaints about your medication, bring them to your doctor's attention.

Anticonvulsant Medications
Generic Name (Brand Name)
- Carbamazepine (Tegretol, Carbatrol)
- Ethosuximide (Zarontin)
- Felbamate (Felbatol)
- Tigabine (Gabitril)
- Levetiracetam (Keppra)
- Lamotrigine (Lamictal)
- Pregabalin (Lyrica)
- Gabapentin (Neurontin)
- Phenytoin (Dilantin)
- Topiramate (Topamax)
- Oxcarbazepine (Trileptal)
- Valproic acid (Depakene, Depakote)
- Zonisamide (Zonegran)
- Phenobarbital (Luminal)
- Rufinamide (Banzel)
- Ezogabine (USA)/Retogabine (EU) (Potiga)

Tranquilizers such as:
- Diazepam (Valium)
- Lorazepam (Ativan)
- Clonazepam (Klonopin)

Besides treating your seizures medically, your doctor can direct you to support professionals. For instance, he or she might recommend a counselor who specializes in coping with epilepsy, or support groups for you and your family. You might also consider consulting a psychiatrist or psychologist who specializes in behavioral medicine (see Chapter 6).

For varying reasons, a small percentage of seizures do not respond to anticonvulsants. In rare situations in which seizure activity is uncontrollable, surgery may be necessary to remove the focal area. If all else fails, you may wish to consider alternative or complementary approaches such as megadoses of vitamin B6, various mineral supplements, and special diets. One specialized dietary program, called the *ketogenic diet* (so named because it results in the presence of high levels of substances called ketones in the body), is one of the oldest forms of therapy for epilepsy.

Complementary Approaches

Biofeedback, specifically heart rate variability (HRV) training, and neurofeedback along with personal Roshi (pRoshi) are considered by some to be effective at controlling seizures (see Chapter 6). Hypnosis and progressive relaxation techniques can help you manage emotional triggers.

Another approach, vagus nerve stimulation (VNS), has been used since the 1990s in the treatment of many different types of epilepsy. A pulse generator similar to a pacemaker is implanted beneath the skin on the chest area. Electrodes are wrapped around your vagus nerve and stimulated at certain current strengths and frequencies to reduce the occurrence and severity of seizures. This technique is frequently used with children who are more susceptible to side effects of antiepileptic drugs that can affect school performance. It is also used with adults. VNS is often not a substitute for antiepileptic drugs but can function to improve the effectiveness of such medications. Newer versions of this technique, called transcutaneous VNS, or t-VNS, are being developed to stimulate the vagus nerve on the skin and will hopefully soon be on the market.

Alternative Approaches

Certain herbs, such as black cohosh, hyssop, and lobelia, are commonly included in herbal prescriptions for people who suffer from seizures. *Cicuta virosa, Helleborus*, and *Natrum sulphuricum* are homeopathic remedies that may be prescribed for seizures that are related to brain injury. However, taking self-prescribed over-the-counter herbs or other remedies may not always produce the desired result, leading to the mistaken conclusion that herbal or homeopathic treatments are not useful. Worse, some herbal preparations may actually contribute to seizures in susceptible people. *Post concussion syndrome* (PCS) and seizure disorders are complex problems. It is therefore crucial to consult with, and use such alternative remedies under the guidance of, a well-trained herbalist or homeopathic practitioner who understands and has worked with seizure disorders and concussion (see "Assessing a Practitioner's Expertise with Concussion," page 85).

PRACTICAL SUGGESTIONS

Living with PCS and its symptoms is no small task. This challenge is greatly compounded if the aftereffects you suffer include seizures. However, there are things you can do to improve your sense of control over this problem—enough so that you can lead a fairly normal life. The following suggestions may help:

- Take all prescribed medications exactly as directed. If you feel a particular medication is causing you problems, consult your physician. *Do not* discontinue a drug or increase or decrease the dosage on your own.
- If you drive, consult your doctor about the advisability of continuing to do so.
- Avoid sports and activities that could be dangerous to you or to others, until your seizure medication and dosage have been regulated.
- Avoid all alcohol. Also avoid caffeine, nicotine, and other stimulants.
- Avoid missed sleep and unnecessary stress—both conditions can trigger seizures.
- Be honest about your seizures. Dealing with your condition in a forthright manner helps to make others more comfortable and can generate valuable support.

Recovery from PTS and PTE due to a concussion is variable. However, there are things you can do to attain optimum wellness. Getting proper medical care, good nutrition, and adequate sleep and rest; keeping physically fit; and avoiding things that may trigger a seizure can help you live a healthier life. Additional support is available from the Epilepsy Foundation of America. For further information, please feel free to get in touch with me via the contact information listed on page 367.

PART 3

MENTAL ASPECTS

INTRODUCTION

◼

SEVEN YEARS AGO, VALERIE WRITES, SHE WAS "STILL ME." AT THAT TIME, SHE was concentrating on helping her husband to set up a business. A quarter-mile from her home, Valerie's car was struck by a vehicle whose driver wasn't looking as he pulled out into the road. Valerie was thrown down across the bench seat of her car. She recalls opening her eyes and finding herself on the floor—she was unaware of having struck her head, but remembers experiencing a flash of tremendous rage. Disoriented and shaky, but with no specific complaints, Valerie was driven home.

The next day, Valerie went to the emergency room because she couldn't see straight and felt confused. The doctor diagnosed concussion, also called *mild traumatic brain injury* (mTBI), with some muscle strain but took no X-rays. Four days later, a general practitioner prescribed Darvocet, a powerful painkiller, and amitriptyline, an antidepressant used as a painkiller. The medications put Valerie in such a fog that she eventually threw them out.

Valerie remembers little about the first year and a half after her accident, but recalls seeing a neurologist who diagnosed *post concussion syndrome* (PCS) and told her that her symptoms would disappear within six months. Her magnetic resonance imaging (MRI) and computed tomography (CT) scan results were normal. However, for two and a half years after her concussion, and occasionally even today, people around Valerie could see her eyes glaze over when lights, noise, or too much information caused sensory overload. Currently, Valerie has trouble remembering what she has just said or done, and she can recall only bits and pieces of the past. Her ability to concentrate and follow through is limited, as is her ability to organize, prioritize, and initiate activities. Her depth perception and visual tracking are impaired, which causes all sorts of dyslexic phenomena, and she has problems with eye-hand coordination. Valerie's concussion also has a strong emotional component that includes irritability, mood swings, and self-doubt—especially concerning memory and judgment.

THE THINKING process involves a number of different components, including how you register information through attention and concentration; how you store and retrieve incoming messages; and how you reason, plan, organize, initiate, comprehend, learn new information, and create new ideas. It also involves your ability to understand language, read and write, and do mathematics.

Many people with PCS encounter a variety of mental effects in the months and years after injury. Part 3 of this book considers the different aspects of your thinking ability and provides information about mental difficulties frequently associated with concussion, along with information about diagnosis and treatment and practical suggestions that can help minimize the effects of such problems.

CHAPTER 18

ATTENTION AND CONCENTRATION PROBLEMS

■

AFTER SUFFERING A CONCUSSION, ALSO CALLED *MILD TRAUMATIC BRAIN injury* (mTBI), Gail, whose story appears in Chapters 7 and 14, struggled with sensory overload caused by her body's inability to regulate incoming sensations such as sound, light, and touch. She walked strangely, because she couldn't tolerate the sensation of her feet touching the ground. If someone touched her elbow, she would jump backward. Ordinary night sounds caused Gail to lie awake, listening to cars that sounded as if they were right outside the window, rather than a half mile away. She was disturbed by the sounds of birds moving in the trees and crickets in the grass. Daytime noise was completely intolerable, as were bright, blinking, or fluorescent lights.

By the third year after her accident, Gail's regulating ability had improved markedly. She is now able to select which incoming sensation she wants to attend to and thus is better able to concentrate. She feels that this improvement is probably the result of conditioning herself to her increased awareness of sound and light. However, she still avoids shopping malls and other busy places.

FOCUSING YOUR attention and concentrating are automatic, spontaneous processes of registering information from sensory and other input. In general, problems in this area go unnoticed until some incident causes you to take notice—for instance, a pot boiling over on the stove. And even these situations are usually chalked up to a faulty memory, rather than to problems with attention.

After a concussion, attention and concentration problems may occur more frequently than before, and your lack of awareness may disrupt your ability to work, maintain social connections, carry out various tasks, or tend to personal matters. A problem like Gail's—an inability to select or filter incoming sensations—can cause actual discomfort, as well as difficulty concentrating.

While it can be hard to live with sudden distractibility or overattentiveness, understanding the nature of your problem and developing a set of management techniques can help immensely.

WHY ATTENTION AND CONCENTRATION PROBLEMS CAN OCCUR AFTER A CONCUSSION

Attention is the ability to focus on a specific message; *concentration* is the capacity to maintain attention to that message. These abilities enable you to select which input from bodily sensations and your surrounding environment you wish to respond to, as well as to shift from one activity or thought to another. It is believed that damage to the upper brain stem and *frontal lobes* (see Chapter 1), or diffuse damage to the body's connections to these areas, can cause permanent changes in your ability to attend to and register messages from your body and the outside world.

TYPES OF ATTENTION AND CONCENTRATION PROBLEMS THAT CAN FOLLOW A CONCUSSION

"Because of sensory overload problems after my concussion, it took me five years to become able to dine in a restaurant or attend a carnival again. Before, I would become physically ill and feel as if I were about to pass out. At home, I had to eliminate background noise before I answered the phone so that I could attend to what was being said. I also needed complete silence when I was writing or working on the computer. To exercise my ability to focus and concentrate, I used the solitaire game that came with my computer. In addition, my family helped me to make lists for shopping and daily routines, which I stored in the computer and retrieved as needed. It was not until I did a year of neurofeedback in my seventh year of recovery that my attention and concentration problems showed marked improvement."

—D.R.S.

Like many brain functions, attention and concentration are dynamic and complex operations. They have three main components: alertness, capacity for attention and sustained attention, and selection. A concussion can affect any or all of these.

Alertness Problems

Alertness is the general readiness that enables you to act upon information from your surroundings, such as sounds, movements, or events. For example, it is alertness that creates awareness that the phone is ringing or that a mosquito has bitten you. Sleep problems (see Chapter 9), which often result from a concussion, frequently impact alertness and awareness. Fatigue, medication, depression, anxiety, and the consumption of alcohol can also dramatically diminish your alertness level—sometimes to the point that incoming information is never registered.

Problems with the Capacity for Attention and Sustained Attention

Your capacity for attention is the amount of information you are able to take in and process at a given moment. For instance, most people can receive and mentally hold on to a seven-digit telephone number long enough to write it down.

Sustained attention refers to the ability to focus and concentrate on a task or thought for a period of time while filtering out other information from your body or from the environment. After a brain injury, you may find concentrating extremely difficult due to fatigue, distractibility, or the fact that you cannot stop your mind from wandering. You may encounter problems with reading, following directions, or even holding a conversation. Also, you may find that you can concentrate on certain things—phone calls, for instance—only at particular times of the day.

Selection Problems

"When I was married, I was on a walk with my husband and was nearly hit by an oncoming car. My husband yelled at me for not moving aside, but in that moment, he forgot that I had problems with attention and selection. Of course I saw the car, but since information I perceived wasn't always registered properly, I didn't respond."

—D.R.S.

The capacity to choose what you wish to concentrate on is referred to as selection. This ability includes all of your senses and occurs spontaneously. Selection has two main parts—filtering, or selecting an experience to focus on, and shifting, or moving your attention from one experience to another. Filtering is what allows you to concentrate on reading the newspaper despite a fly buzzing around you and the noise of neighborhood children at play. If your ability to filter has been affected by your concussion, you can be impervious to things you should notice or overwhelmed by normal background sounds and distractions. Overfiltering can affect your general alertness and awareness of danger signals or distractions, while underfiltering can disrupt your ability to focus. In either case, the result is difficulty completing any task.

Shifting is what allows you to quickly transfer your attention from the magazine article you are reading to a friend calling your name from another room. Problems with shifting ability can cause you to repeat thoughts over and over, or to linger on a topic or problem long after others have lost interest. This particular symptom of shifting problems is called *perseveration*.

Filtering and shifting problems can combine to create sensory overload, which most commonly affects the senses of hearing and sight. Hearing overload can cause sounds to be magnified or make it difficult to understand conversation in a noisy room. Visual overload creates sensitivity to light, especially the fluorescent lighting used in many offices, stores, and other public places. Sensory overload can result in mental fatigue as your mind tries to make sense of all the incoming information. Factors that can contribute to sensory overload include medications, caffeine, hormonal changes, and attention deficit disorders.

DIAGNOSING AND ASSESSING ATTENTION AND CONCENTRATION PROBLEMS

Diagnosing attention and concentration problems can be difficult, because each concussion is unique. You may experience one or a combination of attention problems. Whatever your complaint, you may undergo both formal standardized testing and informal assessments.

A thorough neurological examination and neuropsychological testing should be done to determine your ability to attend to messages, tasks, and situations, and to establish a baseline against which subsequent improvement can be measured. In particular, neuropsychological testing—which compares your current level of functioning to your prior capabilities—can yield important information about specific deficits and possible treatments. A follow-up speech/language evaluation may also be beneficial, to identify strategies and modifications to improve attention and concentration.

Other types of standardized testing may also be done. Tests measuring arousal responses—heart rate, skin temperature, muscle tension, and brain activity—are available but may not be necessary, because most people with PCS can report how they feel or how they perform at school, work, and home. If your responses differ depending on your environment, response testing can pinpoint situations that trigger problems. Tests for sensory overload can be done by an appropriate specialist, such as an audiologist, who can administer an evaluation and a central auditory process test to measure your hearing ability and your capacity for attending to sound.

Informal testing, in the form of simple observations of your functioning, may be done at home, at work, or in the classroom. These informal assessments can take the form of behavioral scales or checklists that contain lists of symptoms to be rated on a frequency scale of 0 to 5. You, or a professional observer, would be asked to assign a frequency to such items as your ability to understand conversation in a crowded room. Informal testing helps to determine how often and under what circumstances you miss being aware of information, become distracted, or experience sensory overload. These assessments help evaluate the character or quality of stimuli or activities that cause you to respond—for example, whether you respond to the intensity of the sound of a clock alarm, or to the duration of the sound.

It can also be very helpful to keep a log recording your difficulties with selection, concentration, or alertness. This will help you to identify and understand the circumstances that pose problems.

TREATING POST CONCUSSION ATTENTION AND CONCENTRATION PROBLEMS

The results of both formal and informal assessments help with the development of a treatment plan pinpointing such things as situations that you should avoid and the best times of day for you to perform problem activities. Naturally, you will want to play an active role in designing a treatment program for your attention and concentration problems. If focusing difficulties sometimes cause you to miss parts of conversations, you may wish to make a digital or MP3 recording of discussions with your neurologist or neuropsychologist about test results.

Proper diagnosis will permit your specialist to identify very specific problem areas—for instance, problems filtering out distracting sounds or movements. There are specific rehabilitation programs available that offer retraining or teach you ways to compensate for such deficits. Your neurologist, neuropsychologist, or local hospital should be able to help you locate a program in your area. Your doctor can also suggest and, if necessary, teach you the treatment methods discussed below.

Conventional Approaches

The type of treatment appropriate for attention and concentration problems is as unique as each person who experiences a concussion. It is important that the methods and techniques developed for you be matched to your requirements. Based on what has been learned through testing and your own observations, you should have some idea of the types of situations that cause problems, and you will probably want to simply avoid them as much as possible, at least for the time being. Cognitive behavioral therapy (CBT) can help you to control your environment and/or to learn ways of coping with those things that cannot be changed or avoided. For example, you may learn to regulate the times of day that you go outdoors. Or you may discover that certain colors cause sensory overload and that simply repainting the walls of your home minimizes the problem. Certain medications, such as methylphenidate (Ritalin) and dextroamphetamine (Dexedrine), can be very effective for attention problems. You may also be able to receive tutoring and additional help from a learning-disabilities specialist. Your local school district should be able to put you in touch with a teacher trained in working with people with attention deficit difficulties.

The process of identifying specific problems and making appropriate changes is not easy. It can take months just to pin down symptoms and triggers. But with patience and the guidance of understanding professionals, you are sure to see progress.

Complementary Approaches

Neurofeedback, which trains the brain to increase alert, or beta, waves while decreasing slower theta waves, has been found to be extremely effective for attention disorders. Hypnosis is also frequently used to help people with post concussion symptoms learn to modify their perception of or reactions to stimuli. LACE (Listening and Communication Enhancement) was specifically designed to help in this area, as was BrainTrain. The EyeQ reading program and Interactive Metronome both have components designed to improve focus and attention. (See Chapter 6.)

Alternative Approaches

Polarity therapy may be helpful in resolving attention and concentration problems, particularly if the practitioner has experience treating your particular symptoms.

Ginkgo biloba, ginseng, super blue-green algae, black cohosh, and suan zao ren are among the herbal preparations sometimes cited as beneficial for mental functioning. Remedies that may be suggested by homeopaths for these problems include *Phosphoricum acidum*, *Helleborus*, and *Calcarea carbonica*. It is recommended that you seek the advice of a qualified herbalist or homeopath who has experience with concussion, rather than experimenting with over-the-counter products on your own. If your physician is unable to provide an appropriate referral, an organization such as the Herb Research Foundation or the National Center for Homeopathy may be able to help. Please email or call me via the contact information on page 367 for further information.

PRACTICAL SUGGESTIONS

"I always carry earplugs and sunglasses to use at the first sign of sensory overload. I also find a baseball cap helpful for reducing overhead stimuli when I shop or travel. In public places, I walk close to walls and keep my attention focused away from crowds. If I am with someone, I walk directly behind them or just slightly to the side so I can focus on the person's feet or back. To go grocery shopping, I make a list of the items I need in the order in which they are shelved in the store. I also select a quiet place to retreat to when I begin to feel overwhelmed. Most important, I try to stay sensitive to the signs of overload, since the problem is easier to handle in its early stages."

—DENA

"I space out tasks that tend to produce overload over the course of the day instead of trying to complete such jobs all at once. I also monitor those senses that are most likely to overload, so that overuse doesn't trigger problems."

—JUDITH

Getting proper rest and regular exercise, avoiding alcohol and drugs (except for those prescribed by your physician), and reducing the stress in your life are the first steps to take in overcoming problems with attention and concentration. Also, it is important to seek relief from post-injury pain, which in itself can be extremely distracting. At home and work, there are a number of commonsense ways to improve your ability to attend and concentrate. These are divided into four groups: environmental modifications, time modifications, task modifications, and social modifications.

Environmental Modifications

When dealing with attention or concentration difficulties, environmental stimuli can play a major role. The following measures can help you to function at your best:

- When working or studying, do so in complete quiet. Keep the radio and the television off whenever you are attempting to focus on an activity. Turn off the ringer on your telephone and let an answering machine take your calls or, if necessary, look into hiring an answering service. Also, turn off your cell phone or put it in "vibrate" mode.
- Consider the lighting, furnishings, seating arrangements, ventilation, visual displays, and colors of your home and workplace carefully, with an eye toward eliminating sensory overload. Clear your desk and remove clutter such as paperwork and pictures prior to beginning a task.
- Remove all nonessentials from bathroom and kitchen countertops. Keep necessary items in clearly marked different-colored containers.
- Use a telephone headset to keep your hands free and help focus your attention during calls.

If your environment interferes with your ability to concentrate on a task, it is reassuring to identify and, to the extent that this is possible, to avoid or change those aspects that trouble you most.

Time Modifications

It is not uncommon for people with PCS to have fairly predictable daily patterns—specifically, good and bad times of day for focusing and maintaining attention. Recognizing and seeking to work within these patterns is one way of coping with the aftereffects of your injury. The following are a few suggestions:

- Keep a log of times and circumstances when you begin to lose your ability to concentrate, and adjust your schedule of activities accordingly.

- Take note of the time of day you perform different tasks, and observe how long it takes you to complete them. You may discover that you perform certain activities better at certain times of day.
- Monitor yourself closely for tiredness. Some signs may include blurry vision, difficulty processing information, or changes in posture. Take frequent work or study breaks, varying the length of these interruptions. Notice how often and for how long you need to take breathers, and then institute a regular practice of doing so. Aim to take breaks before fatigue becomes significant.
- Do what you can to remove time pressures. Minimize stress by allowing twice the time you think you will need to complete any task.

Everyone has times of day when he or she feels most alert. You will find concentrating easier once you begin planning your work activities accordingly.

Task Modifications

After a concussion, it may be necessary to modify certain tasks—even the most basic and familiar—to compensate for deficits in attention and concentration. The following are suggestions that may help:

- Set realistic goals for performing tasks that require attention and concentration.
- Talk aloud as a reminder about coping strategies—for instance, ways to focus on conversation at a party or avoid commotion while shopping.
- Experiment with different ways of paying attention, but avoid added stress by giving yourself permission to fail.
- Investigate computer software programs designed to help with attention and concentration. These are most often created for children, but they can be helpful for adults with attention deficits as well.
- Practice focusing your attention with card games such as Concentration, a matching game that exercises both attention and concentration. Also helpful is working on mazes or sudoku.
- Try coloring, an activity that forces you to focus on shapes, colors, and eye-hand coordination. Puzzles, knitting, and handcrafts require similar concentration.

- Improve your ability to focus when listening by having a friend or family member read aloud to you. Audio books, available for your MP3 or CD player at most public libraries, can also help.
- Prior to beginning a task, break it into small components and focus on just one step at a time. Don't rush through tasks or expect a perfect performance.

For most people, the ability to attend and concentrate varies at times. If you have a pressing work or home project, the above suggestions can help.

Social Modifications

Problems with attention and concentration can affect every aspect of your life, including your social interactions. The following are a number of suggestions that can help you to cope with these new difficulties:

- Ask people to speak slowly when they dispense important information, giving a small bit of information at a time and pausing occasionally so you can process what they are saying. Do not hesitate to ask people to rephrase or repeat their statements, if necessary. Afterward, repeat or paraphrase what you have heard to ensure that you have the correct information.
- Take notes about what is being said, if necessary, or use a smartphone or a pocket digital recorder. Some are voice-activated and have small projection microphones that make them barely noticeable. Request that conversations about important information be held when you are at your least fatigued.
- Be honest and matter-of-fact about your attention and concentration problems. Doing so will help both you and the person you are speaking with feel more at ease.
- If your mind wanders when someone is speaking, try focusing on his or her voice quality or gestures.

Attention and concentration problems that follow a concussion can be disruptive and distressing. However, some of these difficulties diminish over time, and others respond well to treatment approaches that your specialist can recommend, as well as to practical coping techniques. Over time, you will likely discover at least some effective coping methods on your own. As with many other post concussion symptoms, time and support are your best allies.

CHAPTER 19

MEMORY PROBLEMS

■

KIMBERLY, 51 YEARS OLD AT THE TIME, WAS THE ACADEMIC AND EXECUTIVE director of a nonprofit organization. On her way home from work, her car was sideswiped by a vehicle that had run a red light. Her car spun around 180 degrees before coming to a stop. Kimberly was taken to the emergency room, where she was diagnosed with a concussion, also referred to as a *mild traumatic brain injury* (mTBI), and sent home. At work the following day, she experienced a severe headache and dizziness. She also felt confused and couldn't figure out why she wasn't able to perform routine tasks.

Days later, Kimberly saw her primary care physician (PCP) and underwent a battery of tests, including a skull X-ray, magnetic resonance imaging (MRI), a computed tomography (CT) scan, and an electroencephalogram (EEG). All the test results were negative, but Kimberly knew that something was drastically wrong. She asked for neuropsychological testing, but even this turned up no measurable brain damage.

Over a year later, Kimberly was still unable to return to work. She was plagued by headaches, dizziness, extreme fatigue, confusion, and severe short-term memory problems. At times, she couldn't find the research library—a place she had visited several times a week for years. Other times, she would find herself outside the grocery store, unsure of where she was or how to get home. Sometimes Kimberly was sure she was losing her mind.

Carolyn, a Broadway performer, Peter, a hockey player, Dawn, a cyclist, and Ken, a marine, all share something in common with Kimberly. All have had concussions, and all have experienced memory problems as a result. Carolyn was accidentally struck by a falling piece of stage equipment while performing, while Peter was blindsided by an opposing player and crashed into the wall around the ice at a high speed. Dawn's bicycle became entangled with another bicycle, causing her to be thrown over the handlebars. Ken, while deployed, was riding in a jeep when there was an explosion just outside the vehicle. These individuals suffered from various memory problems, from the inability to recall what was said to forgetting where they lived. Actress Carolyn couldn't remember her lines, while Dawn has trouble planning and implementing even the simplest of tasks if she is interrupted. Peter still has no recollection of what happened to him in the hockey rink, while Ken lost the knowledge of how to use his military equipment, including his weapon.

THE ABILITY to store and recall information serves as one of the major criteria for determining the severity of brain injury. Memory problems are the most common and persistent of all neurological consequences of *post concussion syndrome* (PCS), and symptoms can vary from person to person. The types of memory problems that can result from a concussion include more than simple forgetfulness. They can involve the inability to recall events or to digest new information and ideas. The way you remember is also influenced by factors such as attention, organization, motivation, and fatigue, any or all of which may be affected by brain injury as well.

WHY MEMORY PROBLEMS CAN OCCUR AFTER A CONCUSSION

The processes involved in memory are very complex. Your memory is actually a number of interrelated networks for storing and retrieving information. This system allows you to store and recall simple sensory information as well as complex knowledge and personal experiences. Damage to any part of this intricate system can disrupt your ability to categorize, link, and recall recent thoughts and experiences. In turn, if you become unable to recall information, it can become extremely difficult to formulate new ideas or even to act upon old ones.

Post concussion memory problems are believed to result from injury to the front or rear portions of the brain's *frontal lobes*, or to specific areas within the *temporal lobes* and to internal structures such as the *hippocampus* and *amygdala* (see Chapter 1). On occasion, the *parietal lobes* may be involved as well. Memory problems resulting from brain trauma can vary widely in nature and extent, depending on the site, complexity, and severity of the injury.

TYPES OF MEMORY PROBLEMS THAT CAN FOLLOW A CONCUSSION

"When they lived at home, each of my three sons had a different activity schedule. At times, because of my memory problems, I literally 'lost my children.' To help with this problem, I learned to write down their schedules, along with when and where to pick them up. However, there were a few times when I forgot where I placed the written schedule and was unable to recall where my sons were. Naturally, this terrified me."

—D.R.S.

The processes of forming and retrieving memories are complex, involving three distinct phases: registration, storage, and retrieval. The types of memory problems that result from any individual concussion depend on which of these are affected.

Registration Problems

Registration, also called *encoding*, involves the perception of environmental information and sensory input. Sensory impairment, such as that which can result from a concussion, can affect how—or whether—certain environmental messages are perceived. Attention problems (see Chapter 18) also can interfere with the amount of information you are able to register, and the accuracy with which you can do so.

Storage Problems

"I was able to recall everything prior to my concussion, but I had no memory of the accident itself and had difficulty learning and remembering new information. It felt strange to recall certain parts of events so vividly and have absolutely no memory of other parts. When this happened, even hints and cues failed to evoke recall of the incident. It was as if there were huge holes or gaps in my memory."

—D.R.S.

The second phase of memory is *storage*. How you store information is the key to a keen memory. Studies show that relating new material to previously learned information helps to form new pathways between the cells of the brain for more efficient storage of information. There are three types of memory storage: sensory memory, short-term memory, and long-term memory.

Sensory memory is the storage of information that lasts only seconds but leaves a lingering sight, smell, sound, or sensation, such as when a fly brushes against your skin. This type of memory works hand in hand with attention. If you cannot recall the name of someone you were just introduced to, or you cannot recall the phone number just recited by the operator, it is usually inattention that has prevented the information from being stored. However, if you have deficits affecting sensory memory, you may be unable to play back in your mind what you have just heard. In the case of visual images, you may be unable to picture a bit of information. Deficits in sensory memory often go unnoticed. After all, if you don't notice something in the first place, you cannot be aware of not remembering it.

Short-term memory, also called *buffer memory* or *working memory*, is the part of the memory process that receives and recalls chunks of information for up to one minute. Short-term memory is what enables you to integrate previously learned information with new information to form creative or novel thoughts. It is critical to daily living; it is what makes it possible for you to recall where you placed your car keys or checkbook, whether you locked the door or turned off the stove, and whether you have eaten or bathed. In the best of circumstances, short-term memory has a limited storage capacity. This type of memory is the most susceptible to interference from the pain, stress, fatigue, attention problems, and sensory overload that can follow a concussion. For example, if you are interrupted while receiving a bit of information, the thought may be lost.

Long-term memory, also called *remote* or *secondary memory*, differs from short-term memory in duration, capacity, and manner of storage. Long-term memories are information received and held beyond thirty seconds, becoming learned information. Research suggests that the capacity of long-term memory is immeasurable, in contrast to short-term memory's limited capacity, and that the reliving or re-experiencing of memories solidifies their place in long-term storage. There are two methods of forming long-term memory: declarative and procedural. *Declarative memory* is the memory of events and facts, such as the color of someone's hair, a birth date, or information about yourself. *Procedural memory* is the learning of skills, procedures, and motor movement and is often called *motor memory*.

In addition, there are two ways in which those memories are processed: explicit and implicit. *Explicit memory* occurs when you are aware that you are learning material or information. There is intent to acquire the information. For instance, an *explicit declarative memory* would take place when you are at a party and are aware that you're trying to learn someone's name. *Implicit memory* happens when you learn a detail or motor movement and are unaware that you have gained the information. For example, when you become able to balance on a bike while riding, your brain has learned through a variety of networks and hubs the details of what is needed to balance on the bike.

Episodic memory, also called *flashbulb memory*, involves sights, sounds, and details that are connected to an emotional event, such as an accident or recalling exactly what you were doing on September 11, 2001, when you learned of the attacks on the Twin Towers. Memories already stored prior to an injury are called *retrograde memories*, while memories learned and stored after injury are called *anterograde memories*.

Chapter 9 discussed the importance of sleep, especially restorative sleep. This is especially true for the storage of memories. Research on dreaming and memory has shown that new memories are stored in different ways. Non-rapid eye movement (NREM) sleep, in which you do not dream, helps in the storage of declarative memories, such as learning a poem or new facts, while rapid eye movement (REM) sleep, in which you do dream, helps with procedural memory, such as learning the sequence of steps for making a foul shot in basketball.

There have been functional MRI (fMRI) scanning studies done at Massachusetts General Hospital's Athinoula A. Martinos Center for Biomedical Imaging, Harvard University, Washington University in St. Louis, and Stanford University that specifically show where various memories are stored in the brain. As mentioned in Chapter 1, there are many connections, hubs, networks, and locations in the brain that work together to store information. If your concussion causes a disruption or break in one of these locations, storage is either interfered with or made impossible.

After a concussion, long-term memories tend to return in fits and starts. Some may never be fully recovered. In some cases, whole areas of information are lost while related information remains intact. For instance, you may be able to recall that George Washington was the first president of the United States but be unable to recall anything about Abraham Lincoln, even with prompting. This type of long-term memory loss is called the "Swiss-cheese effect."

Usually, after a concussion, long-past memories are the easiest to access, followed by events closer in time to the injury. Verbal memory problems and word-finding deficits can continue for years. Following a concussion, learning new material—which requires attention, organization, and sensory and short-term memory—is often extremely difficult. A common sign of a long-term memory problem is a vague sense that you are reliving a thought or situation, often called *déjà vu*. After a concussion, this may occur because you are unaware that you are actually recalling a past experience.

Retrieval Problems

The last phase of memory is *retrieval*, your ability to access stored information. Retrieval can occur only if both registration and storage have taken place. It is based on cues that trigger your memory of how the information was first registered. Smells, sights, sounds, and emotions, for example, are often linked to memories; this is why hearing an old song can momentarily take you back to the past.

Research shows that information is more easily accessed if you can reproduce the state in which it was registered, either physically or through hypnosis. Any form of stress, fatigue, anxiety, or depression can interfere with this ability. Memory-retrieval problems can range from "tip-of-the-tongue" struggles, to an inability to describe a missing word or thought, to amnesia, or the complete inability to access information. Or, other thoughts may intrude, information may be recalled incorrectly, or messages may be lost among other information.

Forgetting occurs when a particular memory is not accessible. This can mean that the information is no longer stored, or that there is some sort of internal or external interference with the memory. Often, forgetting results from poor organization of information to be stored. For instance, if someone tells you his or her phone number, you need to repeat the number or link it with other information, such as the year you were born or some other familiar number, in order to remember it. Without this step of practice, the information is more likely to be lost. Other considerations in the proper storage and retrieval of information include emotional and psychological factors; the use of certain drugs, including a number of prescription medications, as well as alcohol and recreational drugs; and auditory or visual distractions.

Many people with PCS experience problems with the registration or storage of messages. However, you may not become aware that you have a memory problem until you try to retrieve information at some later point and find you are unable to do so.

Problems with amnesia can also occur following a concussion. There are different types of amnesia. *Retrograde amnesia* affects the ability to recall events prior to a traumatic event—in this case, a concussion. At times, you may recall bits and pieces of certain events, but other memories remain absent. Specific brain functions, such as sensory and motor abilities, can also be affected. *Antero-grade amnesia*, sometimes called *posttraumatic amnesia*, affects the ability to remember events following a concussion or other traumatic event. Neither *total amnesia*, the complete loss of memory, nor *psychogenic amnesia*, a dissociative disorder, is commonly associated with concussion. (A detailed discussion of dissociative disorders will be found in Chapter 26.)

DIAGNOSING AND ASSESSING MEMORY PROBLEMS

A thorough neuropsychological evaluation is the best way to evaluate memory problems. This assessment compares your present level of functioning with your previous abilities (see Chapter 5). From this battery of diagnostic tests, an appropriate treatment plan can be developed, so it is vital that your neuropsychologist explain your results in detail.

TREATING POST CONCUSSION MEMORY PROBLEMS

"When learning new things, I repeat information or write it down over and over until I am able to recall it. New piano pieces are a particular struggle; however, if I record the music on a variable-speed tape recorder, I can practice troublesome sections over and over until I get them right. In my work as a psychologist, I repeat or paraphrase what my patients tell me and immediately write down cues to what is meant. A smartphone or a digital pocket-sized memo recorder, which can hold hours of messages, is also very helpful. Computer games and programs have helped me to sequence and recall information."

—D.R.S.

The appropriate treatment for memory problems depends on the source of the difficulty. If testing determines that you are experiencing problems remembering things because of a failure to register information properly, you will need to focus on improving your ability to direct and maintain your attention (Chapter 18 presents treatment suggestions and practical tips that can help). If you are affected by amnesia, time without stress is the best antidote. Short- and long-term memory problems respond to various approaches, the most common of which are described below.

Conventional Approaches

Time often heals memory loss, and what you eat can also affect your ability to store and retrieve information. It is extremely important to have an anti-inflammatory diet that allows the brain to heal, eliminating refined sugar, corn syrup, and any grains that can be fermented or distilled. An increase of omega-3 from wild salmon and tuna is beneficial. Spinach and other vegetables rich in antioxidants help improve your memory. Coconut, olive oil, and avocado are good sources of fats that help the brain heal and enhance your storage and retrieval capabilities. Drinking water helps the brain, too.

Also imperative is getting a good night's sleep (see Chapter 9 for suggestions). Working with a speech/language pathologist who specializes in brain injury and is trained in remediating cognitive and memory issues can help you learn new methods of storing and retrieving information. Impaired short-term memory function may respond to treatment with certain medications, including methyl-phenidate (Ritalin), a stimulant that can be helpful for attention disorders, and amantadine (Symmetrel), a drug that affects the action of brain chemicals called neurotransmitters and that is sometimes used to treat people with Parkinson's disease. These medications have side effects, but if they are effective, the benefits may outweigh the disadvantages.

Rehabilitation centers often offer programs to help you manage persistent memory problems. One approach is to help you reacquire or improve lost skills through training or tutoring. Another approach is *compensatory intervention*, which teaches you to work around your deficits by learning alternative ways to accomplish specific tasks or behaviors. You are taught how to use your present skills and your innate learning style to recall information. Internal cues such as sensations and thoughts, as well as external cues like color or sound, may be used. The Brain Injury Association can refer you to a center in your area that provides compensatory memory training, or you can get in touch with me for assistance via the contact information on page 367.

Complementary Approaches

Long-term memory loss may be helped by hypnosis, which can be effective at retrieving past memories. Neurofeedback can help the brain to become regulated again and form new neural connections needed for storage and retrieval. There are several computer programs and websites devoted to improving your memory, such as BrainTrain, EyeQ, and Lumosity. Prevagen, a brain health supplement, has been shown to help alleviate memory and sleep problems by binding to calcium cells and reducing damage done by the body's diminished production of calcium-binding proteins. The active ingredient responsible for this work is apoaequorin, a protein found in jellyfish. The regular version of Prevagen can be purchased at a health food store, while a professional, more potent version is sold through medical practices. As always, it is extremely important to consult with your neurologist before using any over-the-counter medication.

Alternative Approaches

Many advertisements state that certain herbs or homeopathic remedies can increase your memory. These over-the-counter products may help, but it is always best to work with a knowledgeable practitioner rather than attempting to self-medicate. Even natural remedies can have serious side effects if not used properly. Depending on your specific needs, a knowledgeable herbalist may recommend a product such as ginkgo biloba, ginseng, super blue-green algae, black cohosh, or suan zao ren for memory improvement. Homeopathic remedies that may be recommended for people with post concussion memory difficulties include *Carbo vegetabilis*, *Silicea terra*, and *Hyoscyamus niger*. If your physician is unable to help you with herbs and/or homeopathics or to provide a referral to a practitioner who can, the Herb Research Foundation and/or the National Center for Homeopathy can help you locate an appropriate practitioner in your area. Feel free to get in touch with me for help or additional information using the contact information on page 367.

Some people have found that taking certain nutritional supplements, such as 50 milligrams of vitamin B6 (pyridoxine) and 100 milligrams of coenzyme Q10 daily, has helped to restore memory. It is important to be aware, however, that excessive amounts of vitamin B6 can damage the nervous system. As with any substance, it is crucial to first confer with your physician to determine what dosage, if any, is best for you.

PRACTICAL SUGGESTIONS

"I suffered a concussion not long after winning a $30,000 academic scholarship, and began to find answering multiple-part questions to be a problem due to short-term memory limitations. Now, each time someone asks me a two-part question, I subtly

touch a fingertip to the table and leave it there as a signal to myself. I answer the first question, then casually say, 'Now, what was the second part of your question?' Once the second question is answered, I remove my hand from the table."

—JULIA

"I find I remember things better with lots of practice. I provide three or four friends with a list of possible questions about material I am committing to memory and ask them to grill me on the information."

—DON

It takes a tremendous amount of energy to think clearly. Extensive periods of thinking and concentrating can cause mental fatigue under the best of circumstances, and will certainly do so in the aftermath of a concussion. Often, a vicious cycle results as you struggle to remember something, discover that you cannot, and then feel even more exhausted.

It is important to bear your new limitations in mind, but equally important not to let your symptoms defeat you. The following are some strategies that can help you register, store, and recall information more efficiently:

- Restrict your use of alcohol. Drinking has a direct effect on memory and cognition. Not only that, but your concussion may have reduced your alcohol tolerance.
- Ask your doctor if one or more of the medications you take may be causing short-term memory loss as a side effect. If so, discuss whether the benefits of the medication outweigh the effects on your ability to remember.
- Stop smoking.
- Reduce your intake of caffeine from all sources, including soft drinks and coffee. Dark chocolate may be the exception, but the greater the percentage of chocolate, the better.
- Have clocks and calendars visible around the house, especially in your bedroom and work areas.
- Categorize and group incoming information in small, concise pieces, such as work-related details, tasks to be done, and phone calls to be made.
- Color-code objects by category or event at home and at work by giving each week a specific color. Using appropriately colored stickers can help you recall

which week a project is to be done, or what week you purchased certain food items. A friend or family member can help you reorganize things.

- Visualize details of your destination and how to get there before leaving home.

- Close your eyes after you set an item down, such as your glasses or keys, and picture in your mind where you have placed it. Then open your eyes and look again to reinforce this image. If you are a tactile person, touch the area; if you use scents as cues, smell the area; and if you are a verbal person, say aloud what you see.

- Make it a practice to finish one task before beginning another. This way, you don't have to remember where you stopped. If this is impossible, use color tags, bookmarks, or notes to yourself as reminders of where you stopped in your projects. A task log can be very helpful.

- Play card games such as Concentration and Memory. These matching games help with attention, concentration, and recall.

- Do memory exercises. For example, have a friend or family member show you pictures, then put the pictures aside and ask you to identify what you saw. Audio programs such as Kevin Trudeau's Mega Memory provide a step-by-step course in improving your memory. Computer programs such as Neurotone's LACE (Listening and Communication Enhancement) are designed for fun but can improve your ability to recall things.

- Experiment to determine your stronger points, memory-wise, and use your strengths to help you recall things. For example, if your visual channel is impaired and you have trouble remembering things you have seen, try touching or smelling things to aid you in creating memories more effectively.

- Use tone and rhythm cues to help you store and recall information. By listening you may be able to store such information as the fact that you vacuumed the living room (a muffled sound), not the kitchen (a sharper sound), or that glasses, not paper cups, go in the dishwasher.

- Consider using a device such as a smartphone, pocket computer, voice-activated recorder, notebook computer, or daily planner to help you keep track of important information.

- Use initial consonants and silly stories, songs, and acronyms to trigger auditory memories, just as advertisers do. For example, you might chant or sing "hat-hamp" to remind yourself to get the hat near the hamper, or "OJ" to remember to buy orange juice at the store.

- Put different scents on different objects to stimulate your olfactory memory—the very first memory used in life. Read up on aromatherapy and explore the different scents that can enhance your recall such as clove, lime, lavender, and lemongrass, or mixed blends such Clarity from Young Living Essential Oils.

- Distinguish work or school materials by covering them in different textures or fabrics. Touch is the second sensory memory used in life, and different surfaces can serve as memory cues.

- Post notes, signs, and checklists to remind yourself what to do and when. A list on the front door can help you remember to turn off the coffeemaker and take your keys, while a note on the bathroom mirror can remind you to floss your teeth before you go to bed at night.

- Set alarms such as kitchen timers, stopwatches, or smartphone apps, with written reminders of what you need to do. Create a daily plan, and review it multiple times throughout the day.

- Use memory enhancement techniques such as chunking, structuring, and associating. Chunking is a method of grouping information, such as remembering 3 bread products, 4 meats, and 1 cleaning supply when you go grocery shopping. Structuring is deciding on proper places for items such as your keys, glasses, wallet, or wristwatch, and being certain always to place things where they belong. If necessary, compile a master list of objects and their locations, and store copies around your house and on your computer, if you have one. Associating is connecting two or more thoughts, because several words are actually easier to remember than one. For example, "Bugs Bunny" and "Daffy Duck" are more easily remembered than if the characters had a single name. In advertising, easy-to-remember examples are "Volvo—Safety" and "Nike—Just Do It."

At best, memory problems are quite frustrating. At worst, they are distressing. Time may eventually heal your recall problems, but devising strategies that employ your personal style of learning and experimenting with different approaches and techniques can help you cope in the meantime.

CHAPTER 20

PROBLEMS WITH REASONING, PLANNING, AND UNDERSTANDING

∎

Barbara was a sixth-grade teacher in Massachusetts. At school one day, a student dropped a basketball down a stairwell. Barbara, who was standing on a lower staircase, was hit on the head and knocked unconscious. She then fell down the flight of stairs. Afterward, Barbara regained consciousness and looked and sounded fine; however, she soon realized that something was very wrong. For instance, she could no longer take care of bill-paying. Ashamed to admit this, she hid months' worth of bills—a fact her family discovered only when their power was shut off. Then Barbara was unable to find the bills she had hidden. Once a highly organized teacher, she found herself unable to function in the classroom, although for a long time she didn't understand why she couldn't work. She simply couldn't judge the extent of her brain injury.

Aside from organizational, memory, and task-management problems, Barbara has trouble with the concept of time. She no longer understands or relates to the passage of minutes, hours, or days. Her old routines are currently impossible, though Barbara has learned to set timers all around her house to help her plan and follow a simple daily itinerary.

Similar symptoms were experienced by Dawn, first mentioned in Chapter 19, in the months after a bicycle accident. While riding, she became entangled with another bicyclist, flew over the handlebars, and was knocked unconscious. She was taken by ambulance to the hospital and released the same day. Within a few weeks, Dawn noticed that her ability to plan and reason were markedly affected. Often, Dawn found herself starting a project, starting another before the first one was finished, and moving on to yet another project before the second was finished. She also had difficulty shopping for groceries and following a recipe. Always an analytical and logical thinker, Dawn now found it difficult to assess a situation and put a plan in place.

RARELY DO we stop to consider how it is that we think, for doing so is as automatic as the beating of one's heart. However, after a concussion, also called *mild traumatic brain injury* (mTBI), even simple tasks can require a great deal of thought, leading people who are unaware of what has happened to suddenly feel incapable or stupid. Activities that require so-called *executive functions*—that is, the ability to reason, make sound judgments, and initiate, plan, or organize—may become virtually impossible, and this can pose a serious threat to independent living.

WHY EXECUTIVE FUNCTION PROBLEMS CAN OCCUR AFTER A CONCUSSION

Problems associated with planning, organizing, initiating, making sound judgments, and understanding (executive function problems) are often linked to injury to the brain's *frontal lobes* (see Chapter 1). However, research suggests that executive functions are complex processes involving several brain areas and affecting many hubs. Therefore, both generalized and localized brain trauma can cause post concussion problems with executive functions. Fortunately, the complete loss of executive function following this type of injury is rare.

TYPES OF EXECUTIVE FUNCTION PROBLEMS THAT CAN FOLLOW A CONCUSSION

"The first time I became aware of my reasoning problems was six months after my accident. We were packing for a trip to the mountains, and my husband suggested that I set out the clothing I needed. A while later, he found me crying, for I had no idea what to do or what to pack. Up to that time, we hadn't truly comprehended the extent of my limitations."

—D.R.S.

The ability to reason and think is not a single process, but an extremely complex network of related processes. Each of the abilities that make up your executive functions depends upon other mental processes to enable you to receive, comprehend, and act appropriately upon information. A problem with any one area can affect your overall thinking ability, just as a problem with one small part of the engine can affect the overall operation of your car. The following are descriptions of some of the higher-level thinking problems that commonly follow a concussion.

Planning Problems

The ability to plan is the capacity for thinking ahead and setting goals, whether for the next hour, the next week, or the next year. Planning is the first step in organizing daily living—you must decide what it is you want to do before you can determine how to accomplish it. Impaired planning ability undermines your ability to set goals, so if you suffer from this problem, you may need to rely on others to make plans for you, or play it safe by avoiding anything other than a repetitive routine.

Organization Problems

"A year and a half after my accident, my husband at the time, believing that I was much better, invited guests for a Fourth of July barbecue. Prior to my concussion, such parties were common events at our house. Now, however, I had no idea what a barbecue was or how to organize one. Happily, this problem has since improved greatly."

—D.R.S.

Organization is the ability to determine how your daily plans are going to be accomplished. For instance, if you are planning dinner, you must first decide what foods will be included, whether you need to take anything out of the freezer, whether a trip to the store is required, and when to start preparing each of the different dishes included in the meal so that they are all ready at the same time. Together, planning and organizing require skills in concentration, memory, problem-solving, and sequencing (putting or recalling events in order, or breaking a task into necessary steps). If you have problems with organization, you may encounter difficulty giving directions or breaking down a task. If you cannot track and sequence the past, present, and future, it will seem as if time has been altered or become nonexistent—as if you have somehow lost time. Often, the emotional result is a general feeling of anxiety, which can further impair your ability to organize, as well as aggravate your post concussion symptoms in general.

Initiation Problems

Initiation is the ability to carry out the tasks you have set for yourself—the ability to translate thoughts into activity. Even if you are able to plan and organize, a concussion may leave you unable to initiate the actions you have planned. To family and friends, this can look like a motivational problem, but an inability to initiate is in fact unrelated to energy level or ambition. Rather, the injury may have left your brain unable to take even the most specific and detailed thought and turn it into activity.

Problems with Processing Information

This phase of executive function is the lightning-quick combination of a multitude of new pieces of sensory information with existing knowledge. A concussion can affect the speed, duration, and accuracy of the integration, and later interpretation, of such input. Such a processing delay can cost you precious minutes in reaction time, perhaps leading to injury. For instance, you might not know to immediately remove your finger from a hot stovetop if there is a delay or other problem in processing the incoming signal of heat. Or a clear message may lead to an inappropriate response, such as yelling "Fire!" in a crowded theater and then wondering why you are in the middle of a riot.

Comprehension Problems

Comprehension is the ability to make sense out of processed and registered information—for instance, grasping the meaning of subtle humor or a complex story line in a movie. After a concussion, you may miss these messages. You may also be unable to understand verbal directions, commands, or questions, and be unable to make sense of maps and signs. In extreme cases, this problem can take the form of *visual agnosia*—the inability to recognize familiar objects or surroundings—causing the person with *post concussion syndrome* (PCS) to get lost inside his or her own home or become unable to recognize family members.

Decision-Making Problems

Even mild problems making judgments and decisions can affect all aspects of your thinking. Everyday activities such as cooking, shopping, or driving may suddenly become impossible if you ponder at length what used to be split-second decisions—such as knowing not to begin cooking an elaborate dinner when it is already 7 p.m. After a concussion, you may find yourself making business decisions that you later regret. Judgment problems stem from four sources: awareness, selection, memory, and emotions. Obviously, if you have a problem with awareness or attention, you may overlook information that is needed to make a sound decision, such as the cost of an item you are considering purchasing. If you cannot focus or remember, you will also have problems making choices that are appropriate. If you are upset or anxious, this too will interfere with your ability to make accurate and appropriate decisions.

Judgment difficulties range from mild to severe, and they affect concrete behavior, such as exercising caution at a stop sign, as well as higher-level problem-solving. Many people with post concussion symptoms deny their decision-making problems at first for fear of appearing incompetent or stupid, but colleagues, family members, or friends often provide insight by pointing out gross errors in judgment.

Learning Problems

After a concussion, you may retain and use many of your old skills but be unable to acquire and use new information. For example, you may be extremely proficient at using a computer program you learned prior to your injury but, despite weeks of training, fail to master even the basics of a new program. Even though you may not have any muscular or motor problems, you may also encounter difficulty learning new physical activities, such as a dance step or basketball move.

Self-Monitoring Problems

Self-monitoring is the ability to identify your errors while executing a plan and being able to modify or correct them. Difficulty with self-monitoring can look like carelessness and result in compromised safety or an inability to complete tasks accurately. This can create roadblocks to career advancement or even the loss of a job.

Problems with Creativity

Creativity is the process of developing new and original thoughts, plans, and solutions to problems. Researchers believe that the creative process begins in the right hemisphere of the brain. Of course, it is very difficult to form new ideas if your executive thinking skills have been impaired by a concussion. You may misjudge the appropriateness or feasibility of an idea, or simply have trouble focusing on or remembering different facets of your thoughts. In addition, you may have trouble organizing and following through with the creative process, which means that you cannot act on novel ideas that do occur to you.

DIAGNOSING AND ASSESSING EXECUTIVE FUNCTION PROBLEMS

A thorough examination by a neuropsychologist trained in PCS, along with a cognitive evaluation by a speech/language pathologist (see Chapter 5), is the best method of evaluating deficits in reasoning, planning, and understanding. This series of tests compares your current level of functioning with your previous abilities and can pinpoint specific problem areas. The results will enable you and the specialists involved in your care to develop a treatment program for your individual needs. A quantitative electroencephalogram (qEEG) looks at specific areas of functioning and can pinpoint where the brain is dysregulated and/or whether the brain is able to communicate from one region to another.

Hormones, which can affect your executive functioning, may have been disrupted or altered during your concussion. It is important to consult your primary care physician (PCP), a gynecologist, and an endocrinologist to ensure that problems with reasoning, planning, or understanding are not also due to hormonal changes.

TREATING POST CONCUSSION EXECUTIVE FUNCTION PROBLEMS

"I lost some of my sense of time and never knew how many minutes elapsed when I was talking with someone. I learned over the years to watch the clock when talking and to ask friends to let me know when they have to hang up the phone. Also, as the mother of three teenagers, I did a lot of driving. I learned to clock my trips ahead of time and write a schedule of places to be and the travel time involved. Preparing a schedule also enabled me to ask for help recalling things or places I had forgotten."

—D.R.S.

Trusting others is the first step toward recovery from the reasoning, planning, and understanding problems that can surface after a concussion. It is important to allow friends and family members to help you, and to let go of the idea that you alone know what is best. The following are some approaches that your doctors may recommend.

Conventional Approaches

In many cases, executive function problems improve with time. While alcohol and recreational drugs may give a false sense of being able to think better, these substances actually interfere with healing and thought processes. Drugs and alcohol also contribute to fatigue and, in some cases, seizures.

There are medications that are reported to improve executive function and cognitive processing, such as donepezil (Aricept), rivastigmine (Exelon), amantadine (Symmetrel), levodopa (Sinemet), modafinil (Provigil), and some tricyclic antidepressants (Elavil, Endep, Pamelor, Aventyl, and others). All of these medications can potentially impact the central nervous system (CNS), which includes your brain and cognitive ability. It is extremely important to read about possible side effects before taking any medication. Eating a diet rich in "good" fats such as olive oil, and omega-3 foods like wild salmon, and also eliminating sugar, can benefit your ability to reason, plan, and understand with the only side effect being overall good health. Vitamin B complex and coenzyme Q10 are also noted for helping to boost cognitive ability. When choosing the best foods and vitamins for your particular circumstances, it is wise to consult with a dietitian or nutritionist with a specialty in brain injury.

Getting restorative sleep is also extremely important to repairing and improving your reasoning, planning, and other executive functions (see Chapter 9). Because chronic post traumatic pain (PTP) can affect your ability to sleep and think (see Chapter 15), it is important to review the recommendations in these two chapters to help you create a plan to repair the affected cognitive skills.

Most rehabilitation hospitals offer treatment programs to help remediate deficits in executive functions in the form of cognitive therapy done by a speech/language pathologist. These programs help you develop skills to compensate for your inabilities, and teach you to use the skills you have retained more effectively. In general, five main areas are emphasized: awareness, goal formulation, planning and organization, initiation, and self-regulation (the ability to monitor your problems by yourself). You are taught how to identify problems and select solutions, and learn to review options and to sequence parts of a task. You are shown various compensatory strategies and trained to identify and correct errors in thinking and reasoning. In addition, you learn how to avoid distraction and effectively use support. Each concussion is unique, but you and the rehabilitation staff will soon learn which techniques work best for you.

Complementary Approaches

In the recovery of executive functions, biofeedback and neurofeedback are exceptional at helping the brain to become regulated again and form new neural connections needed for reasoning, planning, and understanding. Your specific difficulties in these areas can determine which of the various approaches of biofeedback and neurofeedback are best for you—from traditional methods, LENS (Low Energy Neurofeedback System), Z-score training, BrainAvatar, Neuro-Field, personal Roshi (pRoshi), and the Bio Acoustical Utilization Device (BAUD), to heart rate variability (HRV) training. (See Chapter 6 for descriptions of the wide variety of methods available.) There are also several computer programs and websites devoted to improving executive function skills, such as Interactive Metronome, BrainTrain, EyeQ, and Lumosity. Also, hyperbaric oxygen therapy, or HBOT (see Chapter 6), has been found to be very helpful in the recovery of executive functions.

Alternative Approaches

Bach Flower White Chestnut can help with repetitive thinking (when you keep thinking the same thoughts over and over again). There are a number of herbal and homeopathic products advertised that are reported to help you think clearly and accurately. To determine what might be appropriate for your specific post concussion executive function problems, it is best to consult with a Bach Flower practitioner, an herbalist, or a homeopathic practitioner who is experienced in these areas. Your physician, the Herb Research Foundation, or the National Center for Homeopathy should be able to provide referrals to the type of practitioner or practitioners you need. An herbalist may suggest such products as ginkgo biloba, anise, blue cohosh, or chuan xiong. The homeopathic remedies *Staphysagria*, *Phosphorus*, *Arnica*, and *Natrum sulphuricum* may also be recommended.

PRACTICAL SUGGESTIONS

"I use a digital watch to help with my awareness of time. Each beep reminds me that another hour has passed, and the alarm feature helps keep me on time for appointments. On trips, I carry a timer as a supplement to my watch."

—PATRICIA

"My efforts to organize my home have concentrated in the kitchen. Lists of contents are posted on cabinet doors, and I keep a blueprint in a drawer for reference. My refrigerator and pantries are inventoried, and I update the list every time I remove or replace an item."

—ELIZABETH

"I keep three different-colored book bags packed for school, and my husband reminds me of what day it is and which bag I need that day. I have an assistant who helps me to grade papers, and I color-code folders containing class notes, exercises, and exams before storing them in master folders labeled for each of my fifteen class sessions."

—MARY BETH

"I combat my reasoning and organization problems by carrying a Day-Timer appointment book and pen everywhere I go. I also write a task sheet outlining what needs to be done to start and finish each day, and I rely strongly on a watch with an hourly beep and several alarms."

—CHRIS

If you have had a concussion, you may face much more of a challenge as you go about your work and home life. It helps to take each day as it comes, accepting that your ability to reason, plan, understand, and learn new things may sometimes fluctuate. The following are some ways to minimize the disruption caused by executive function problems:

- Acknowledge that your brain has been damaged, and that this will affect your life. Accept the fact that learning new things, making appropriate judgments, and other tasks are now difficult for you, and remind yourself that mental disability is not the same thing as a lack of intelligence.
- Tell others of your need for quiet during work periods. If no distraction-free area exists at home, use a study carrel or reading room at your local public library.
- Discuss with your employer ways to provide you with a place in which you are able to do your work. This type of accommodation is required under the Americans with Disabilities Act.

- Check to see whether your insurance company will cover the cost of a home health aide to help with everyday tasks, such as meal preparation, that you are unable to do because of executive function problems.
- When your thoughts become disorganized, seek out a peaceful place. A church, park, or courtyard on a college campus can be an excellent place to "regroup."
- Build a support system to help you deal with daily frustrations. This can include therapists, your friends and family, a brain injury support group, and/or an online bulletin board.
- There are many digital devices and applications to help you improve your ability to sequence sights and sounds. These aids allow you to repeat bits of information until you grasp the meaning of what is being presented.
- Use a timer to relieve anxiety about forgetting tasks or appointments and to help with time management.
- Make notes via a digital recorder, smartphone, electronic tablet, daily planner, computer, or notebook, to help with short-term memory, planning, and organizing problems.
- Ask someone else to take charge of bill-paying for now. There are also computer programs, such as Quicken, that can help to guide you through this task. In addition, most financial institutions provide the ability to do your banking online.
- Allow more time than you think you will need to learn new tasks. Be patient, and deal only with today's problem.
- Be willing to put aside tasks that prove too difficult for now. Chances are, you will be able to learn (or relearn) needed skills later.
- Work at regaining your perception of time by noting how long everyday tasks take. Or put a friend or family member in charge of a timer and practice guessing at how long you have been engaged in different tasks.
- Call your local school district's special education chairperson for information about rehabilitative games and activities. Find out if a specialist is available to do private tutoring.
- If you have children, observe how they learn best. This can help you to develop your own learning strategies.
- Use board games such as Monopoly, Scrabble, and Clue, and card games like Go Fish, gin rummy, and poker, which develop planning, sequencing, and judgment skills. The more you practice, the better your skills will become.

- Ask your local software dealer about various programs from the Learning Company and BrainTrain that encourage the development of thinking skills.
- Set realistic goals for improvement. Your doctor or rehabilitation therapist can help you do this.
- Use a smartphone or your current phone's calendar system, which enables you to set alarms, modify schedules, set repetitive events, and alert others to what you are doing. Not only can you track appointments, but many apps help you organize the content as well.
- Expect splinter areas of recovery. For example, you may find you are able to read with comprehension before you regain your social skills.

Problems with your ability to reason, plan, and understand can significantly affect your frustration level and your ability to work and maintain social relationships. While recovery from executive function problems can be slow and erratic, it helps to know that there is a valid reason for your sudden deficits. It is also reassuring to know that professional assistance is available to supplement the coping strategies that you develop on your own or learn from others.

CHAPTER 21

SPEECH AND LANGUAGE PROBLEMS

■

J OHN, A 45-YEAR-OLD CAR SALESMAN FROM NEW HAMPSHIRE, WAS A PASSENGER in a car involved in a rear-end collision. When the police arrived, they asked the questions necessary to complete the accident report. John was more talkative than usual when responding, but to his amazement, he had great difficulty retrieving the words he needed for his answers.

A few weeks later at the car dealership, John's boss took him to task for his declining sales performance. While they were talking, the boss realized that John's manner of speaking had changed dramatically—that the once-articulate salesman sounded less sophisticated than before and was peppering his speech with nonsense words. John, however, was aware only of a slight word-finding problem.

As months went by, John's language difficulties increased. His family physician referred him to a psychiatrist, believing that stress was the culprit. Meanwhile, John's job performance became so poor that he was laid off, and his anxiety about finances and his now-obvious language problem made matters even worse. Eventually, John decided to seek another medical opinion, which led to neurological testing and the discovery that his word-retrieval problem was due to a concussion, also called *mild traumatic brain injury* (mTBI). John is still unemployed, but he is working with a speech/language therapist to try to regain his former verbal skills.

SPEECH PROBLEMS, or difficulties using the tongue, lips, palate, and larynx to produce sounds, are a common enough occurrence in everyday life. So are deficits in the ability to use and understand language. However, problems of this kind rarely appear suddenly, as they can following a concussion—a circumstance that can easily overwhelm you if you must suddenly scramble at home and on the job to compensate for mysteriously absent verbal skills.

WHY SPEECH AND LANGUAGE PROBLEMS CAN OCCUR AFTER A CONCUSSION

Several areas of the brain help to govern your ability to form words, express yourself, and understand spoken language. Even microscopic nerve-cell damage in one of these areas can disrupt your ability to process the auditory stimuli that precede and accompany verbal communication. Injury to the lower left hemisphere of the *frontal lobe* can damage *Broca's area*—one of your speech centers—and hamper articulation (the ability to pronounce speech sounds) and fluency (the ability to combine sounds and words smoothly). If other parts of the frontal lobe bear the brunt of the blow, both your ability to concentrate on what you are saying and your attentiveness to the conversation of others may be affected. In general, you may be less able to use or understand verbal or written communication.

Damage to *Wernicke's area*, located in the upper left hemisphere of the *temporal lobe*, can impair your ability to hear and interpret spoken words. You may have trouble understanding language and thus speak nonsense words out of context to the conversation. Language problems can also result if undetectable tearing or stretching of nerve-cell fibers hampers your powers of concentration and your ability to store and retrieve information. In addition, right temporal lobe damage can cause difficulties with nonverbal communication, which involves gestures, body posture, facial expressions, and eye contact.

Damage to the frontal lobes, particularly the *prefrontal cortex*, can impact conversation skills. People with executive functioning impairments often present with vague, nonspecific comments and difficulty adding details to a conversation, and may also be observed to have difficulty with the initiation of questions or comments, verbal organization, and the ability to stay on topic (topic maintenance).

TYPES OF SPEECH AND LANGUAGE PROBLEMS THAT CAN FOLLOW A CONCUSSION

"Before my concussion, I spoke in a rapid-fire fashion and was fond of embellishing my speech with lots of vivid analogies. Afterward, I spoke slowly, deliberately, and in a noticeably concrete manner. While this tendency has faded over time, I still sometimes use a word or expression incorrectly. I also have an intermittent word-retrieval

problem. Interestingly, my son Craig has a learning disability that is characterized by a similar word-finding problem. These days, we communicate beautifully! He says, 'Mom, may I have one of the yellow things on the shelf?' and without hesitation, I walk toward the bowl of bananas."

—D.R.S.

"I spent two days trying to come up with the English word for melanzana. I could see the eggplant and picture it in recipes, but could think of only its Italian name. If I continue to picture an object without asking someone or looking it up, the name will eventually come on its own. Stuttering happens most when I'm thinking and can't keep up with the speed of the conversation. I've learned to stay relaxed, slow down my tongue, and let things catch up."

—ELIZABETH

The types of communication difficulties related to concussion can be as different in form and degree as in origin. Whatever your deficit, it is likely to have an impact on every aspect of daily living. To help you better understand your sudden struggles with speech and language, the most commonly encountered problems are described below.

Speech Problems

There are three main types of speech problems that occur after a concussion: verbal apraxia, dysarthria, and dysfluency. *Verbal apraxia* is characterized by the inability to produce purposeful sounds or words on command, even though there are no muscular problems that would interfere with speech. This problem can cause you to sound as if you are stuttering, or as if you are having problems with word-finding.

Dysarthria is often characterized by problems with the muscle movements needed to form, or articulate, words. It can also affect pronunciation of spoken sounds. *Dysfluency*, better known as stuttering, takes the form of hesitant, stammering pronunciation of the beginning sounds of spoken words. Usually, there are a number of "false starts," as you repeatedly utter the initial sound or syllable of a word, but the rest of the word fails to follow. Or you may involuntarily draw out single sounds for several seconds as you attempt to summon the rest of the word. Dysfluency after a concussion is most often seen in people who stuttered as children, though it is not known why such an injury can cause stuttering to resurface.

Language Problems

Aphasia is an impairment in the ability to understand or express words or their nonverbal equivalents. There are many different types of aphasia, but most fall into one of three categories: expressive, receptive, and mixed.

Expressive aphasia involves problems with spelling, sentence structure, verbal reasoning, and/or the rate of speech. The most common type of expressive aphasia is known as *Broca's aphasia*, or *nonfluent aphasia*. With this type of aphasia, a person is able to understand language but unable to produce speech fluently. Instead, words are spoken in a telegraphic manner (with fewer than three or four words per sentence) using single words and gestures to convey meaning. Small words, such as articles (*a, an, the*) and prepositions (*of, from,* etc.), are typically omitted. For example, a person with Broca's aphasia talking about a plane trip might say, "Plane . . . me . . ." and spread his or her arms like wings to make the point. Broca's aphasia also involves the inability to repeat or write things that are heard.

Another characteristic of expressive aphasia is when people utter *neologisms*—grammatical confusions, inappropriate words, and nonsense words substituted for real words. *Anomia*, another form of expressive aphasia, renders a person completely unable to name familiar objects, almost as if he or she were suddenly required to converse in a foreign language. A lesser form of this problem is *dysnomia*, which causes you to grope for words that you know but simply can't think of. "It's on the tip of my tongue" and "You know, the whaddayacallit" are statements characteristic of people with word-retrieval problems.

Wernicke's aphasia includes both *fluent aphasia* and *receptive aphasia*. Fluent aphasia is a type of expressive aphasia that results in speech that is properly pronounced, grammatically correct, and effortlessly produced. However, it is often rapid, excessively wordy, and lacking in meaningful content.

Receptive aphasia denotes problems with reading, interpreting, and comprehending spoken language. This problem affects the understanding of the meaning of spoken and written words. Your ability to articulate words may be unaffected, but even though you may be able to recognize the conversation of others, you may be unable to comprehend it, almost as if they were speaking a foreign language. Or you may be able to comprehend, but find yourself struggling to process one aspect of what is being said and missing much of the subsequent conversation. You may also engage in a great deal of meaningless verbalization.

Conductive aphasia is characterized by halting speech with word-finding pauses and concrete rephrasing of words. *Perseverative speech* involves remaining on a topic or the uncontrolled repetition of words, phrases, sentences, or ideas.

Paraphasia is a type of receptive aphasia characterized by the substitution of parts of words or syllables for real words. *Alexia*, another form of receptive aphasia, is the inability to understand written language. *Dyslexia* involves difficulties with reading (more about this can be found in Chapter 22). *Mixed aphasia* is a problem with both the comprehension and expression of language.

DIAGNOSING AND ASSESSING SPEECH AND LANGUAGE PROBLEMS

Successful verbal communication requires that several neurological events occur simultaneously. A malfunction in any facet of the intake or transmission of nerve impulses can have a far-reaching effect. Because the result can be frightening, frustrating, and a significant handicap to job performance and everyday functioning, it is wise to investigate the cause of any speech or language deficits that follow your concussion.

Your primary health care provider may recommend magnetic resonance imaging (MRI) or a computed tomography (CT) scan, though these tests usually yield negative results in concussion cases. (See Chapter 5 for a detailed discussion of these procedures.) You may wish to ask about an electroencephalogram (EEG), which can be significant if it shows a slowing of brain waves in the temporal lobe. You will probably be given a referral to a neurologist, and you should ask for a neuropsychological assessment as well. This evaluation should be able to pinpoint the underlying source of speech or language difficulties, and provide a starting point for the formulation of a rehabilitation program.

Evaluation by a licensed speech/language pathologist will be able to assess your speech, language, and cognitive abilities. There are a variety of assessments to detect, for example, spontaneous speech, speech comprehension, naming, reading, writing, and repetition of words. There are other tests that assess and evaluate how you understand and process language. Also, a speech/language pathologist can help you evaluate your cognitive skills—in particular, attention and memory, both fundamental to functional communication.

TREATING POST CONCUSSION SPEECH AND LANGUAGE PROBLEMS

Articulation and stuttering problems that are aftereffects of a concussion often disappear on their own within three months. Language deficits may fade more slowly and require additional help. What follows is a look at conventional, complementary, and alternative approaches to resolving communication problems that are slow to correct themselves.

Conventional Approaches

If your neurologist feels that intervention is indicated because of your lifestyle or the degree of your speech or language impairment, therapy with a speech/language pathologist is likely to be the first step. This type of therapy helps you learn to work around your deficits, stimulate or retrain your brain's speech centers, and monitor the redevelopment of your verbal skills, as needed. Psychotherapy may be suggested to help you cope with the frustration of feeling misunderstood and being unable to express yourself. Family counseling can also be helpful as a means of promoting patience and understanding, and of teaching strategies for assisting the person with speech-related post concussion symptoms.

Complementary Approaches

Electromyography (EMG) biofeedback can be very effective for improving speech (it teaches you to identify and recognize individual muscle movements in and around your mouth), while neurofeedback can help find the dysregulated brain frequencies for stuttering or word retrieval (word-finding). Hypnosis can be very effective for improvement in articulation and stuttering. Hyperbaric oxygen therapy (HBOT) can be very useful in cognitive and language repair. Acupuncture by a licensed acupuncturist has been shown to improve articulation.

Alternative Approaches

There are no established alternative treatments for expressive or receptive language problems. However, polarity therapy has been known to help stuttering in some cases. This hands-on technique should be applied by a trained polarity therapist. The American Polarity Therapy Association should be able to refer you to a practitioner in your area. Or, you can contact me via the information listed on page 367 for assistance.

PRACTICAL SUGGESTIONS

"I found that by reading aloud for one hour every day, slowly repeating any words I stumbled on, I was finally able to say them correctly without stuttering. I used humor a lot, too. When I stuttered really badly on a word, I would grin and add, 'That's easy for you to say!' or even, 'Just call me Porky.'"

—JULIA

At home and at work, you can become practiced at analyzing your speech or language problems. Do you seem to struggle the most when you are fatigued or pressed for time? Are your thoughts disorganized, or does your problem seem to be purely physical? Examining all aspects of your struggle to communicate can point the way to helpful coping strategies, such as those that follow:

- To relax yourself and cut down on stuttering caused by stress, try inhaling deeply through your nose and exhaling through your mouth.
- Eliminate distractions to conversation. Your speech will flow more smoothly and you will have an easier time with comprehension if you talk in a quiet place.
- Gain a measure of control over stuttering by reading aloud to yourself, using a recorder and headphones. Start slowly and gradually increase your speed so that you learn to recognize—and then avoid—the point at which you start to stutter.
- Ask a friend or family member to give a prearranged signal when you are going off on a tangent or failing to make sense in conversation. A friend can also stand by at social gatherings to supply key words that escape you.
- Be honest about your problem both at work and at home. This will help you avoid embarrassment and promote patience and understanding in people who might otherwise judge you harshly.
- Temper any tendencies toward outspokenness for now, and avoid becoming involved in friendly debates. Doing so will save you a great deal of frustration.

- Try to visualize an elusive word as if it were written on a chalkboard, or try to hear the word in your head. If you still cannot retrieve the word, describe it or substitute another.
- Use a computer to communicate. Helpful software is widely available, including children's language games and programs and the *American Heritage Dictionary*'s word-finding feature.
- Explore drawing, music, dance, journal writing, and the theater as ways to help redevelop your language skills. Being inventive can help you think of many activities that stretch your ability to express yourself.
- Consider working with educational card and board games geared toward students of English as a second language (ESL). Contact the special education department of your local public school system for specific suggestions and other helpful ideas.
- Practice synonyms and antonyms to help expand your vocabulary.
- Watch movies with the sound turned off for practice interpreting gestures, expressions, body movements, and other forms of nonverbal communication.
- If your problem is an expressive one, consider learning American Sign Language as a temporary means of restoring your much-needed ability to communicate.

It is difficult to accept sudden deficits in speech or language, and very humbling to have to rely on others to help you communicate appropriately. It often helps to look at your verbal deficits as a transient symptom rather than a permanent disability. By seeking professional assistance and family support, developing strategies that work for you, and being realistic about occasional setbacks, you will pave the way for certain improvement in your speech and language skills. Also, there are online rehabilitation services that provide telerehabilitation due to advances in speech therapy and teleconferencing software. All that is needed is a standard computer and a broadband connection. However, many of these services are not designed for your specific needs and can actually hinder your recovery. On the other hand, there are interactive software, smartphone applications, and patient/team conferencing that are directed toward the goal of complementing inpatient and outpatient rehab for TBI.

CHAPTER 22

ACADEMIC PERFORMANCE PROBLEMS

■

JOE, A 22-YEAR-OLD MECHANIC, WAS A WRITER AND AN AMATEUR MUSICIAN. AT work one day, he was struck on the top of the head by a wrench. The young man's head ached and he complained of dizziness, but he was back on the job the next day. A few weeks later, Joe suddenly lost his ability to read music. And though he could write both spontaneous and dictated text in a perfectly normal manner, Joe found copying music or written passages to be strangely difficult. His struggles were compounded by a sense of despair. It took time and a great deal of patience, but Joe's reading and writing skills have shown significant improvement. Five years later, Joe has returned to his beloved music—a hobby he once feared he would have to abandon.

Nancy, a high school basketball player, was struck in the side of her head by a ball passed accidentally after the coach had stopped play. She continued to practice, thinking nothing of the impact; however, when she returned home that day and tried to study, the words on the page made no sense, to the point that she was unable to work. Nancy's symptoms increased the next day, and she was taken to the doctor and closely monitored. At the doctor's recommendation, Nancy stayed out of school for several days, resting at home and revamping her diet to eliminate sugars and processed foods. With an improved nutritional intake and a few days' rest, Nancy was able to return to school. She resumed sports months later after meeting the requirements of post-injury testing for concussion, also called *mild traumatic brain injury* (mTBI), by her doctors and athletic trainer. She was also given special accommodations to complete her schoolwork over time as her brain healed. Today, Nancy continues to be a fine athlete and an excellent student.

GIVEN THE wide range of possible aftereffects of *post concussion syndrome* (PCS), you shouldn't be surprised if you find yourself faltering academically following an accident of this type. You may struggle to understand or perform calculations. Or you may encounter reading comprehension problems, spelling difficulties, or a diminished ability to write. Naturally, such conditions have an adverse effect on school or job performance, and are likely to trouble you at home as well.

WHY ACADEMIC PERFORMANCE CAN SUFFER AFTER A CONCUSSION

Your brain is an intricate organ that governs the multitude of skills that are part of academic competency. As you would expect, the academic deficits that can surface after a concussion vary, depending on the site and extent of nerve-cell damage within the brain. With reading, writing, spelling, or math problems, the location of injury is believed to be the area between the back of the left *parietal lobe* and the left *occipital lobe* (see Chapter 1). Problems with the recognition of faces and symbols, social relationships, dancing, and creative expression are believed to originate in the corresponding area of the brain's right hemisphere.

If the *temporal lobe* is affected by a concussion, some degree of short- or long-term memory loss often occurs. If this happens, you may encounter related problems with word and letter identification, reading comprehension, or remembering and applying the principles of phonics. If the back of the brain received the impact, the occipital lobe may be injured. This part of the brain oversees vision and recognition. Problems with eye movement and eye-hand coordination can result, as can difficulties with perception and with recalling words.

TYPES OF ACADEMIC PERFORMANCE PROBLEMS THAT CAN FOLLOW A CONCUSSION

"I was an avid reader prior to my accident, plowing through some 3,000 words per minute with 90 percent comprehension. Suddenly, I couldn't read simple instructions! Sometimes I could see the letters but had no idea what the words were or what they meant. At other times, I could read and understand, but couldn't recall what I had read just a few minutes before. My math skills were affected, too. I was shocked to find that I—a former cost-accounting instructor at a local college—was unable to perform computations and fathom monetary values. It was four and a half years before I could go to lunch with a friend and calculate my share of the bill!

This ability was retained until I had another concussion, after which my reading level once again went from 3,000 words per minute to 285 words per minute. This time, it took over a year to regain my former level."

—D.R.S.

The brain trauma caused by a concussion has the potential to diminish a number of academic skill areas, and can be linked to certain specific deficits in reading, writing, spelling, and math. The problems of this type that are encountered most often are described below.

Reading Problems

Reading difficulties can stem from several different sources. If your concussion has interfered with eye movements, you may struggle to focus or have trouble tracking—that is, following the text from one line of print to the next. If your memory has been affected, you are likely to have trouble recognizing letters or words and retaining the information you have just read. Or you may encounter a processing difficulty such as *dyslexia*, which can cause misperception of letters and letter sequences, misidentification of words, and an inability to distinguish text from its background. You may also have problems following visual sequences and doing puzzles.

Alexia, as mentioned in Chapter 21, is also called "word blindness," and is another processing problem that makes you unable to recognize letters or words. As a result, printed words appear as meaningless groups of marks or symbols on the page. When the letters are eventually understood, the person is able to read the words. *Agnosia alexia* is the complete inability to understand written words, a result of damage to the left occipital lobe.

Writing Problems

Writing problems can be muscle-related, resulting in problems with fine motor movement (the movement of your fingers, hand, or wrist) or coordination. Depending on the location of your concussion, you may also have trouble coordinating your eyes and hands, which makes copying extremely difficult.

Dysgraphia, another writing disability, results from injury to the parietal lobe that disrupts the transmission of nerve impulses between the hand and the brain. As a result, you are unable to perform the motor movements necessary for legible handwriting. If you are suddenly dysgraphic, you may be unable to recall what letters and numbers look like, or how to reproduce them.

Agraphia is a nerve-disconnection problem that interferes with your ability to get your hand to write legibly—or at all, in some cases. Another writing problem is *agitographia*, which is characterized by very rapid writing movements that cause letters, words, or parts of words to be distorted or omitted.

Spelling Problems

Spelling difficulties that follow a concussion can have several causes. If your visual memory has been impaired, for instance, you may find yourself forgetting what certain words—or even certain letters of the alphabet—look like. Auditory memory problems can adversely affect your "sounding-out" skills by interfering with your recall of letter sounds, word sounds, and the rules of phonics. *Alexia agraphia* is a disability marked by an inability to identify and reproduce letters, words, and numbers. This condition completely undermines any attempts at spelling.

Problems with Math

You may find that your ability to use and understand numerals, mathematical symbols, musical notes, and other symbols has been diminished as a result of your PCS. This disorder, called *asymbolia*, can cause you to struggle to comprehend prices, sizes, measurements, and other everyday numerical concepts. Another skill impairment, *dyscalculia*, affects your ability to add, subtract, multiply, and divide—both on paper and in your head. Visual memory problems, another common occurrence as part of PCS, can diminish your recall of the rules behind fractions, decimals, percentages, and other higher-level math concepts. You may also have challenges understanding mathematical word problems because of working memory and abstract language problems.

DIAGNOSING AND ASSESSING ACADEMIC PERFORMANCE PROBLEMS

While deficits in reading, writing, spelling, or using numbers are easy to recognize—and, when they appear suddenly, to link to a concussion—it can nevertheless be difficult to determine the exact source of such problems. Impaired writing skills, for example, can stem either from problems with your hand muscles or from parietal lobe damage. Mathematical disabilities can originate in the left or the right side of the brain. In addition, your diminished skills may stem from a combination of problems—say, impaired eye-hand coordination combined with visual memory loss—rather than from injury to just one area of the brain.

If your concussion has left you with academic problems, your physician or other health care provider should refer you to a neuropsychologist for evaluation. You will be interviewed, examined, and given a battery of tests to assess various cognitive and academic skills and compare them with your previous level of functioning. The results should determine the nature and extent of your problems and point the way toward treating and overcoming your deficits.

TREATING POST CONCUSSION ACADEMIC PERFORMANCE PROBLEMS

"I could hold a pen, but could not get my hand to make the writing movements I wanted it to make. Yet I could operate my computer with little difficulty. This helped me to record my thoughts and feelings, communicate, and learn to read again. Later, when I could write again, I found that gesturing with my other hand helped me to improve my spelling. I also took a multisensory approach to spelling, tracing words in sand and asking family members to write on my back with their fingertips."

—D.R.S.

Time is a great healer of academic problems caused by a concussion, since most problems improve in the first six months. However, since skills of this nature are often needed on the job—and are always required to perform at-home responsibilities—most people with a concussion are reluctant to simply wait out the recovery process. Happily, help is widely available.

Conventional Approaches

There are special study strategies and other therapeutic activities that can help you improve or regain faltering academic abilities. First, it is important to change your diet and get restorative sleep. Eating more protein, such as foods rich in omega-3, and eliminating cane sugar is essential. The brain needs to repair itself with good nutrition and restorative time, which can only happen through sound sleep (see Chapter 9). If necessary, you can also be helped to find ways to circumvent deficient skills. A speech/language pathologist, learning-disabilities specialist, or other special educator can help you set reasonable goals throughout your recovery, suggest materials and exercises, and work with you to help you attain these goals. Your doctor, the local school district, or a nearby rehabilitation hospital should be able to refer you to a specialist trained to work with people who have a brain injury.

There are many specific treatment techniques that may be used, depending on your particular problems and individual learning style. For instance, if you learn best through tactile input, or feeling things, a program to remediate calculation problems would involve the manipulation of materials to teach the skill through sight and touch.

Occupational therapy may be recommended, especially if you need to overcome visual or small-muscle impairments or learn new techniques for dispatching troublesome tasks at work. In addition, psychotherapy and family counseling can help you cope with the feelings of frustration and despair that can stem from finding yourself with suddenly diminished academic abilities.

Complementary Approaches

Acupuncture has helped in this area, along with neurofeedback, which can help the brain become re-regulated in the specific areas related to academics. EyeQ is a computer-based program specifically designed to improve reading speed and comprehension, while BrainTrain, another computer program, helps in many areas of reading, comprehension, and memory. Cogmed is yet another very effective approach.

Alternative Approaches

Reiki, polarity therapy, and Qi Gong can be very useful in improving specific areas of academic performance. There are particular Bach Flowers, herbs, and homeopathics that also may help. Over-the-counter methods are not as effective as consulting with a Bach Flower practitioner, naturopathic doctor, or homeopathic practitioner, who can develop a program especially designed for you and your unique issues.

PRACTICAL SUGGESTIONS

"My solution for dealing with the problem of transposing letters and numbers was to spend time entering recipes and gardening notes into the computer. There has been

very noticeable improvement, which has stayed, for the most part. I also discovered that my concentration was affected by various musical backgrounds, and that I seemed to concentrate better with Mozart and classical jazz."

—ELIZABETH

While you put your doctor's or practitioner's advice to work against faltering academic skills, you can also take steps on your own to make life easier during your recovery period. The tried-and-true suggestions that follow can help you get started:

- Make grocery lists from supermarket circulars and compare the costs of various items. This not only exercises your numerical skills, but it also allows you to do comparison shopping ahead of time and at your own pace.
- Use a smartphone or computer to store ideas, lists, schedules, reminders, and notes about just-read material. When your memory fails you, the computer can recall the needed information (and, unlike a piece of paper, won't be mislaid).
- If writing is a challenge, consider dictation-to-text applications, like Dragon Dictate. Other computer programs can help with the organization of written information.
- Most computer browsers now include options for changing fonts, colors, and type sizes, and also include text-to-speech functions.
- Carry a calculator with you at all times to help with difficult math calculations and money management.
- Read information more than once. If text is lengthy, break it into smaller pieces and read small chunks of information at a time.

It is distressing to suddenly lose your ability to enjoy a novel, compose a letter, take notes, or do math computations. Problems of this nature that result from a concussion often fade over time; however, it makes little sense to simply wait out the recovery process. Instead, be honest about the skill areas that trouble you, be aggressive about finding the right professional assistance, and concentrate on formulating helpful strategies and shortcuts to offset your disability. Your take-charge efforts will spark faster improvement and do wonders for your state of mind as well.

PART 4

EMOTIONAL ASPECTS

INTRODUCTION

■

TWENTY-EIGHT-YEAR-OLD BETTY, AN OPERATING ROOM NURSE FROM ANDOVER, Massachusetts, was involved in a crash with an eighteen-wheel truck. Several ambulances arrived at the scene, but Betty felt fine and insisted that she was okay. In fact, one of her friends took her out for breakfast and then drove her home.

At first, the only symptom Betty noticed was severe muscle pain. Later, when she complained of irritability, crying spells, and mood swings, doctors said her emotionality was a reaction to her discomfort. It was not until five or six months later, when Betty began experiencing sensory overload and blackouts, that she was referred to a neurologist. Within minutes, the neurologist diagnosed *post concussion syndrome* (PCS).

In the years that followed, Betty experienced emotional instability and feelings of sadness and grief. For a time, she saw a clinical psychologist at a local rehabilitation hospital. In addition, she joined the hospital's support group for people with concussions, also called *mild traumatic brain injuries* (mTBI), which helped a great deal. At present, Betty is back at work on a part-time basis. She recently had her third child and is enjoying life, though she is still recovering from her concussion.

PART 4 of this book deals with the emotional and psychological aspects of PCS. In some ways, the psychological aspects are more complicated than either the physical or mental aspects. First of all, emotional and psychological symptoms can be more difficult to recognize and describe. If you are having headaches, for instance, you will probably know immediately that something is wrong and why the problem is occurring. With emotional and psychological symptoms, this is not always the case. To begin with, you may have trouble recognizing that what you are experiencing—say, frequent bursts of anger—is not an ordinary emotion but a sign that something is wrong. Then, once you do identify an emotional or psychological symptom, you may find it difficult and/or embarrassing to discuss this with your physician.

Further complicating the situation is the fact that many emotional and psychological symptoms can have more than one underlying cause. Sometimes they result directly from injury to the brain; other times they may be a secondary reaction to brain trauma. They can also be a side effect of medications prescribed for post concussion symptoms, or they can represent an exacerbation of a previously existing psychological disorder.

Take the example of depression, which can result from several conditions. It may be caused by injury to the *frontal lobe*, a part of the brain involved in mood. Or you may be unable to continue working and, as a result, feel depressed. Or, if you have migraines or cluster headaches following a concussion, your doctor may prescribe a beta-blocker as a preventive, and the beta-blocker may cause depression as a side effect. Finally, if you had occasional mild but manageable depressive episodes prior to your injury, you may find yourself facing major depression afterward. Thus, any one of four different scenarios—or any combination thereof—can lead to the same result. In addition, some emotional and psychological symptoms can cause and/or be part of others. For example, depression can cause reduced sex drive, which can in turn lead to difficulty in personal relationships.

If you think this sounds confusing, you're right—it can be, but Part 4 will provide you with some direction. The most common emotional and psychological effects of a concussion are considered here in four groups: post-injury reactions, mood and behavior problems, the magnification of preexisting psychological disorders, and grieving. However, you should keep in mind that, as described above, it is possible for a single symptom to have more than one cause, and as such to have a place in more than one of the four groups.

With the assistance of health care practitioners who have experience in treating concussion, it should be possible to identify the underlying cause of your distress. The good news is that for most of these problems, there are treatments that can help.

CHAPTER 23

POST-INJURY PSYCHOLOGICAL REACTIONS AND POST TRAUMATIC STRESS DISORDER (PTSD)

■

WYOMING RESIDENT CINDY WAS INVOLVED IN A MINOR AUTO ACCIDENT. THE impact caused her to bump her head, but based on her appearance and behavior, police at the scene told her she could go home. Weeks later, Cindy resigned from her job, which had suddenly become quite stressful. But at home, things were no better. Cindy, who had always been careful about money, began to lose bills or fail to pay them on time. She was unable to balance her checkbook. She decided to try her hand at cosmetic sales, and bought $3,500 worth of skin- and hair-care products without a single customer. At night, she would wake up from a sound sleep, drenched in perspiration and feeling jittery and upset.

Eventually, Cindy took a new job, but it lasted only two weeks. She couldn't put her finger on the problem, but things in her life just didn't feel right. At yet another job, Cindy's work pace was pitifully slow. She was afraid to answer the phone, was unable to make decisions, and found herself getting up in the middle of the night to tackle unfinished work. Convinced that she was going crazy, Cindy sought professional help, only to discover that she was having a psychological reaction to a concussion.

LIFE EXPERIENCES, whether normal or out of the ordinary, create physical and psychological stimulation that summons responses from both body and mind. Upon failing a test, you might flush with embarrassment and feel defensive or guilty. Faced with losing a job or relationship, you may tremble and sweat and feel awash in self-reproach. These reactions show that circumstances have pushed you beyond your tolerance level and that your defenses have been activated. It should not surprise you to learn that psychological reactions can easily be triggered by the physical and emotional upheaval of a concussion.

WHY POST-INJURY PSYCHOLOGICAL REACTIONS OCCUR

Much as your immune system kicks in as a response to a deep cut or an infection, the circumstances and aftermath of brain trauma ignite psychological responses. Physical and emotional pain that exceeds your personal threshold can make you feel nauseated or numb, or even cause you to faint. Such physical reactions are often part of psychological upheaval.

Psychological responses also commonly involve emotional, cognitive, or behavioral elements. Emotional elements may include denial, avoidance, anxiety, emotional numbness, and/or feelings of grief or guilt. Cognitive reactions may take the form of rationalizing, blaming, and/or being judgmental. Behavioral elements may include aggressiveness, expressions of anger, withdrawal, diminished abilities, lack of control, and overwhelming sadness. In many cases, behavioral responses develop into physical symptoms such as headaches, ulcers, chest pain, sleep problems, or suppression of the immune system.

Extraordinary life experiences, including such unexpected and traumatic occurrences as fire, assault, sports or recreational injury, automobile accidents, and combat often lead to post traumatic stress. The same is true of a concussion. This can be experienced immediately as acute stress, or as a delayed response months or even years later.

WHAT POST-INJURY PSYCHOLOGICAL REACTIONS ARE LIKE

Post concussion symptoms are often experienced as a personal disaster. You may have feelings of defeat, frustration, and inadequacy. In addition, you may suffer anxiety over your sudden lack of control over things and the sense that you have failed yourself and your family.

When your mind and body are out of harmony or balance (neurologically dysregulated), a distress signal is sent to indicate danger to you. This may take the form of pain. To avoid feeling this pain, your mind's or body's reaction is to shut down through an initial reaction of numbness. Following this shutdown phase is another set of responses called the "fight/flight/freeze" mode. At this point, some people choose the "fight" option—that is, they take the offensive as a way of dealing with concussion aftereffects, displaying such responses as verbal or physical aggression, angry outbursts, and blaming others. Others choose "flight"; their psychological response is to withdraw, flee, or psychologically defend themselves against the realization of sudden personal changes. This withdrawal can take different forms, including physical withdrawal (such as literally running away from an accident scene), denial (refusing to believe the injury happened), rationalization (coming up with an explanation of its cause), or guilt (blaming oneself). A person exhibits "freeze" behavior by becoming overwhelmed by the fear that something is wrong and becoming emotionally, and sometimes physically, paralyzed and unable to function.

In most situations, psychological responses are not displayed in separate parts, but as a mixture of reactions. For instance, if you were injured in a sports contest or an automobile accident, it might be emotionally easier for you to express feelings of anger at the player who injured you or at the other driver (aggressiveness) and to insist that the collision was his or her fault (rationalizing and blaming) than it would be either to acknowledge that you might be to blame or to focus your thoughts on the disabilities you now face. This is especially true if such an acknowledgment might be painful—say, if alcohol or drugs were involved, or if a loved one was injured while you were behind the wheel, or if you must deal with a permanent physical disability of some kind.

WHAT IS POST TRAUMATIC STRESS DISORDER (PTSD)?

Another possible response that can occur in conjunction with PCS is post traumatic stress disorder (PTSD), the signature of injury from violence such as combat, assault, domestic abuse, and auto accidents. With this syndrome, you find yourself involuntarily reliving the traumatic experience in your mind. You may also experience nightmares, feelings of overwhelming helplessness and anxiety, nervous alertness, distractibility, and depression. If you also have amnesia, instead of experiencing intrusive memories and flashbacks, you may experience emotional or bodily sensations evoked by sounds, colors, temperatures, or other stimuli that are in some way related to the accident. For instance, cracking ice might be upsetting because it mimics the sound of breaking glass. The reactions to PTSD may be heightened if the disaster was life-threatening and caused you to feel overwhelmingly vulnerable.

Whatever direction psychological reactions take, feelings of guilt and shame over the inability to live life as before are common. These emotions can leave you isolated, reproachful, and filled with self-doubt. They can be compounded by a prior history of coping problems, which makes psychological distress more likely, or by the malaise that accompanies chronic fatigue.

DIAGNOSING AND ASSESSING POST-INJURY PSYCHOLOGICAL REACTIONS AND PTSD

Not all psychological reactions are severe or long-lasting enough to require professional intervention. But because brain trauma, depression, and denial can cloud your judgment, and because the range of potential emotional and psychological symptoms that can occur in the aftermath of a concussion is so broad, you may not be the best person to assess your own situation.

For the most accurate and objective diagnosis and assessment, you should consult a mental health professional who has training and experience in both trauma and brain injury. Symptoms such as aggression, depression, and suicidal thinking or ideation (formulating a plan of action) can be the result of organic brain injury (more about this in Chapter 26), a post-injury psychological response, and/or PTSD. In order to get proper treatment, it is extremely important to know what is behind your symptoms. (See page 291 for a comparison of PCS, PTSD, and grief reaction.)

To properly diagnose whether the psychological reaction to your concussion is PTSD, it is important to be seen by a neuropsychologist with training in both PCS and PTSD. A battery of tests is done over a six-hour period to tease out whether what you are experiencing is a result of prior mental health issues, injury to the brain, or your brain's reaction to severe trauma. Another method of assessment is a quantitative electroencephalogram (qEEG) done by a neuropsychologist, psychophysiologist, or certified specialist in qEEG (see Chapter 6). A qEEG measures the function of the brain, comparing you to a database, similar to the way a blood test compares your blood to what is considered normal. In addition, it is important to be evaluated by an endocrinologist, as a major part of PTSD involves changes in cortisol levels. An endocrinologist can determine how your concussion and the related trauma have affected you.

TREATING POST-INJURY PSYCHOLOGICAL REACTIONS AND PTSD

As mentioned above, post-injury psychological reactions do not necessarily require treatment, while PTSD does. Professional help is certainly indicated if reactions become severe and/or prolonged enough to interfere with daily living, which does occur with PTSD. But even if your post-injury reactions are not that severe, you may find treatment to be very beneficial for your recovery and for your life in general.

Because these problems are often multifaceted, treatment through a team approach is usually recommended. Depending on your circumstances, your neurologist may refer you to a neuropsychologist, a psychiatrist, a psychologist, and/or a psychopharmacologist. You may also receive assistance from a clinical social worker, a rehabilitation counselor, and, if needed, a case manager. Patient and family counseling and training can be very effective. In addition, spiritual or religious counseling and prayer can be very helpful in the most difficult moments.

Conventional Approaches

Nutritional changes, specifically the increase of vitamin C and omega-3 from wild salmon and sardines, are very helpful in stabilizing cortisol levels. Your doctor may recommend medication to help you cope with post-injury psychological reactions. Antidepressant medications such as sertraline (Zoloft) and fluoxetine (Prozac) have been used effectively in the treatment of anxiety associated with PTSD. Depending on your symptoms, there are a number of other medications, such as anticonvulsants, mood stabilizers, and alpha- or beta-blockers, that may help. The exact medication or combination of medications appropriate for your needs will depend on the nature and cause of your problem, as well as on your own biochemical makeup. To ensure that you obtain proper care, medication, and dosages, it is wise to see a psychopharmacologist who specializes in PCS.

Cranial electrotherapy stimulation (CES) is a medical device approved by the Food and Drug Administration for insomnia, depression, and anxiety. Exercise of any type—from gardening, dancing, Zumba, and water therapy to taking a walk in your neighborhood—really helps the brain to become more regulated and brings you to the present time, which helps with symptoms of disassociation and flashbacks. Therapeutic massage has been found to be beneficial in relieving the psychological symptoms of a concussion. Beyond helping your muscles to relax, massage therapy may stimulate the blood flow to the brain, aiding in the healing process.

Psychotherapy can be extremely valuable for coming to an understanding of, and working through, psychological reactions to injury. Cognitive behavioral therapy (CBT) can help you to modify your thought patterns, change problem behavior, and deal with psychological trauma. Both eye movement desensitization and reprocessing (EMDR) and hypnosis have a long history of effectiveness with resolving PTSD. (See Chapter 6 for a complete discussion of these therapeutic approaches.)

These types of therapy should be conducted by a licensed psychologist, psychiatrist, social worker, or counselor certified in these modalities. For the therapy to be effective, it is crucial to find an appropriate medical or mental health care provider. This person should be compassionate, caring, well trained, and experienced with your type of problem. Finding the right person may be difficult, especially in less populated areas where the supply of well-trained people may be limited. With telemedicine and Skype, however, the possibility of finding the right person increases. Ultimately, it is vital for your outcome to find someone who believes you can get better and is willing to work with you.

In addition to one-on-one therapy, support groups work well for brain-injured people. Group work is not recommended for people with symptoms of PTSD until they have received some individual counseling, because hearing of other people's traumatic situations may result in a traumatic reaction in someone who has not first acquired coping skills and strategies to handle their reactions. There are four basic types of support groups. The first, a self-help group led by a trained facilitator, can educate a person with PCS and his or her family as to who he or she has become. The second type of support group is informational in nature and invites outside speakers and others to make presentations on relevant topics. A third, more therapeutic type of support group provides a trained counselor who helps members deal with their emotions and progress through the various stages of grieving and healing. The fourth type, more often used in cases of severe and moderate brain injury, serves as a training group for family members involved in home health care. A local rehabilitation center or the Brain Injury Association should be able to furnish information about support groups in your area. For help with this, you can contact me via the information listed on page 367.

Complementary Approaches

Both acupuncture and acupressure are very effective at stabilizing the energy system. The difference is that while acupuncture uses fine needles, acupressure uses finger pressure on the body, hands, feet, or ears, to release blocks in the flow of *qi*, or vital energy. There are books to guide you in this practice, although ideally you should consult with a licensed acupuncturist before trying to treat yourself.

Other energy balance systems include Thought Field Therapy (TFT) and Emotional Freedom Techniques (EFT). Energy psychology, originated by Dr. Fred P. Gallo, has specific methods for treating trauma that are very helpful. Bilateral sound therapy, similar to EMDR, is also beneficial. A wide variety of biofeedback and neurofeedback methods and equipment, such as the Othmer method, LENS (Low Energy Neurofeedback System), Z-score training, Neuro-Field, and personal Roshi (pRoshi) are effective at returning the reactive part of your brain to a state of regulation (see Chapter 6). When there is severe trauma affecting the limbic system (see Chapter 1), HeartMath's emWave heart rate variability (HRV) training system is extremely helpful at calming the mind and body.

Alternative Approaches

Reiki, Qi Gong, and polarity therapy, which help bring the mind and body into better harmony, can help you deal with psychological reactions to your concussion. Polarity therapy should be provided by a trained practitioner. To ensure proper treatment, inquire about the practitioner's level of training and whether they have worked with people with PCS and PTSD. The American Polarity Therapy Association should be able to provide a referral to a polarity therapist in your area. For further information, you can email or call me via the contact information on page 367.

There are herbal and homeopathic preparations that can be beneficial for some post-injury psychological reactions. Other types of alternative treatments that may help your symptoms include aromatherapy and flower essence therapy. Aromatherapy, the use of aromatic essential oils distilled from plants, can be used to help calm and relax you or to boost your energy level. For example, clary sage is often used for its calming effects, ylang-ylang for relaxation, and cypress for increased energy. Roberta Wilson's *Aromatherapy for Vibrant Health and Beauty* provides specific, easy-to-follow instructions for using this art to treat both physical and emotional conditions.

Unlike essential oils, flower essences do not employ scent. They are closer in nature to homeopathic remedies—highly diluted preparations that contain the imprint of plant energy. Flower-essence therapists believe that the life force of the various flowers can affect both body and mind. Edward Bach, an English homeopath and physician, is the most noted theorist and practitioner of flower-essence therapy. Bach Flower Star of Bethlehem is specifically used for trauma, and White Chestnut for racing thoughts (repetitive thinking). However, to determine what is right for you, it is best to consult with a qualified Bach Flower practitioner, herbalist, or homeopath who specializes in PCS and PTSD. At first, some post-injury psychological symptoms may seem easy to identify and treat; you know if you are feeling sad, anxious, or whatever. But as with headaches, the underlying causes can vary widely, so remedies of any kind should be used with care. If you are depressed, for example, taking the wrong product could cause a more severe depression. If your physician is unable to help you or to refer you to an appropriate practitioner, the Herb Research Foundation or the National Center for Homeopathy should be able to help. Contact me for help with this via the information listed on page 367.

PRACTICAL SUGGESTIONS

"Pets tend to reteach us uncomplainingly how to touch when you scratch their ears, 'shake hands,' or pet them. I used my cats as my first therapists—they would move out of arm's reach to get me to realize that I had done the petting too roughly."

—LIANNE

There is a satisfying sense of control inherent in finding ways to speed your recovery from any post concussion symptom. The suggestions below may help you cope with the psychological aftermath of your injury:

- View informative DVDs. The Brain Injury Association offers a helpful one about concussion and PCS. Another DVD, which debuted as an ABC Sunday Night Movie, is called *Stranger in the Family*. The Brain Injury Association can help you secure a copy of this DVD as well.
- Look into interactive communication networks for computers. There are bulletin boards, chat rooms, and forums through social media such as Facebook and LinkedIn, as well as websites such as Neurotalk.org, Brainline.org, and Braintrauma.org where a wide range of people with similar problems can find support. However, bear in mind that what you read online may not necessarily be true, and that some people who post on these sites may not have information that is applicable to your specific needs.

- Pursue a sport or hobby that brings a feeling of accomplishment or comfort. Consider unstructured activities such as gardening or painting that encourage expression and emphasize your personal strengths.
- If you don't already have one, consider getting a pet. Research has shown that pet owners recover faster than those without animal companions. Any type of pet is suitable, provided you can care for it properly. The type you choose should depend on your capabilities and housing situation. Many locations have rent-a-pet and foster pet programs for those who cannot own or provide full-time care for a pet of their own.
- Depending on your needs, there are assistive pets that are specially trained to work with people with TBI, PCS, and PTSD.
- Avoid activities that require organizational skills and memory, or whatever skill you are having trouble with. Cooking, for instance, is likely to highlight shortcomings in thinking skills and can be extremely frustrating.
- When you feel anxiety or frustration mounting, nip it in the bud by taking a bath, going for a walk, doing yoga, dancing, singing, counting to ten, or using relaxation techniques like deep breathing.
- Avoid the use of alcohol or cigarettes to calm yourself. These substances might seem to help in the short term, but they can cause further injury to your body and make many post concussion symptoms worse.
- Do not attempt to medicate yourself with over-the-counter drugs, herbal remedies, or homeopathics. Overuse or improper dosages may cause further complications; therefore, do not rely on what works for others.
- Before using any self-medication, it is extremely important to consult with a physician, naturopath, or certified herbal or homeopathic practitioner with extensive knowledge of PTSD and TBI.
- Consider spiritual counseling and/or a church-, temple-, or mosque-based support group. Most houses of worship offer or can refer you to some kind of community support group.

You will surely discover additional ways of coping, adjusting, and regaining your sense of purpose and self. As you recover from your post concussion symptoms, an understanding mental health specialist can be a great source of strength. It is vital to keep searching until you find such a professional. Remember: the road you are on is not an easy one, but you need never travel it alone.

CHAPTER 24

ALCOHOL, DRUG, AND SUBSTANCE ABUSE

C HAD, A 24-YEAR-OLD, HAD BEEN A SUBSTANCE ABUSER FOR SEVEN YEARS. After an automobile accident, it was found that he had been driving under the influence of so many drugs that the hospital and lab were never able to identify them all. His car was a wreck, and so was he. He had had similar substances in his body for years, so his brain never had a chance to recover between episodes. As months and then years passed after the car accident, Chad self-medicated the chronic pain from his injuries with fast food, sweets, and alcohol, along with various prescription medications such as Suboxone. Most, if not all, of his symptoms of *post concussion syndrome* (PCS), such as problems with sleeping and recalling information, have continued for years. In order to deal with his depression, Chad continues taking recreational drugs and Suboxone.

Stories like these among young adults are not unusual and are even more prevalent among warriors returning from combat. Some may have had preexisting marijuana or alcohol habits or began using those substances while deployed. However, the majority of returning military personnel with alcohol or drug problems never abused substances until they returned home. For many, alcohol is the substance of choice for self-medication of chronic pain and the symptoms of post traumatic stress disorder (PTSD), particularly flashbacks.

Athletes will occasionally use one or more performance-enhancing substances, such as steroids, believing that there will be an improvement in their physical and/or mental ability. However, there is impact to the brain as a side effect. In conjunction with a concussion, also called *mild traumatic brain injury* (mTBI), medications prescribed for pain management, including Oxycontin, Vicodin, and medical marijuana, may also be abused. When the brain is in the resulting state of disarray, it craves foods that compound this effect, such as candy, sweets, and highly processed food items that only add to the injured brain's inability to function. When this happens, there are major problems with sleep, and restorative sleep becomes virtually nonexistent, potentially leading the athlete to self-medicate even further. The result is a vicious cycle of self-destruction and continued symptoms of PCS.

IT IS known that worldwide, the majority of auto accidents, assaults, and injuries are in some way related to the use of alcohol, recreational drugs, and medications such as Benadryl or Ambien. It is very important to read about the possible side effects of medications you are taking. Also, the duration of post concussion symptoms and one's ability to recover are directly related to the practice of self-medication with alcohol, comfort foods, recreational drugs, and the overuse of prescribed medication.

DIAGNOSING AND ASSESSING ALCOHOL, DRUG, AND SUBSTANCE ABUSE

There are many medical and mental health professionals who specialize in diagnosing and treating alcohol, drug, and substance abuse. In addition, there are specialized rehabilitation hospitals and clinics for this purpose. It is important to find substance abuse professionals who also have training in PCS, so they can properly diagnose and evaluate your needs for recovery. They will look at any family history of dependence and addiction, along with your own history, in conjunction with the type of concussion you sustained.

TREATING ALCOHOL, DRUG, AND SUBSTANCE ABUSE

There are numerous approaches to the treatment of substance abuse, some of them conventional methods, and others complementary or alternative. The following techniques and approaches have been shown to be very effective.

Conventional Approaches

Many rehabilitation hospitals and clinics offer day programs for the treatment of substance abuse, while others are residential facilities at which you stay for days or months to help you recover. The Department of Veterans Affairs, for example, has specialized programs for recovery from alcohol, drug, and substance abuse. It is crucial to make sure that the program you select also works with PCS. Alcoholics Anonymous (AA), Narcotics Anonymous (NA), and Overeaters Anonymous

(OA) are the major self-help groups that address self-medication, dependency, and addictive issues while providing support and one-on-one sponsors to help you with your recovery. There are also sponsors and recovery programs available online to help you get started. Prayer, consulting with clergy, spiritual and prayer groups, and nonreligious humanitarian support have all been a great source of comfort and guidance to those who want to recover.

The first step toward recovery is to acknowledge addiction. Brain mapping is a method of assessment that helps you to negate the stigma of addiction, accept the existence of biological traits or markers, and see the actual damage to the brain. The second step is withdrawal from self-medication. Detoxification can take many forms, and it is best to undergo this process with a trained professional and/or support group that will help you confront the denial of your abuse. There are medications, such as naltrexone, disulfiram, acamprosate, buprenorphine, and others, that can enhance your success with recovery.

Complementary Approaches

Acupuncture can be very helpful in treating substance abuse, as can hypnosis. Hyperbaric oxygen therapy (HBOT) has also been found to be effective. Both biofeedback and neurofeedback can help locate the area of the brain that is being impacted and correct the dysregulation that exists from the abuse and PCS. If these methods are used first, the client is helped to identify the physiological experience of cravings or PTSD anxiety that may present as "panic," and for which doctors may prescribe additional medication, making the problem worse. The use of heart rate variability (HRV) will help to identify sympathetic nervous system dysregulation and teach you how to increase your parasympathetic system, lowering respiration, pulse, and blood pressure. The Low Energy Neurofeedback System (LENS) and NeuroField, used by a clinician who is well tuned in to his or her client's situation and needs, have also been shown to be very helpful.

Alternative Approaches

Also helpful in treating substance abuse are Reiki, polarity therapy, neuromuscular training, massage, detoxification of heavy metals (identified from hair analysis), and nutritional programs designed to decrease inflammation. Exercise, as well as Qi Gong, has been shown to be effective, as well. Specific Bach Flower Remedies, herbs, and homeopathics for recovery and the relief of symptoms are beneficial when used properly. It is best to consult with a certified practitioner to get the best results.

PRACTICAL SUGGESTIONS

- Admit and accept that you have an alcohol, drug, or substance abuse problem.
- Realize that you will not recover from your concussion until you stop abusing substances, including sugar, foods that convert to an alcohol, and highly processed foods.
- Search for a recovery program that best fits your personality.
- Find and join a support group in which you feel welcome and comfortable.
- Exercise at a level and frequency that you find manageable and helpful.
- Take up one or more new hobbies to help you feel productive.
- Spend time out of doors enjoying nature; for instance, take a walk in the woods or on the beach.
- Find a mentor who will support both you and your family.

Your concussion may or may not have been initially related to alcohol, drug, or substance abuse. However, if it was, you and your family must realize that for your brain to recover and become regulated again, you have to cease your intake of substances. If you have found yourself using alcohol, drugs, or substances to self-medicate the symptoms of PCS, it is important to acknowledge that you are not helping your brain heal. Instead, you are masking your symptoms and interfering with your brain's ability to recover. It is crucial to stop your intake of alcohol, drugs, or substances, for only when you do will you have a chance to truly recover. Only you, for your sake and the sake of your loved ones, can stop, find a recovery program that fits you, and stick with it. This will allow your brain to heal and become more regulated and lead to direct improvement in your symptoms of PCS.

CHAPTER 25

MOODS AND BEHAVIOR

■

KEVIN, A 40-YEAR-OLD MASSACHUSETTS MAN, SUSTAINED SEVERAL CONCUSSIONS, also called *mild traumatic brain injuries* (mTBI), in his youth due to football injuries. He recalls only one that seemed to affect him—he was knocked unconscious during a game and diagnosed in the emergency room as having suffered a mild concussion. He was discharged and taken back to the game, but on the school bus ride home, other students noticed a change in Kevin's behavior. Normally soft-spoken and passive, the boy began swearing a lot and acting rowdy and confrontational. In the locker room the next day, he put his fist through a safety-glass door in an unexplained surge of anger. At the time, no one related Kevin's uncharacteristic behavior to his brain injury. The aggressiveness abated, and he did not display this type of outburst again during his youth.

As an adult, Kevin struck his head again after stumbling over one of his child's toys. The injury seemed minor, but in the days that followed, the old rage returned. At work, Kevin started a fistfight with a man who was vying with him for a parking space. Another time, he flung a cup of coffee across the room when his secretary didn't pour it correctly. At home, he was verbally abusive of his loved ones. Once, he put his fist through the wallboard during an argument.

Eventually, Kevin's uncontrollable anger cost him his job, his girlfriend, and his relationship with his parents. When he sought help, he was diagnosed as having a concussion and told that his aggression was a result of repeated blows to the head. Since then, Kevin has received medical treatment and psychotherapy. This, along with his participation in a brain injury support group, has been very effective. Kevin is now working again, has begun a new romantic relationship, and has repaired the ties to his family.

FROM THE time we are children, we are taught that behavior defines a person, and that it is imperative to exercise control over our actions and reactions. If you lose this restraint, suddenly and without apparent cause, it can be terrifying both to you and to your loved ones. It has been shown that mood and behavior changes of this type can have a physical basis—that brain trauma can affect your moods and undermine your ability to check impulses and contain anger. However, you can reestablish self-control and avoid the long-term consequences of inappropriate behavior by understanding why this can occur and by educating yourself about corrective measures.

WHY MOOD AND BEHAVIOR CHANGES CAN OCCUR AFTER A CONCUSSION

The brain's *frontal lobe* helps to govern personality. As a result, a concussion that causes damage to this area can significantly affect your moods and behavior. The frontal lobe also serves as a braking mechanism; it helps to make you aware when anger is building and allows you to exercise control over your responses. Trauma to the frontal lobe can therefore cause a malfunction in your ability to inhibit aggression.

When there is a head injury, the *temporal lobe* is frequently damaged. However, the damage may sometimes not be apparent for ten or twenty years. As described in Chapter 17, a concussion that causes damage to the temporal lobe sometimes leads to seizures, or irregular discharges of nerve-cell activity. Marked behavior changes—specifically, increased hostility and a lack of control over angry outbursts—can be manifestations of temporal lobe seizure disorder.

TYPES OF MOOD AND BEHAVIOR CHANGES THAT CAN FOLLOW A CONCUSSION

"Before my auto accident, I was a calm, patient person who could cope with stress and handle many situations at once. One year after my accident, there was an incident that made me think I was going crazy. I was in a conversation with my teenage daughter and I suddenly flew into a rage. Shrieking, 'I can't take this anymore!' I threw papers and my pocketbook ten feet into the air. Then I turned and kicked the back door with such force that I almost broke it."

—DEBBIE

Over the years, you have developed a sense of appropriateness regarding such emotional displays as tears, anger, or yelling. This learned ability to react in a manner befitting the circumstances is critical to social acceptance as well as to the building of relationships. A frontal or temporal lobe injury can interfere with this ability and trigger marked behavior changes. The following are some of the most common problems people with *post concussion syndrome* (PCS) experience:

- *Intolerance.* After a concussion, you may find yourself unable to deal with even minor changes in your environment or daily routine without experiencing frustration and, possibly, reacting with unreasonable, almost childish anger.
- *Apathy.* This symptom, which is characterized by extreme indifference and little or no outward emotion, often exists as a function of depression, but it can also be associated with large bilateral frontal lobe lesions.
- *Misperception of time or events.* A concussion can affect your grasp of time, as well as your ability to focus on and assimilate the goings-on around you. Either of these conditions can ignite fear and frustration, which commonly manifest themselves as impatience, extreme irritability, and seemingly self-centered behavior.
- *Difficulty sustaining relationships.* Close personal interactions involve some degree of patience and give-and-take. However, the demanding, clingy, or hostile behavior wrought by your concussion can quickly erode the fabric of relations with friends and family.

If you undergo a measurable personality change after a concussion, you may be diagnosed with *organic personality disorder,* also called *organic personality syndrome.* This disorder is often characterized by emotional lability (sudden, intense shifts of emotion), impulsivity, suspiciousness, quickness to anger, and frequent verbal outbursts. In other cases, it may manifest itself as listlessness, inattentiveness, and extreme self-involvement. A heightened sensitivity to sound, medication, and alcohol is very common among those affected by this syndrome. Other possible symptoms include excessive talkativeness, immature or otherwise inappropriate social behavior, physical aggression, impatience, poor judgment, eating and drinking problems, distractibility, uncontrollable crying, irritability, excessive dependency, uncontrollable rage, unrealistic optimism, denial of problems, indifference, and violent outbursts.

DIAGNOSING AND ASSESSING MOOD AND BEHAVIOR CHANGES

It can be difficult to determine whether behavior changes that follow a concussion are caused by brain trauma, post-injury psychological reactions, post traumatic stress disorder (PTSD), or a heightening of preexisting psychiatric problems. For instance, if you are only marginally able to cope with feelings of anger before suffering a concussion, an insult to the brain might further limit your ability to control feelings and behavior, leaving you unable to deal with even small changes in bodily sensations or your environment. Often, the inability to cope is manifested as extreme frustration, anger, and impatience, which can be seen as self-centeredness. In such a case, it is not the symptom itself—the anger—that is a direct result of the injury. Rather, the insult to the brain has limited your ability to control the expression of anger.

As mentioned in the previous section, it can also be difficult to distinguish between the apathy that accompanies organic personality disorder due to a brain injury and the depression seen in a personality disorder, and that which characterizes depression. (Read more about depression in Chapter 26.) As a further complication, behavioral symptoms and other injury aftereffects, such as attention, concentration, and reasoning deficits, can mimic each other. For example, impulse buying may look like impulsivity, but it may also come about because the selection of appropriate merchandise has suddenly become an ordeal. Similarly, what looks like paranoia may result directly from brain injury, or it may be an individual's response to, say, having the family relieve him or her of bill-paying responsibilities.

Neuropsychological testing is the best means of evaluating the behavioral component of PCS, because this battery of tests can distinguish between preexisting personality traits and post-injury reactions in the assessment of symptoms. The other three methods of evaluation are the quantitative electroencephalogram (qEEG), functional magnetic resonance imaging (fMRI), and the single photon emission computed tomography (SPECT) scan. These types of testing enable the specialist to tailor treatment to the patient, pinpointing the need for speech and language therapy, cognitive therapy, neurofeedback, psychotherapy, or consultation with an audiologist or ophthalmologist. Moreover, neuropsychological testing determines whether rehabilitation (working to restore previous levels of functioning) or compensation (learning ways to live with your deficits) is the appropriate goal.

A test may also be done to rule out malingering (faking illness or injury to achieve some type of gain). This can be very valuable because you may find people questioning whether your post concussion symptoms are real—especially where legal and insurance-related processes are involved. For example, many people with PCS have found themselves suspected of insurance fraud. The test for malingering provides additional information that can help to demonstrate to insurers, employers, or attorneys that your symptoms are real.

TREATING POST CONCUSSION MOOD AND BEHAVIOR PROBLEMS

"The emotional instability brought on by my concussion left me feeling out of control. Whereas I rarely cried prior to my accident, I found myself weeping and becoming extremely irritable for no apparent reason. Concerned about the possibility of depression, I called a psychologist who had known me for years and who was also trained in neurology. He urged me to relate my symptoms to my neurologist, who in turn determined that my problems were being caused by atypical migraine activity in my brain. He prescribed a beta-blocker, and within twenty-four hours, all my mood and behavioral symptoms disappeared."

—D.R.S.

Behavioral symptoms that follow a concussion—specifically, mood swings, short-temperedness, and lack of behavioral control—are likely to decrease over time unless a complicating factor such as a seizure condition, PTSD, or a preexisting psychological disorder is present. In the meantime, there are steps you can take to help control your symptoms and hasten the recovery process.

Conventional Approaches

The first step in treating mood and behavioral problems is to find a behavioral neurologist. This area of neurology specializes in organic personality disorder. If such a specialist is not available where you live, seek out a psychopharmacologist who has experience treating people with PCS. This practitioner may suggest various medications, such as anticonvulsants, mood stabilizers, antidepressants, or beta-blockers. It is extremely important to note that as a result of your concussion, you may be more sensitive to the side effects of medications. Anticonvulsant medications may be used to suppress temporal lobe seizure activity that can interfere with your regulation of behavior. Beta-blockers can be similarly effective, and are also useful for helping to control your emotions.

Psychotherapy, specifically cognitive behavioral therapy (CBT), may be recommended to help you learn to manage frustration and make lifestyle modifications to ward off negative behavior. For instance, you may have to restrict your activities and keep socializing to a minimum until you regain emotional and behavioral control. Role-playing and psychodrama are psychological techniques that can help you learn to control outbursts and inappropriate responses.

Complementary Approaches

Behavioral medicine and health psychology—in particular, hypnosis, energy psychology, Thought Field Therapy (TFT), biofeedback, and behavior-modification techniques—can be very effective at teaching relaxation. One specific method is heart rate variability (HRV) training. The various types of neurofeedback are very helpful in pinpointing the areas of the brain where the emotional dysregulation is occurring and helping it to become regulated again.

Alternative Approaches

Reiki, Qi Gong, and polarity therapy can help you to regain a sense of emotional balance. These therapeutic-touch techniques should be performed by trained professionals.

There are also over-the-counter herbal and homeopathic remedies that promote relaxation and even-temperedness, including Bach Flower Remedies. You should exercise caution with such products, however, because they are designed for use by the general public, not for controlling mood or behavior problems that can accompany PCS. If you wish to try alternative remedies, it is best to consult with a qualified herbalist, Bach Flower practitioner, or homeopath, preferably one who has knowledge of organic personality disorder and PCS. With this training, the practitioner can tailor a prescription to your unique symptoms and situation. The Herb Research Foundation and/or the National Center for Homeopathy may be able to help you locate an appropriate practitioner in your area. Or, feel free to contact me for assistance, using the information listed on page 367.

PRACTICAL SUGGESTIONS

"Physical exercise was instrumental in helping me cope with psychological pain. Not long after my accident, for instance, I was told of the death of a patient I had seen that last day on the job. In turmoil, I walked over two miles until I was able to come to grips with my powerful reaction."

—D.R.S.

WHILE PROFESSIONAL treatment is critical to your recovery from any post concussion symptom, there is also much you can do on your own to regain a sense of control over your moods and behavior. The following suggestions may be helpful:

- Inform your friends, family, and coworkers about your difficulties with behavior control. Explain to them that any inappropriate behavior you display is temporarily beyond your control and is not to be taken personally. Enlist their support and efforts to shield you from situations that tend to trigger inappropriate responses.
- Ask someone you trust to let you know with a prearranged hand signal, facial expression, or special word when they see you beginning to act out.
- Suggest to coworkers and those close to you that they leave the room rather than confront you when you behave objectionably. Discussion can follow later, when you are calmer.
- Apologize for inappropriate responses. While your behavior is not your fault, it is important to acknowledge that you have been irritable, abusive, or insulting.
- Control verbal outbursts by stopping, breathing deeply, and thinking before you speak. A behavioral therapist can help you learn to do this.
- Avoid people and places that annoy you, until you learn methods of controlling your behavior. Understand that normally negative reactions will be greatly intensified by your post concussion symptoms.
- Ask family members and friends to help you respond appropriately by alerting you when a trigger topic must be introduced. For example, "Mary, I know this will be upsetting, but I need to talk about something."
- Remember the effects that inappropriate outbursts have on your family and friends. They, too, are suffering as a result of your injury.

Injury to the brain frequently produces changes in how people feel and react. However, these symptoms are often overlooked. Many people assume that behavioral and mood changes such as excessive anger must be related to a post-injury psychological reaction rather than to the brain injury itself. This can result in crucial delays in obtaining appropriate treatment.

If you, your friends, or members of your family have any questions about mood and behavior changes that occur after an accident or brain injury, obtain a second opinion from a behavioral neurologist or psychopharmacologist with expertise in PCS. There is help available.

CHAPTER 26

PSYCHIATRIC DISORDERS

■

CAROL, A 24-YEAR-OLD MISSISSIPPI WOMAN, HAD A HISTORY OF CLINICAL depression. Her problems had necessitated several hospitalizations over the years, but she had made significant progress. Then, on the way home from a routine appointment with her psychiatrist, Carol was involved in a minor car accident. X-rays were taken at the emergency room, but Carol's injuries were slight and she was sent home.

Days later, severe headaches, memory loss, and uncharacteristic irritability compelled her to see her family physician. Carol also found herself dwelling on thoughts of suicide, but chose not to mention this to either her doctor or her psychiatrist. Based on the symptoms she did discuss, Carol's physician diagnosed a concussion, also called *mild traumatic brain injury* (mTBI), and suggested that the young woman consult a neurologist. Before she could do so, however, Carol tried to kill herself and was subsequently hospitalized at a local psychiatric facility.

THE AFTEREFFECTS of a concussion, called *post concussion syndrome* (PCS), are pervasive, influencing not only your physical health but also your emotional well-being. The connection between brain trauma and one's emotions is extremely complex. As we have seen, emotional reactions can result either directly or indirectly from brain injury. This is not the case with psychiatric disorders. Brain injury does not *cause* psychiatric disorders as such, but it can magnify a pre-existing problem to the point that your ability to function may be jeopardized. To further complicate matters, symptoms of psychiatric disorders can sometimes mimic those of PCS, making the true nature of the problem difficult to determine.

TYPES OF PSYCHIATRIC PROBLEMS
THAT CAN FOLLOW A CONCUSSION

To better understand psychiatric disorders, you need to know how they differ from post-injury psychological reactions, post traumatic stress disorder (PTSD), and organic personality disorder. In post-injury psychological reactions and/or PTSD, your moods and behavior are a response to outside influencing factors. With organic personality change, your moods and behavior are the result of injury to the brain. In contrast, psychiatric disorders are due to heredity, developmental factors, biochemical imbalance, and/or other factors not yet identified.

Some people, like Carol, have had psychiatric symptoms under control through medication and psychotherapy prior to their concussion. In other cases, symptoms of a specific disorder in an individual's family's history may not become apparent until after his or her concussion. In either situation, psychiatric symptoms are often heightened by a concussion, and they can become severe if there is injury to the brain area that controls moods and psychological reactions. Carol, for instance, had been diagnosed with clinical depression resulting from a chemical imbalance. Her accident caused her depression to worsen to the point that she attempted suicide. The most commonly seen psychiatric disorders that may be worsened by a concussion are described below.

Anxiety Disorders

The anxiety disorders include both generalized (chronic) and acute anxiety (panic attacks) and phobias. As discussed in Chapter 23, anxiety is a common reaction in the immediate aftermath of a concussion, but it can also become a chronic problem that lasts beyond the reaction phase, particularly if you suffered from any degree of anxiety disorder prior to your injury. Phobic disorders are experienced as great anxiety and irrational fear triggered by specific objects or situations. Common examples include *agoraphobia* (fear of open spaces), *claustrophobia* (fear of closed spaces), and *acrophobia* (fear of heights), but virtually anything can be the object of a phobia.

Mood Disorders

Mood disorders are characterized by extreme changes and variations in moods, from depression (profound sadness) to mania (utter elation). There can also be "mixed mood state" with pressured speech but dysphoric (anxious or depressive) mood. Depression is by far the most prevalent psychiatric disorder among people with PCS. In fact, depression occurs fairly frequently among persons with virtually any type of chronic health problem, and it can lead to a kind of vicious cycle in which depression aggravates your disabilities, which leads to even deeper depression, and so on.

As described in Chapter 23, a temporary depressive reaction is a common occurrence among people in the immediate aftermath of a concussion, as they adjust to the impact that the injury has had on their lives. Clinical depression is longer lasting and more severe than this, and has physical as well as psychological components. Symptoms of clinical depression can include disruptions in your sleep/wake cycle; changes in appetite, with resulting weight loss (or, in some cases, weight gain); pervasive apathy and fatigue; a near-total loss of motivation; loss of sexual interest; an inability to experience pleasure, even from previously enjoyable activities; and thoughts of suicide. Fatigue related to depression is different from fatigue that is a direct result of a concussion, which is described in Chapter 7. With depression-related fatigue, you wake up exhausted and remain exhausted throughout the day. In contrast, with PCS fatigue, you wake up alert and become exhausted as the day progresses due to cognitive overload and/or physical activity.

Another form of clinical depression can be caused by long-term pain resulting from a traumatic event such as an auto accident. In this situation, it is believed that the signal of and/or a biochemical reaction to ongoing pain triggers depression. If depression is accompanied by persistent bodily pain—such as constant headache, neck, and/or facial pain—for which no physical or psychological cause can be found, you may be diagnosed with clinical depression caused by chronic pain (see Chapter 15).

Manic-depressive disorder (known to professionals as *mixed-type mood disorder* or *bipolar disorder*) involves extreme changes in mood, from deep depression to unrealistic elation and/or hyperactivity and back again. The symptoms of this disorder are sometimes confused with the emotional mood swings that can follow brain injury (see Chapter 25) or severe personal trauma (see Chapter 23).

Obsessive-Compulsive Disorder

This disorder causes you to feel an uncontrollable need to perform a particular activity over and over again. Some of the compulsive activities most commonly seen include eating, drinking, shopping, gambling, hand-washing, and collecting or checking on things. If you have obsessive-compulsive disorder (OCD), your symptoms are likely to become worse after a concussion.

Sometimes the coping mechanisms people with PCS use in response to attention and short-term memory problems can be confused with symptoms of OCD—for instance, keeping things in strict order so that you can find or remember them. This can make a correct diagnosis difficult.

Personality Disorders

A personality disorder is an enduring pattern of exaggeration of an ordinary personality trait, such as a tendency to be self-centered or withdrawn. These exaggerations are considered disorders because they lead to behaviors that interfere with daily living and the maintenance of normal relationships.

In most situations, personality disorders are a result of developmental factors. Often, however, similar behaviors can be explained by brain injury, as seen in *interictal* behavior (see Chapter 17) or organic personality disorder (see Chapter 25). Types of personality disorders include the following:

- Antisocial (having disregard for others and their rights)
- Avoidant (withdrawing from social interaction)
- Borderline (impulsive and intrusive)
- Compulsive (having perfectionist traits)
- Dependent (emotionally needy)
- Histrionic (excessively emotional and attention-seeking)
- Narcissistic (emotionally aloof and lacking remorse)
- Paranoid (overly suspicious)
- Passive-aggressive (behaving placidly, then becoming hostile)
- Schizoid (socially detached)
- Schizotypal (having acute problems or unusual mannerisms that can interfere with social relationships)

Persons with personality disorders often do not think there is anything wrong with them, and feel their behavior is normal. Friends, family members, and coworkers are more likely to notice the existence of a problem and encourage the individual to seek treatment. In most cases, when personality disorders seem to appear after a concussion, the problem was actually present before the injury in a minor or mild form, and it emerged in response to the stress of the injury and its aftermath.

Psychotic Disorders

Psychotic disorders are disorders that are characterized by a split with reality. Symptoms can include delusions, hallucinations, judgment problems, and complete emotional withdrawal, as well as an inability to think clearly or to perceive reality. Probably the best known of the psychotic disorders is *schizophrenia*, which is typified by the symptoms listed above under schizoid and schizotypal personality disorders, as well as by inappropriate (or absent) emotion and marked memory problems. Most cases of psychotic disorders that appear after a concussion are due to a worsening of previously mild and manageable symptoms, rather than the development of an entirely new illness.

Dissociative Disorders

Dissociative disorders are complex, poorly understood psychiatric disorders in which a person loses conscious awareness of memories, ideas, and feelings—in some cases, even his or her own identity—and becomes unable to recall these things. Types of dissociative disorders include *multiple personality disorder* and *psychogenic amnesia*, or memory loss that is a psychological response to emotional stress. With this type of amnesia, the greatest memory loss is in response to events that were sources of emotional anguish, rather than physical trauma. Like many psychiatric disorders, dissociative disorders most often are not a direct result of brain injury, but can be made worse by it.

Somatoform Disorders

The term *somatoform disorder* refers to the presence of physical complaints for which no physical explanation can be found. Sometimes there are observable symptoms such as seizures, strokes, paralysis, chest and abdominal pain, fibromyalgia, blindness, vomiting, bloating, or back pain. Other characteristics of somatoform disorder can include imagined defects in appearance; an alteration in physical function suggestive of illness, such as dizziness, headaches, vague chronic pain, or vision problems; and preoccupation with sickness and injury. Like dissociative disorders, somatoform disorders can be exacerbated by PCS. These disorders are difficult to recognize, given that patients often wonder why doctors cannot find anything wrong with them. These patients truly believe in the symptoms they think they have and are able to convince others that the symptoms are real, even without corroborating clinical or medical evidence. It is not uncommon to see an immediate family member become an unknowing enabler of the patient's symptoms. Such patients can trick even the most experienced clinician and are best diagnosed by witnessing an episode and ruling out organic conditions. Once organic conditions are ruled out by an electrocardiogram (EKG), electroencephalogram (EEG), magnetic resonance imaging (MRI), or computed tomography (CT) scan, a neuropsychological evaluation with response bias (a test for malingering) and personality testing is of enormous importance. Many of these behaviors are deeply rooted strongholds from remote emotional abuse. They are difficult to treat and may mislead a clinician. With a trusting therapeutic counseling relationship and through an increase in the patient's insight, the behaviors can become more manageable and, in turn, the patient's quality of life can be improved.

Factitious Disorder and Malingering

These two disorders have many features in common. *Factitious disorder* involves intentionally faking some type of illness by inflicting injury on yourself or by pretending to have symptoms that suggest illness, even though you do not stand to gain anything (except, perhaps, a doctor's attention) by doing so. *Malingering* also involves falsifying illness or injury, but with the aim of achieving some sort of benefit, such as being able to avoid work, military duty, or criminal prosecution, or to gain financial compensation. Both of these disorders can become worse following a concussion.

Disorders of Infancy, Childhood, or Adolescence

These disorders include problems stemming from intellectual disability, autism, and developmental delays, as well as behavior problems and gender-identity and eating disorders. Virtually any of the many types of problems that fall into these categories can be worsened by PCS.

DIAGNOSING AND ASSESSING PSYCHIATRIC PROBLEMS

A trained professional can easily diagnose certain prior or underlying psychiatric disorders, such as schizophrenia or psychosis, as being separate from PCS.

However, this is not the case with obsessive-compulsive disorder, mood disorders, and other psychiatric problems. Symptoms of these disorders can mimic those of other problems related to PCS. It is therefore vital that your mental health care practitioner consider your pre-injury personality as part of the diagnostic evaluation. A neuropsychological evaluation (see Chapter 5) is the best source of this information.

If you, a friend, or a family member suspects that you may have a psychological disorder that has been made worse by a concussion, you should consult with a psychiatrist or psychologist who specializes in brain injury and who can make the critical distinctions needed for correct diagnosis. Fatigue, for instance, can be an aftereffect of injury or a symptom of depression. Vague chronic pain can signal physical injury, injury in the area of the brain that perceives pain, a somatoform disorder, malingering, or an emotional reaction. An experienced professional can conduct appropriate testing and assess substance abuse, behavior problems, denial, and other emotional reactions.

TREATING POST CONCUSSION PSYCHIATRIC PROBLEMS

There are a number of unique difficulties associated with the treatment of PCS-related psychiatric problems. To begin with, because of the very nature of these problems, the first and most necessary step toward finding appropriate treatment—recognizing that something is wrong and that some type of help is needed—is often more difficult than it is with other types of disorders. Friends, family members, or coworkers often realize that there is a problem before the affected individual does, and it may take some time to convince him or her to accept the possibility. Then, too, in the past, many mental health professionals were hesitant to treat brain-injured people because they mistakenly believed that such people were unlikely to show significant improvement. In addition, little research has been done on treating patients with combined neurological and psychological problems. In fact, therapists trying to provide such treatment often experience many of the same emotions—especially frustration and hopelessness—that plague their patients.

Nevertheless, there are a number of conventional, complementary, and alternative approaches to treating psychiatric disorders. Those that have been found to be the most successful for people with PCS are described below.

Conventional Approaches

In general, psychiatric disorders respond best when traditional psychotherapy and cognitive behavioral therapy (CBT) are used along with appropriate medications. A psychopharmacologist (a psychiatrist who specializes in using drugs to treat psychiatric disorders) can work with you to determine the medication and dosage appropriate for your specific problem. Clinical depression is often best treated through a combination of psychotherapy and nonsedating antidepressant medications, such as fluoxetine (Prozac) or sertraline (Zoloft). Behavior modification is also useful for treating disruptiveness, compulsiveness, eating disorders, and other manifestations of emotional difficulty.

Complementary Approaches

Both biofeedback and neurofeedback are used to treat depression, anxiety, compulsive behaviors, and autism. There is limited success with personality disorders. Hypnosis is very effective with dissociative disorders. Acupuncture is also very helpful.

Alternative Approaches

Reiki, Qi Gong, and polarity therapy are extremely effective against depression, anxiety, and compulsive disorders. It is important that these types of therapy be performed by trained practitioners with an understanding of both psychiatric disorders and PCS.

Certain over-the-counter herbal preparations and homeopathic remedies advertise that they can diminish depression, agitation, and other symptoms related to psychiatric disorders. Before you purchase any such product, it is important to realize that having both PCS and a psychiatric disorder creates an extremely complex situation. It is crucial to locate an herbalist or homeopathic practitioner who is willing to work with your psychopharmacologist and/or mental health professional (and vice versa). Such a team can properly evaluate your circumstances and specific needs, discuss types of products and dosages, and select the herbal or homeopathic remedies that are best for you. If your primary care physician (PCP) is unable to provide you with an appropriate referral, organizations such as the Herb Research Foundation and/or the National Center for Homeopathy may be able to help. For information or assistance with this, feel free to contact me using the information on page 367.

PRACTICAL SUGGESTIONS

When it comes to psychiatric problems, treatment under the guidance of a mental health professional is the surest route to recovery. However, there are a number of things you can do to speed up the process on your own and enhance your chances for a successful recovery. Here are some helpful ideas:

- Honestly acknowledge the fact that you have a problem and assume responsibility for it. Unless you do this, you will not be able to bring about the changes you need to get well.
- Insist upon working with a compassionate mental health professional who has an understanding of brain injury and its effects on psychiatric disorders.
- Join a self-help or support group. Your local hospital or community mental health center can put you in touch with the appropriate parties.
- Participate in group therapy with an understanding mental health professional.
- Seek online one-to-one support through forums or computer bulletin boards.
- Be aware that help for people with chronic psychiatric issues is becoming more widely available as hospitals and clinics recognize the need for such services.
- Consider seeking the comfort of a religious or spiritual group.
- Allow yourself to be receptive to the guidance and encouragement of family and friends.
- Look into National Alliance on Mental Illness (NAMI) support groups.

While psychiatric problems can be very distressing, it can be reassuring to know that most individual symptoms are not physical effects of your PCS. Instead, your injury has only heightened a preexisting condition. Today, with consistent and proper medical and psychological care, most psychiatric problems are treatable. By finding the right approach and investing time and effort in recovery, you can significantly reduce the grip that psychiatric problems have on your life.

CHAPTER 27

GRIEVING

■

I N HIS YOUTH, 52-YEAR-OLD JACK HAD BEEN A STAR IN THREE SPORTS: TRACK, football, and baseball. After college and a stint in the Marines, he became a law-enforcement officer in Massachusetts, a job he held for over twenty-three years.

One June day, Jack was struck by a car and thrown over ten feet. He was unconscious for only a few minutes, and could recall everything about the accident by the time medical assistance arrived. At the local emergency room, the headache and dizziness Jack complained of were attributed to a concussion, also called *mild traumatic brain injury* (mTBI). Eventually, Jack was also diagnosed as having post traumatic stress disorder (PTSD).

Since his accident, Jack has repeatedly sought help for stuttering, fatigue, and depression. Several medical and mental health professionals have treated Jack for specific problems related to his *post concussion syndrome* (PCS), but he is still far from well. Now retired from the police force, Jack spends most of his days in bed. Even counseling by a priest has failed to improve his attitude toward his problems. Surprisingly, neither Jack's priest nor any of the specialists who have treated him has ever mentioned the possibility that his recovery has been stalled by grief over his loss of self.

GRIEVING IS a normal process that relieves sorrow and allows us to adjust to loss. Many people think of grieving as something that happens only after certain specific events, such as the death of a loved one, but it occurs in response to other types of loss as well. For instance, as you grow older, you periodically mourn the loss of the younger person you once were. This is part of the process of adjusting to advancing age. If you experience a life-changing event like PCS, grieving the loss of the person you used to be is not only normal, but is actually a necessary part of recovery.

GRIEVING THE LOSS OF SELF

"In the past, I took my photographic memory for granted. In twenty years of doing psychotherapy, I never took notes during a session, but later could recall every detail of the sessions that occurred that day. After my concussion, it was difficult to acknowledge that I had total amnesia to certain events that occurred in my life. What I did know was that in one brief second on a beautiful March day, my previous life seemed to have died."

—D.R.S.

The concept of *self* is complex. It is made up of two parts: the real self and the capacities of the self. According to psychologists, the structure of the real self consists of self-image (how you think of yourself), self-representation (how you present yourself), superordinate self-organization (how you feel and present yourself over time), and the total self (who you really are). These aspects interact with one another. For example, you may think of yourself as a good worker, which may be the case, and you may hope that others think so, too, which they may not. With the development of the real self come the capacities of the self, which include creativity, intimacy, aliveness, assertiveness, and commitment—all of which enable you to develop thoughts, be caring, feel enjoyment, and pursue your dreams.

The sense of self is not fully developed until adulthood. It is gained through work and through social relationships, especially family relationships and assuming the role of caretaker. At different points in your life, usually spurred by lifestyle, career, or physical changes, you will relinquish a former self-image and move on. This natural process can be drastically altered and/or accelerated by circumstances such as the loss of employment, a natural disaster, a close encounter with death, or a personal disaster.

A concussion is experienced as a personal disaster. If your injury has robbed you of some of your ability to function at work or at home, this can have a crushing effect, because for most people, one's occupation is a prime source of purpose and gratification in life. In addition, you may feel less able to interact with your family, socialize, and pursue hobbies. After a concussion, you may have to face the possibility that you will never be as you once were. This experience constitutes a loss of self, and loss of self triggers grieving.

EXPERIENCING THE GRIEVING PROCESS

Healthy grieving can be more prolonged, pervasive, and complicated than you may realize. While not all grieving follows the same pattern, certain phases have been observed often enough to be recognized as typical. In most cases, the phases of grieving include the following:

- *Denial of the loss.* This phase includes being truly unaware of losses—or, in the case of PCS, deficits. You may firmly believe that you are no different from before.
- *Anger.* This phase often manifests itself in expressions of rage and bouts of aggression over the injustice of the loss.
- *Bargaining.* Here, you try to set terms that will change the eventual outcome—as in, "If I do [fill in the blank], things will be different."
- *Disorganization.* At this stage, you feel confused and have difficulty ordering your thoughts and behavior.
- *Despair.* This phase involves the loss of hope that things will ever be any better.
- *Depression.* Here, you experience emotions of hopelessness, inadequacy, and worthlessness. You may have eating and sleeping problems, exhibit anxious or withdrawn behavior, and even think of suicide.
- *Acceptance or resolution.* At this phase, you acknowledge your limitations and feel comfortable knowing that life can continue.

In the immediate aftermath of your injury, you may experience shock, numbness, or bewilderment. Emptiness, remorse, waves of crying, and attempts to regain what you have lost often follow in the ensuing weeks or months. Overall, you may feel sad and unable to experience pleasure—alternating, perhaps, with tense, restless anxiety. You may even notice one or more physical symptoms, such as sleep disturbances, loss of appetite, headaches, back pain, shortness of breath, heart palpitations, indigestion, dizziness, or nausea. In an attempt to prevent painful feelings, you may distance yourself emotionally from friends and family.

Clearly, grief has many depression-like symptoms (see Chapter 26), and depression can sometimes accompany grieving. A person experiencing normal, healthy grieving, however, does not usually have the general feeling of worthlessness typical of a depressed person, and he or she may demonstrate episodes of lighter moods interspersed with depressed feelings—circumstances not seen in clinical depression. However, the depression-like symptoms of grieving can last as long as several years, until you can finally consider your loss without feeling overwhelming sadness and you have begun to invest energy in other thoughts and activities.

Working through grief and letting go is difficult, but it can be made less so by redirecting your energy to such activities as learning new skills, volunteering your services, or being a support person for another brain-injured individual. Gradually, you will begin to acknowledge and accept a new identity, which will allow your grief to fade into memory. However, if you merely stifle or obstruct your grief, the result may be pathological grief—a paralyzing sadness that lasts longer than a year, with no movement toward recovery from the loss. In most cases, pathological grief is characterized by continuing denial of reality or preoccupation with death and dying in general.

The greater your perceived loss of skills and abilities, the more extensive your sense of loss will be. Compulsively successful, high-achieving intellectual people, for instance, often experience a powerful loss of self if their thinking ability is even very slightly impaired. Very independent people, who are seen by others as leaders, caretakers, or sources of guidance, may be devastated if they become unable to live up to their previous self-reliant image. Young adults between the ages of 18 and 22 are tremendously affected by grief after a concussion. Psychologists believe this is because, at that age, a person has acquired a self-image but has not yet had the opportunity to establish a sense of achievement or purpose. In contrast, older people have already enjoyed the accomplishment of some of their life goals and so tend to grieve less. Children also tend to be less affected by grief, probably because they are unable to recall functioning at another level. They therefore have less trouble blending PCS-related deficits into their self-perception.

RECOGNIZING GRIEF

Grief over the loss of self is something every brain-injured person goes through. However, grieving often is not recognized for what it is because the resulting distractibility, anger, fatigue, and other signs can be masked by or confused with the symptoms of PCS or PTSD (see Table 27.1 for a comparison). Also, lack of insight, which may make you unable to correctly evaluate the impact your

TABLE 27.1. IDENTIFYING THE SYMPTOMS OF GRIEF

The process of grieving the loss of self that follows mTBI is often unacknowledged, and its symptoms are often confused with those of Post Concussion Syndrome (PCS) or Post Traumatic Stress Disorder (PTSD). The table below offers a comparison of the typical symptoms associated with these three conditions.

SYMPTOM	PCS	PTSD	HEALTHY GRIEF
Amnesia	Yes	Yes	No
Anger	Yes	Yes	Yes
Lack of awareness	Yes	No	No
Concentration problems	Yes	Yes	Yes
Depression	Yes	Sometimes	Sometimes
Despair	Yes	Yes	Yes
Disorganization	Yes	Yes	Yes
Distractibility	Yes	Yes	Yes
Dizziness	Yes	Sometimes	Sometimes
Lack of emotion	Yes	Yes	No
Fatigue	Yes	Yes	Yes
Headaches	Yes	Sometimes	Sometimes
Isolation and withdrawal	Yes	Yes	Yes
Poor judgment	Yes	No	No
Nightmares and flashbacks	Yes	Yes	No
Personality changes	Yes	Yes	Sometimes
Attempts to regain previous self-image	Yes	Yes	Yes
Short-term memory loss	Yes	Yes	Sometimes
Sleep disturbances	Yes	Yes	Yes
Ultimate acceptance/ resolution	Yes	Yes	Yes

symptoms are having on your life, is a typical aftereffect of PCS. Unfortunately, the recognition of grief as a possible cause of post-injury behavior has eluded many physicians and mental health professionals, as well as concussion survivors themselves. Many doctors tend to attribute symptoms of grief following a concussion to the physical consequences of the injury.

Understanding that there are emotional components to your loss of self is critical to winning family support and obtaining appropriate professional guidance. All too often, loved ones say things like "Control yourself" or "Think how lucky you are to be alive." They may mean well, but statements like these only perpetuate grief. The eventual resolution of your grieving can come only with sympathy, patience, the acknowledgment by you and by others that you are a different person from before—and, most important, with time.

Within the medical community, there is still much ground to be covered in this area. The idea of grieving following a concussion has been largely overlooked by doctors; even the most highly trained psychotherapists sometimes may lack knowledge about brain injury, much less about grieving the resultant loss of self. It pays to keep looking, therefore, until you find a professional who understands the sadness and mourning you feel.

WORKING THROUGH GRIEF

"I often think of myself as a house that was hit by a hurricane and then restored. The concussion destroyed portions of the house. The years of rehabilitation were like adding new lumber and materials onto the original design. To all appearances, the restored house is the same, but it is not. It is a composite of the old and the new. I look and sound similar to my old self, but I'm really a blend of the old and the new. In the years after my concussion, I did a lot of grieving, and I learned to accept who I am now."

—D.R.S.

Grieving is an emotionally painful but necessary part of life. Fortunately, there are a number of approaches that can assist you as you pass through the stages of the grief process. There are now therapists who specialize in grief work who can enable you to recognize and express your fear and sadness in a safe environment, without worrying about how your feelings may affect loved ones or how they might respond. Assisting rather than resisting grief will allow you to come to terms more quickly with your new situation.

Grief therapy is tailored to several variables, including developmental factors, the circumstances of your injury, your pre-injury personality, and previous experiences you may have had with denial of your grief by support people in your life. Optimally, the therapist you choose should have previous experience working with patients grieving the loss of self due to injury (he or she need not have specific expertise in PCS). Your primary care physician (PCP), a local rehabilitation facility, or the nearest VA hospital should be able to refer you to a qualified specialist. As with any mental health professional you choose to work with, it is important that you feel completely comfortable with your therapist.

On a practical, everyday level, simply recognizing and accepting the grieving process can do a great deal to make it easier to bear. As you undergo the grieving process, you may find the following suggestions helpful:

- *Acknowledge the reality of your loss.* Ignore any expressed or implied messages from doctors, family, or friends to "snap out of it" or "get a grip." You cannot get on with your life until you grieve, and you cannot resolve your grief unless you recognize that your concussion has made you a new person.
- *Identify and express your grief.* Therapy will help you to experience the pain and intense feelings that accompany the loss of self.
- *Commemorate your loss.* After the death of a loved one, the grieving process is aided by religious or cultural rituals and customs. Some people with PCS have found it helpful to honor the memory of past accomplishments by collecting mementos of their old selves and burying them—whether literally or figuratively.
- *Acknowledge your ambivalence.* You may well have conflicting feelings about your concussion. Sometimes you may view your survival as a second chance, while at other times you may see it as nothing but a burden. Such mixed feelings are normal, but if you do not recognize them, this inner conflict can pose a considerable barrier to the resolution of your grief. Instead of denying conflicting feelings, work toward a balance between positive and negative feelings about your new self and put them into perspective.
- *Learn to let go.* Ultimately, you must withdraw your emotional investment in the person you once were, in order to go forward with your life. Realize that the person you are today is not a poor substitute, but a composite of your old and newly acquired selves.
- *Move on.* Resist viewing yourself as a tragic figure whom life has dealt a cruel blow. Relinquish plans and dreams that revolved around your former self and rethink your goals based on your present strengths and abilities.

While the recognition of your loss is a painful process, it is important to work toward emphasizing the good qualities you still possess. With guidance, you can bridge the gap between your pre- and post-injury selves, and emerge with strength, motivation, a redefined creative side, and a restored sense that life has meaning. It hurts to accept the reality that you may never completely recover, and both recovery and grieving can be slow processes. Once you give yourself permission to grieve, however, you will find the going much easier.

PART 5

RECOVERING

INTRODUCTION

∎

GEORGE AND PAULA AND THEIR TWO CHILDREN, KEVIN AND SUSAN, WERE involved in a five-car collision in Georgia. They underwent X-rays and computed tomography (CT) scans at the local emergency room, all with negative results. In the weeks and months that followed, however, each was troubled by symptoms that included dizziness, headaches, memory problems, excessive fatigue, and difficulties with reading and concentration.

George, the first to seek help, was diagnosed with *post concussion syndrome* (PCS) and was told to take a few weeks off from his job as a computer programmer. Paula, a second-grade teacher, also sought medical assistance after she was told by her principal that her speech was unclear and that she seemed confused and disorganized. On a neurologist's advice, she took a leave of absence from work. Meanwhile, their children, tenth-grader Kevin and fifth-grader Susan, were having trouble at school. Their grades plummeted, and Kevin's behavior became quite aggressive. Susan seemed withdrawn and visibly depressed. Officials at both their schools recommended psychological evaluation and family counseling.

During the next three years, both George and Paula took early retirement from their jobs. Their children's problems, which by now included substance abuse, continued. They attempted therapy several times without success, and the future looked bleak—until Paula began to attend meetings of a brain injury support group. Here, for the first time, she realized that many of her family's problems could be linked to their car accident, and that her lack of insight was probably a function of her own injury.

Five years after the accident, the family was reevaluated. A team of specialists developed rehabilitation programs for each family member, a step that turned their lives around within a year. George is now self-employed, Paula has returned to teaching, Kevin is a community-college student, and Susan is on the high school honor roll. The family mourns the five years they lost, but, for the first time in many months, they can look forward to the future.

RECOVERY FROM a concussion, also called *mild traumatic brain injury* (mTBI), is a complex process. Part 5 of this book deals with different aspects of recovery, including rehabilitation, financial issues, the problems of living with someone with PCS, and concussion outcomes. The path toward wellness may be a rocky one, but the information provided in the following chapters can make the going easier for you.

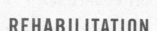

REHABILITATION

■

ELLIE, A 20-YEAR-OLD LONG ISLAND COLLEGE STUDENT, WAS ON HER WAY TO meet a friend for dinner when, for no apparent reason, her car went out of control. Ellie never really lost consciousness after the accident, but she remembers nothing about the first two weeks she spent in the hospital, bruised beyond recognition from her numerous physical injuries.

Ellie underwent numerous computed tomography (CT) scans, spinal taps, and electroencephalograms (EEGs) before doctors reached a diagnosis of concussion, also called *mild traumatic brain injury* (mTBI). When she was discharged after three weeks, Ellie was paralyzed on one side of her face, blind in one eye, and deaf in one ear. She had significant memory loss and no sense of smell, and her right eye turned inward. No one knew the extent to which Ellie might recover, yet she was not told that there were rehabilitation services that could help her. On her own, Ellie pursued psychotherapy and medical assistance. With determination and the help of a wonderful support system, the young woman was able to return to college after only eight months. She made the dean's list and won a merit scholarship, and is now a graduate student. Recently, she married a longtime friend.

NOT ALL people with a concussion are as fortunate as Ellie. While this young woman and her family were able to focus their energies on her recovery, many people who have suffered such accidents, returned from combat, or have had a sports injury lack the necessary direction, financial wherewithal, and family support to devote themselves to recovery. Instead, they may be left with an innocent-sounding diagnosis, unexpected problems at home and on the job, and little or no information about programs that can help them live a quality life once again. However, the right rehabilitation program can take a person a long way toward recovery.

WHY REHABILITATION SERVICES ELUDE
MANY PEOPLE WITH PCS

"Despite the fact that one of my neurologists was based in a rehabilitation facility with a concussion section, and another was located near a hospital with an entire inpatient unit for concussion, I realized only later on that coordinated rehabilitation services were available to me. After my accident, I was treated with various outpatient therapies, and I was making progress. But then I had a setback that left me with right-side weakness, slurred speech, poor judgment, problems with thinking and remembering, and intense pain in my right arm, shoulder, neck, and upper back. After lengthy testing, a neuropsychologist asked if I would consider rehabilitation. In fact, he was amazed that none of my previous doctors had ever suggested this service or informed me that it existed for people with my type of injury. Once I knew, I began to explore new avenues to ensure my ongoing recovery."

—D.R.S.

There are brain injury rehabilitation programs worldwide that vary in treatment and services. The majority of these are designed for people who suffer moderate or severe brain injury and were directly referred to the hospital where they first were seen. This is not the case for the majority of people with a concussion, because most do not require hospitalization, and those who do are usually admitted only for treatment of bodily injuries. As a result, the symptoms of brain injury, which may surface one at a time, are most often addressed on an outpatient basis—sometimes by several different doctors, and often by doctors who lack training in the complexities of this type of injury.

Overall, a person with PCS is frequently left to piece together his or her own recovery program—a process that can be significantly hampered by some of the very skill deficits that make rehabilitation necessary, such as difficulties with organization, memory, and judgment. Do-it-yourself rehabilitation can certainly be successful, but it lacks the cohesiveness and sense of security offered by a coordinated team approach.

WHY REHABILITATION MAY BE NECESSARY AFTER A CONCUSSION

Not all individuals who sustain a concussion require rehabilitation. It may be that outpatient treatment of symptoms is enough to bring about marked improvement and enable you to return to work and other everyday activities within a reasonable period of time. On the other hand, you may find that your job performance and daily living skills are so greatly affected by PCS that changes in your daily routine are necessary. Or you may be so consumed by the aftereffects of your injury that your life lacks fulfillment. You may suffer chronic pain, debilitating fatigue, or have specific impairments that just are not improving.

If any of these is the case, the team approach adopted by many rehabilitation hospitals may be the best means of improving your quality of life. Rehabilitation may involve working on an outpatient basis with one or more of the following specialists: a neurologist, a neuropsychologist, a physiatrist, a psychologist, a physical therapist, an occupational therapist, a speech/language pathologist, and a vocational therapist. In facilities that have a pain unit, pain-management techniques may also be taught.

Good places to start when looking for a rehabilitation program are CARF (the Commission for Accreditation of Rehabilitation Facilities), the Sports Concussion Institute, the Center for Integration of Medicine and Innovative Technology, and the Department of Veterans Affairs, which can direct you to the nearest facility that offers team services for outpatients. You can contact me via the information on page 367 for help with this. Otherwise, you may have to piece together a program on your own, a task that can be overwhelming.

FINDING THE RIGHT REHABILITATION PROGRAM

Just as each concussion and case of PCS differs, rehabilitation programs for people with PCS vary. In some localities, there are specific concussion units; in others, you might be eligible for vocational rehabilitation, counseling, and/or physical or occupational therapy services. Getting into an appropriate program is not always easy. Although federal regulations prohibit the use of a patient's age as a factor in determining eligibility for rehabilitation services, there have been instances in which people have been turned away from programs because of their age. Many programs have long waiting lists, and some have residency require-ments. In addition, you may be refused admission to a program if it is determined that your disability does not substantially handicap your daily living or job skills, or that rehabilitation services will not improve your employability. Most rehabili-tation programs require some evidence (from the type of injury and your initial moves toward recovery) that your condition is likely to improve.

Medical insurance coverage may also be a factor. Some insurance companies will pay for participation only in rehabilitation programs that have contractual arrangements with them. If you are in a managed-care plan, it is helpful—indeed, it may be necessary—to get your primary care physician (PCP) to assist you in getting into an appropriate rehabilitation program.

Before you sign up for any rehabilitation program, you should become as informed as possible about all aspects of the program and the services offered. (See "Factors to Consider When Comparing Rehabilitation Programs, page 303," for suggested questions to ask to help you evaluate rehabilitation programs.)

Whatever your particular circumstances, it is wise to remember that rehabili-tation is time-consuming and requires a strong physical and emotional commit-ment. Just as you might seek a second medical opinion, it is advisable to shop around for the program best suited to your specific needs. After all, different programs have different success rates in different skill areas. The following sug-gestions can help you take an active role in this important part of your recovery:

- Have a diagnostic assessment done to determine which of three major areas—physical, mental, and emotional capabilities—require rehabilitation.
- Ask your neurologist or neuropsychologist for program recommendations. (Be aware, though, that you and your doctor may differ in your opinions as to the necessity of rehabilitation.)
- Ask for program referrals from your disability or insurance company.
- Contact the Brain Injury Association to determine whether your state or province has its own brain injury organization. Request referrals from both groups.
- Visit recommended facilities in person. Do not rely on brochures or tele-phone descriptions.
- Ask to speak to families who have used the programs you are considering (but remember that facilities will likely offer names of satisfied customers only).

- Consider both nearby facilities and more distant ones. Location may be a factor if you cannot drive, but transportation arrangements can often be made if a faraway program is better suited to your needs.
- If your insurance company limits your choice of facilities, explore the possibility of using a nonparticipating facility anyway, if you feel strongly that it is the best for you. Insurance companies occasionally do extend coverage to outside programs. This can happen if your insurance coverage is very good and the injury requires very specific or high-quality care. If you were hospitalized, there are nurses with case management or liaison experience who are following your case in the hospital and have the necessary knowledge to advocate for you when speaking to an insurance adjuster. It is possible for an adjuster to make a decision that would permit you to receive a service not ordinarily granted by the insurance company that could improve or hasten your recovery or require fewer insurance resources in the long run. This is called negotiating out of contract and is rare, but still possible. If your request is refused, ask the out-of-network facility about working out a reasonable payment program.
- Be aware that home rehabilitation programs exist for people who are immobile. The Brain Injury Association can help you locate such a program.
- Attend local brain injury support groups and ask whether other members have been in rehabilitation. Ask for details about any programs you learn of.
- If you are receiving workers' compensation, let your case manager take an active role in getting you the help you need. Remember, he or she wants you to return to work successfully.

Factors to Consider When Comparing Rehabilitation Programs

The goal of rehabilitation is to enable you to resume your normal everyday activities. You will make the most rapid progress toward this goal if the program you choose is a good fit for you and your needs. The following are some questions to ask when considering a rehabilitation program:

- *Will rehabilitation be done on a one-to-one or group basis?* Depending on your diagnosis, a combination of the two may be better than one or the other.
- *Are the members of the interdisciplinary team full-time staff members or consultants?* People who are supervised by personnel within the hospital are best.

- *Will more than one therapist or team member be working on my program?* The team approach is preferable as a means of getting a full range of care.
- *How often would I have to go to the facility?* Your allowed number of days of rehabilitation services may be limited by your insurance coverage.
- *Who would make decisions about my progress?* Ideally, the team and program manager or rehabilitation physician will make decisions at team meetings, aided by you and your family members.
- *What is the cost of the program?* It is wise to compare the costs of comparable programs.
- *Is transportation provided by the facility for outpatient services?* If so, what type is available? Are there mileage limitations?
- *Does this facility offer all of the services that are recommended for my care, including speech, vocational, educational, physical and/or occupational therapy, as well as psychotherapy and case management?* If not, can they contract out to other outpatient service providers?
- *Is case management available for both inpatient and outpatient treatment?* This service can be extremely important to the success of your rehabilitation.

The answers to these questions will help you to determine which facilities are best suited to your needs. It is very important for you and a trusted friend or family member to make personal visits to programs under consideration, rather than making decisions based only on telephone interviews. Once you have chosen the right facility for your situation, ask to see the patients' rights list published by that facility. Use this information to help yourself. Many institutions also have lending libraries that afford access to books, articles, MP3s, CDs, and DVDs about concussion.

It CAN take as long as two to three months to determine your specific rehabilitation needs and locate the most suitable program, but this is time well spent. The uniqueness of every instance of PCS and the many personal circumstances that can affect recovery make the selection of your program a most important decision.

MANAGING THE REHABILITATION PROCESS

"Four years after my accident, I tried the Burdenko method of water therapy. The developer of this method is Igor Burdenko, Ph.D. The therapy is based in the water

and on land and emphasizes balance, coordination, flexibility, endurance, speed, and strength. Burdenko therapy did for me what four years of weights, Nautilus training, swimming, aquatherapy, medication, and alternative treatments had not been able to do: it enabled me to negotiate stairs without pain, kneel without falling, walk without staggering, and begin to rebuild lost muscle tone. In fact, a few months of the Burdenko method put me back on my bicycle for the first time since my accident."

—D.R.S.

When you enroll in a rehabilitation program, you should be assigned a case manager to coordinate your insurance and medical care, and to work with your lawyer when needed to seek reimbursement for costs not covered by insurance. If your job skills have been severely affected by your PCS, you may also be assigned a counselor to assist you in reentering the job market.

Diagnostic assessments will be required by any rehabilitation program you choose. Your test results will help specialists pinpoint the exact services that are needed. If you have had previous testing done on an outpatient basis, you may be able to save time, money, and needless duplication of tests by providing the rehabilitation facility with these records. Home and workplace assessments may also be done to evaluate your support system and see whether changes are needed in your physical environment. Then a personalized program will be developed according to test and assessment results. Therapists will be assigned, and specific goals and time frames will be defined. Be aware that there may be skills that cannot be regained through rehabilitation. If this proves to be the case, you will be taught other ways to do these things, as well as methods of coping with your limitations.

It is important to get to know the people involved with your case. Communication between you and the various specialists, and between the specialists and your outpatient doctors, will help you achieve your goals more quickly. Sometimes, home instruction may be advised, either at the hands of a staff member or a friend or family member who has been trained by the rehabilitation team.

Your team can also assist your employer or school system in making adaptations designed to improve your effectiveness on the job or in the classroom. In the United States, the Americans with Disabilities Act (www.ada.gov/q&aeng02 .htm) requires employers to make reasonable adaptations to allow disabled persons to work. For instance, an occupational therapist can help set up an appropriate work site and get a computer programmer to make a special program to suit the writing needs of a person with post concussion issues. If you live outside the United States, there may be a similar program in your country.

Naturally, there are a vast number of rehabilitative approaches that may be used. The appropriate techniques vary from patient to patient. The formulation of your rehabilitation program will be based on your specific needs. It may include speech/language therapy to improve communication skills; occupational therapy to help with organizational skills; physical therapy to improve mobility; and psychological services to help you cope with all of the changes that have taken place in your life. Some rehabilitation programs provide driver-evaluation programs to assess your physical and emotional readiness to resume driving.

Rehabilitation programs are meant to help you resume a normal daily life after significant injury. While rehabilitation is not always necessary after a concussion, and may not even come up in consultations with your PCP, these types of programs and specialists do exist to help you. In many cases, the right rehabilitation program can eliminate confusion, minimize frustration, and accelerate your recovery process.

CHAPTER 29

FINANCIAL ISSUES

■

VALERIE, WHOSE STORY APPEARS IN THE INTRODUCTION TO PART 3, LIVES IN Maryland, a state whose insurance laws mandate a minimum of $2,500 to a maximum of $10,000 in personal injury protection (PIP) for every driver. This insurance is meant to cover the policyholder's initial medical expenses in the event of an automobile accident. The assumption is that an injured party can sue to recover expenses above that amount if necessary. Valerie—like most of the 98 percent of Marylanders who purchase only minimal PIP coverage—never considered that $5,000 might be inadequate. She discovered this only after her accident. Valerie also didn't realize that being injured in an accident might make it impossible for her to obtain medical insurance—until a sharp premium increase forced her to cancel an existing medical policy after her accident. For three years, she was repeatedly denied replacement coverage, until a lawyer suggested that she purchase open-enrollment insurance. This is a costly and very limited type of hospitalization and catastrophe coverage that cannot be denied to anyone, regardless of preexisting conditions. Valerie says that the benefits provided by this policy are a disappointment, but at least it covers most catastrophic hospital bills—a concern due to her family medical history.

Valerie sees herself as a victim of the auto accident that ended her artistic career, and also as a victim of the legal and health care systems that were supposed to help her. She is lucky to have a family that has been able to assist her financially. Even so, she has at times thought about moving with her husband to his native Italy, where the government-run health care system would afford her better care than she has received in the United States.

Post concussion syndrome (PCS) carries with it two main financial issues: lost wages due to layoff, firing, or a change in employment; and medical bills for the extensive services that are often needed after an injury like a concussion, also called *mild traumatic brain injury* (mTBI). This chapter examines both of these issues and gives advice concerning the types of financial help that may be available to you, as well as suggestions for dealing with reductions in income, and tips to help you cut through the red tape that so often surrounds the insurance process.

LOST WAGES

Obviously, after an injury like a concussion, a certain recovery period is usually required before you can return to work. In some job situations, it is possible to take a medical leave of absence with pay. In others, you may be paid during your recuperation from illness or injury only to the extent of accumulated sick and vacation time. If you are self-employed or have no employer-provided benefits, you may not be able to get any paid time off at all.

Regardless of your employment situation, you may attempt to return to work during your recovery, only to discover that your ability to function on the job is not what it was prior to injury. You may see the need to take a different job that calls for less intellectual processing, for example, or you may even have to stop working—at least for the present. Many people with PCS end up losing their jobs because their work performance doesn't measure up after what their employers consider a "reasonable" period of time. Others leave voluntarily or abandon a business rather than face daily frustration and embarrassment.

The result is that many people with PCS find themselves earning less money after injury than before. Meanwhile, normal household expenses remain more or less constant and medical bills mount up rapidly. Because it is often impossible to predict how fully you will recover from your concussion, or how long recovery will take, it is important to know how you can obtain financial compensation to help you with your expenses.

TYPES OF COMPENSATION

"Before my accident, I had a successful two-office psychology practice. Fortunately, I carried overhead insurance to cover fixed expenses such as rent, utilities, phone bills, advertising, managerial and secretarial help, and my answering service. I had income disability insurance and, because I was also an employee of my corporation, workers'

compensation coverage. My overhead insurance covered my business expenses until I was able to close my offices, and, because my accident occurred as I was returning to my home office from visiting a patient, I also qualified for workers' compensation benefits. I was required to undergo four separate neuropsychological examinations and several consultations with an independent physician, but for the first four years, the workers' compensation agency was cooperative, congenial, and efficient. Then policy and personnel changes brought a rude awakening. Bills were delayed for months and then paid only in part, many more evaluations and tests were required, and my new claims representative hinted that many of my expenses would no longer be covered. I was forced to seek legal counsel."

—D.R.S.

The possibility of compensation for lost wages and medical bills is determined by the circumstances of your concussion. As you read in Chapter 4, these injuries most commonly result from auto accidents, sports and recreational injuries, falls, blows to the head, assault, or blast injuries. If your concussion occurred in a car accident, financial support may be provided through automobile insurance. If your injury happened on the job, you can seek assistance through workers' compensation. Liability and health insurance usually cover sports and other injuries that take place on school premises; homeowner's insurance, health insurance, or, in some cases, government assistance may cover injuries that happen at home. Some states have victims' compensation laws that provide for financial assistance for persons injured as a result of physical assault.

Dealing with insurance companies and/or government agencies can be one of the most difficult and frustrating aspects of a concussion. Payment for injury is a billion-dollar business that employs thousands of doctors, attorneys, investigators, consultants, and office personnel. When you become involved in this system, you become a case number in a huge maze. It is important to bear in mind that just because you have been the victim of a TBI, you do *not* have to become a victim of bureaucracy and corporate decisions. Remember that insurance companies are in business to make a profit, and that these institutions deal daily with people who want to take advantage of the system. As you pursue your case, you are likely to encounter delays, tremendous amounts of paperwork, and a certain lack of sensitivity to your needs, so it is important to enlist someone—a family member, a trusted friend, or someone from the Brain Injury Association (www.biausa.org)—to be a personal advocate who will work with you on your behalf. In addition, it is often advisable to secure the services of an attorney. (See "Finding the Right Attorney," page 314, for help in your search for appropriate legal counsel.) In this section, we will look at the various possibilities for financial compensation.

Automobile Insurance

Automobile insurance is designed to deal with responsibility, liability, and medical aspects of a car accident. In some states, a determination must be made as to who was responsible for causing an accident before a claim for compensation can be settled. Traditionally, damages are paid by the insurer of the party determined to be at fault. Many states have sought to simplify this process by passing so-called no-fault insurance laws. Under no-fault insurance, each person's policy covers expenses incurred. If it can be established that one party is more than 50 percent at fault in the accident, his or her insurance company then assumes full financial responsibility.

Health Insurance

If your concussion occurred as a result of a fall or sports injury, your medical expenses may be covered under your health insurance policy. However, if your injury occurred during work, workers' compensation, not your health insurance, will cover it. The extent of payment depends on the type of policy you have, the coverage it provides, and the amount of mandatory copayments, if any. Many policies require you to choose doctors and medical facilities from among those participating in the health plan, which may mean choosing from among health care providers who lack specific training or experience in treating PCS. In most situations, health insurance companies resist paying for care provided by practitioners outside their own networks, even though this can have a negative effect on the recovery process. However, a health maintenance organization (HMO) or preferred provider organization (PPO) may allow outside consultations if you can prove that your health needs cannot be met otherwise.

The first step in arranging for care outside your health plan network is to consult your primary care physician (PCP). If he or she agrees that there is no one in the managed-care network to help you, then he or she should make a referral to an appropriate person outside the network. If your PCP refuses to make an outside referral because he or she will be penalized financially for doing so, you can see a doctor of your own choosing. In this situation, however, you will have to pay the outside doctor's cost yourself. You should then consult with your lawyer about including this bill in your settlement.

Available coverage and services usually depend on the health coverage you or your employer held prior to your accident, or what is covered under workers' compensation or the other party's policy. Some policies cover occupational therapy, chiropractic, accupuncture, and psychological services; some do not, or have strict limits on such coverage, including not covering neurofeedback treatment. Only in the past few years has alternative insurance that covers such services as Reiki and polarity therapy, become available.

Government Programs

There are a number of different government programs that may provide benefits to people with PCS: Medical Assistance (Medicaid), Medicare, Social Security Disability Insurance (SSDI), Supplemental Security Income (SSI), and Department of Veterans Affairs programs.

Medical Assistance is a combination state- and federally funded program. Eligibility depends on your financial and medical needs. Depending on your state, there may be restrictions on coverage, including the types of treatment, equipment, and medication covered. Medicare pays for medical services for persons who are age 65 or older, or who have received Social Security Disability Insurance (see below) for at least two years.

SSDI is available to individuals whose disability occurred within five years of their last employment and who were employed for a required period of time. If you are a widow or widower and have become disabled, you may be eligible for this benefit if your deceased spouse would have met the employment criteria. There is no set salary or income required for this benefit. If you do not qualify for SSDI, you and your dependents may be eligible for the SSI program. This program is available to individuals with disabilities who have never been employed or who became disabled before they contributed to the Social Security fund through employment for a sufficient amount of time. It is also available to those with little income and few resources. It is important to investigate, since SSI has an income requirement.

If you need help in applying for any of these government benefits, call your local Social Security office, listed in the government section of your local telephone directory or online. They can give you guidance and assistance in the application process. However, you should be aware that getting this type of help can be difficult and time-consuming, and that eligibility requirements for certain benefits are subject to change in the future—most likely in the direction of becoming more restrictive. Nevertheless, you should not be discouraged if your claim is rejected at first. With your doctor's support, persistence, and an appeal or two, you may ultimately succeed in obtaining benefits.

In most states, there are VA hospitals with physicians on staff who are knowledgeable about brain injuries. If you served in the armed forces and have become disabled, you may be eligible for wage or medical assistance. Contact the nearest office of the Department of Veterans Affairs, listed in the government section of your local telephone directory or online, to determine whether you qualify and learn how to apply.

In addition to these nationwide programs, some states also have programs available to injured people who are 18 years of age or younger. The Brain Injury Association can advise you of state or province programs for which you may be eligible. If you are disabled and have minor children living at home, you may qualify for benefits under Temporary Assistance for Needy Families. This program is administered throughout the United States, and different states have different names for it. Eligibility requirements and benefits also vary from state to state. For specific information about benefits that may be available to you and how to apply for them, contact your state or local social services department.

One thing is more or less constant when dealing with any government agency: getting adequate care can be difficult because you must meet stringent requirements and deal with a fair amount of red tape and paperwork in order to benefit from government programs. In addition, the coverage provided is limited. In some states, outpatient services in particular are strictly limited. If you encounter problems filling out Medical Assistance or Medicare claims, you or your personal advocate can contact other doctors and medical facilities, a social service worker, or your state legal-aid service for help in expediting your claim.

Workers' Compensation

"About ten years ago, I got a job as an assistant to a film director and his actress wife. Six years later, while checking the gate where I worked, I fell down onto the driveway. I was taken to the local hospital. My apparent injuries were two teeth protruding through my upper lip. In the weeks that followed, I experienced various symptoms of concussion, such as smelling phantom smells, feeling cold, and having problems with articulation, memory loss, confusion, and poor judgment. I was contacted by a

workers' compensation representative, who suggested I see a neurologist. My doctor diagnosed me as having PCS. The claims person at workers' compensation suggested that I go home and rest. After a month, I felt better and attempted to resume working. However, I soon discovered that I could no longer perform the needed duties. I eventually quit my job.

In the years that have followed, I have been assigned several claims adjusters; however, no treatment was provided for my PCS. I finally realized that I needed to hire an attorney to represent me. After years of waiting, I recently had neuropsychological testing done, but I am still awaiting appropriate rehabilitative treatment for my concussion."

—MISSY

If your concussion was employment-related, you are probably covered by workers' compensation laws. The time frame and procedure for filing vary from state to state, and the process itself can be tiresome and frustrating, so it is advisable to contact an attorney or a Brain Injury Association advocacy program for assistance. Under workers' compensation laws, you may be entitled to receive a percentage of your pre-injury earnings as well as payment for medical expenses. Before being approved for benefits, you will probably be required to undergo an evaluation by a specific medical professional under contract to the workers' compensation insurance carrier. This person's opinion may determine whether certain services will be covered and/or if existing services should be continued. If the insurance carrier's physician feels that particular services are not necessary, the carrier may stop paying for those services. If you disagree with the doctor's evaluation, you can get a second opinion and go to court to argue your side. Meanwhile, if you need the service under dispute, you must pay for it yourself or run up a bill.

Even payment for treatment approved under workers' compensation can be delayed, sometimes for long periods. It is not unusual for doctors to refuse to accept workers' compensation patients because of the paperwork, minimal payment, and other obstacles. Don't give up, however. The Brain Injury Association should be able to help you locate a qualified practitioner or practitioners who accept such patients.

Victims' Compensation

If your concussion occurred as a result of a violent crime or physical assault, you may be entitled to compensation for lost wages and medical expenses through a state victims' compensation fund. Your lawyer, the local legal-aid society, or the office of your state's attorney can tell you whether there is such a fund in your state. The rules and requirements for receiving compensation from victims' funds differ, but in most states, a claim must be filed within a specified period of time. It is therefore important to find out what is needed and to get the necessary forms filled out as soon as possible after your injury.

Disability Insurance

Many companies supply income or disability insurance as part of an employee benefit package. Disability coverage pays a percentage of your previous wages while you are disabled, though exactly what percentage and for how long depends on the individual policy. The maximum dollar amount is not likely to approach the amount you previously earned, but it can help if you are unable to work. If you have this kind of coverage, your employer can advise you of the proper filing procedure. If you are self-employed and have private disability coverage, you will have to file a claim with the insurance company on your own. You may want to ask a family member or your attorney to work on your behalf to obtain the needed compensation.

FINDING THE RIGHT ATTORNEY

It is often advisable to hire an attorney to help you through the process of securing compensation for your injury. Without legal help, this process may be exceptionally difficult for a person with PCS, who looks fine but whose poor judgment places him or her at an enormous disadvantage before the process is even started.

To help locate an attorney with expertise in PCS, ask your state or the national Brain Injury Association if they have a referral list, or ask your health care professional for help. If you are in a brain injury support group, ask other members whose services they have used or whom they would recommend. Be cautious of lawyers who advertise on television. Claims of experience with injury cases are no guarantee that an attorney is necessarily the right choice for you.

Depending on where you live, you might be able to locate more than a few lawyers who are specialists in personal injury or workers' compensation and who have an understanding of TBI. Once you have compiled a list, you should arrange to interview each candidate personally. This is extremely important, not only to ascertain a prospective lawyer's expertise but also to ensure that you feel comfortable with him or her. Because your concussion may cause you to have problems recalling information, consider bringing a digital recorder, notepad, or friend or family member to the interview.

The following are questions to ask an attorney that can help you determine whether he or she has the background necessary to properly represent you after a concussion:

- *How many cases similar to mine have you been involved with as the principal attorney over the past three years?* Though the numbers may vary, it is important that the lawyer has had concussion clients for whom he or she has won settlements.
- *What percentage of your practice is devoted to cases and injuries similar to mine?* This too may vary, depending on where you live, but it can be a good indication of an attorney's experience with PCS cases.
- *What were the results in terms of settlements or verdicts in the last five cases that you handled involving injuries similar to mine?*
- *Could you furnish a list of prior concussion clients?*
- *How many seminars or conferences have you attended over the past two years involving presentations on injuries similar to mine?* Ideally, your lawyer will have attended more than two such seminars.
- *How many articles have you written over the past three years involving any aspect of injury similar to mine?* It is desirable for your chosen attorney to have written at least one.
- *Would you explain the process you follow in handling a case like mine?*
- *Do you have consultants with expertise in PCS?*
- *What kinds of problems might occur in the settlement process?*
- *Will you personally work on my case, or do you have an assistant? If an assistant will be used, does that person have experience with concussion and PCS?*
- *Will you personally be representing me in court? If not, who will? Does that person have expertise in concussion?*
- *What are your legal fees?* Generally, there are three types of fee arrangements: hourly fees, flat fees, and contingency fees. In most states, lawyers obtain a contingency fee—usually 33 percent—for auto accidents, and a fixed rate for workers' compensation settlements. The client does not pay the lawyer; rather, payment is received by the lawyer only if the client is awarded a monetary settlement.

Auto Insurance

Following a concussion, your choice of legal representation can be crucial to obtaining appropriate financial compensation for your injuries. Time invested in locating an experienced attorney will be time well spent.

There are three types of damage compensation that you may qualify for after an auto accident:

1. *Special damages.* These provide reimbursement for your past and future medical expenses and compensation for lost wages. You may also be eligible for reimbursement for what you could have earned if you had not been injured.
2. *General reimbursement of damages.* This is compensation for emotional pain and suffering caused in your daily life.
3. *Punitive damages.* Punitive damages may be assigned by the court if an insurance company fails to issue a reasonable settlement on a valid claim.

Most automobile insurance policies cover damages that someone else has caused you and have liability coverage to protect against both bodily and property damage. This will pay for damages you may cause someone else. Depending on what state or province you live in, there may be fault or no-fault laws. Regardless of these laws, you may have PIP, which can cover loss of wages and/or medical payments. A similar type of coverage, called MedPay, is for medical bills. Your insurance agent can provide specifics about the coverage afforded by your policy. Depending on where you live, you may also be able to purchase additional insurance to protect yourself against accident or injury caused by an uninsured or underinsured motorist. This is known as Coverage U.

Following an accident, your first step should be to call your insurance agent—the same day, if possible. If you have sustained injuries from an auto accident and are at fault or being sued, the insurance company will assign one of its own lawyers to act in your behalf. If you are seriously injured, it is imperative that you retain private counsel even though your insurance company will not necessarily advise you to do so. It is extremely important to do this as quickly as possible. Do not wait until a settlement is offered.

It is also crucial that your attorney and your personal advocate look at any proposed settlement with your or the other party's insurance company before you agree to it. Remember that symptoms do not always arise immediately after a concussion and that your injury may have affected your judgment. Carefully consider any lump-sum settlement with your attorney and physician before accepting such offers. Many offers come with the provision of surrendering compensation for future medical care. You do not know if your post concussion issues will be accepted by other insurance, and your accident insurance may be your only resource for some time to come. Caution and legal counsel are always advised.

PRACTICAL SUGGESTIONS

"I have saved a lot of time and energy by filling out the personal data section at the top of a blank medical form and then making photocopies of the entire form so that only the date and signature need to be added in the future."

—RITA

"I highly recommend learning to interview professionals to ensure that you are seeking help from appropriate sources. Also, make photocopies of every application, form, and cover page that you submit to agencies and insurance companies. If you need to reapply or be recertified for benefits in the future, you can simply copy the previous form."

—ELAINE

"I was fortunate in that I had insurance and that I was able to cover my bills—unlike many people with PCS, who have to choose between paying medical bills and feeding their families. To help me cope with seemingly uncaring bureaucratic personnel, I found comfort within my local brain injury support group, from my psychotherapist, and from the many caring friends I made through social media."

—D.R.S.

The process of filing for compensation for lost wages and medical expenses can be long and frustrating. The suggestions that follow can make things a bit easier:

• Be organized. Keep a daily diary, beginning with the events that led to your injury. Keep all your medical records in one file, and create another file for records regarding your accident. List names of witnesses, emergency personnel, and doctors, and keep detailed notes about your symptoms. If necessary, ask a friend or family member for assistance with this.

- Document all telephone conversations relating to your accident by keeping a log. Include the date and time of each conversation, the name of the individual you spoke to, and a summary of your conversation.
- If you hire a lawyer to help you secure compensation for your injury, send him or her copies of your telephone log and all written correspondence relating to your accident and its aftermath. If your lawyer does the paperwork, keep notes of (or digitally record, with permission) your conversations with him or her.
- Find a good mental health therapist who has had experience with concussion. If your health and recovery begin to be affected by your experiences with health care providers, insurance companies, and government agencies, talk to your therapist about this.
- If strained finances prevent you from locating a mental health therapist, contact the Brain Injury Association or a nearby hospital's mental health clinic for assistance.
- Seek out a support group. Call the Brain Injury Association to see whether there is a concussion group in your area. Also find out whether the Brain Injury Association can put you in touch with an advocate to assist you with money issues.
- If you have access to a computer, explore online forums on Facebook, social media, and bulletin boards. Discussing your problems with other people with PCS can be extremely helpful. If you do not own a computer, check to see if your local public library makes computers and Internet service available to patrons.

Some people with PCS may neither have insurance nor qualify for government compensation or assistance programs. It may be that your employer does not offer health insurance or other benefits, or perhaps you are self-employed and you cannot or choose not to buy disability or medical insurance on your own because it simply costs too much. You may have lost your job after suffering a concussion, and with it, your insurance—just when you need it most. Or you may be able to work part-time, but even though you do not qualify for employer-provided benefits, you earn too much to qualify for government assistance. Meanwhile, your household and medical bills continue to pile up. While a long-term solution may seem elusive, there are a few options to consider in these circumstances:

- Switch roles with your spouse. If you are the breadwinner, discuss the possibility of your spouse taking on more work hours or, perhaps, a second job.

- Change your lifestyle. Do what you can to prevent your household bills from becoming unmanageable, including selling your home or other assets if necessary. If needed, ask a trusted family member or friend to do an overall budget inventory to see what you are actually spending on things. Then you can discuss ways to scale back your spending and develop a reasonable budget to live on.

- Be honest about your situation with creditors, doctors, and your landlord or mortgage banker. You may be able to negotiate payment plans that are easier to meet.

- Allow friends and family to help. Doing so can be embarrassing, but accepting heartfelt assistance can get you through a very difficult time.

- Consider living with your parents, in-laws, or other willing relatives for an established period of time.

- If your children require assistance, contact your local mental health facility about free counseling and other services in your area.

- Contact the Brain Injury Association (www.biausa.org). Laws are always changing, and new options for financial assistance may become open to you. In addition to providing advocacy and other services, the association monitors such developments.

- Check with religious organizations in your community about funds and services available to people in need. They may offer, or know sources of, basic necessities such as food and clothing at no or reduced cost.

- Ask your doctor or advocate about programs for obtaining prescription medications at reduced prices. Some pharmaceutical manufacturers offer such benefits to qualified persons.

- If you need a lawyer, check with your local and state government about free legal services available to people who qualify. Also, some attorneys dedicate a certain amount of their time to offering free, or *pro bono*, legal services. In some situations, these arrangements may not be necessary, since legal fees are usually collected as part of a settlement.

- Consult your bank about services that can advise you about managing your money and obtaining credit while you recover.

- If your financial situation is truly unmanageable, consider filing for personal bankruptcy. This decision should probably be considered a last resort, and it should be made with great care and under an attorney's guidance. However, bankruptcy can sometimes be the right choice, particularly if your debt is overwhelming.

Financial concerns are a very real part of coping with post concussion symptoms. The way money issues are dealt with can dramatically affect your final outcome. Not only do you need money for daily living expenses, but after a concussion, you are also likely to need money to finance a rehabilitation process that can last for some time—in some cases, for years. It is not always easy to navigate the maze of red tape and paperwork required, but help is available to most people with PCS through commercial insurance, health insurance, government assistance, workers' compensation, and victims' compensation. When coping with monetary difficulties, it helps to remember that you are not alone. Consult trusted family members or friends, an attorney with expertise in concussion, and/or the Brain Injury Association, and allow yourself to accept their advice and assistance.

CHAPTER 30

LIVING WITH SOMEONE WITH POST CONCUSSION SYNDROME (PCS)

◾

JEFF, THE HUSBAND OF GAIL FROM CHAPTER 7, SAYS THAT LIVING WITH A PERSON with *post concussion syndrome* (PCS) takes patience . . . patience . . . patience, because the person you love isn't the same anymore. Jeff describes his wife as an incredible person who used to give 120 percent to her work, her family, and making a home. She was consistent and dependable, and very tolerant and understanding. The impact of Gail's injury on the family—their daughters were 5 and 3 years old at the time—was like someone turning off the lights, Jeff says. The unpredictability of her symptoms, the frequency and extent of her anger, and her difficulty handling more than one activity at a time are what cause him and the children the most frustration. For a long time, the older daughter wouldn't admit that Gail had been in a car accident. She is now getting psychological help, as well as support from Jeff's parents, who live nearby and help out often. The younger daughter also has been traumatized.

Jeff estimates that Gail has now returned to 85 percent of her old self. She has taken a job as a crossing guard and is gradually exhibiting more normal behavior. But the family has to live with the unpredictability of Gail's symptoms and eventual outcome, and that takes patience . . . patience . . . patience.

A CONCUSSION, also called *mild traumatic brain injury* (mTBI), affects everyone whose life is touched by the injured person, particularly family and friends. How these important people are affected, and the way in which they respond, can affect the individual's recovery process and eventual outcome.

EMOTIONAL RESPONSES

My family loves me for what I was, and protects what I am.
My friends cherish what I was, and often forget what I am.

I remember who I was. I want to find out who I am.

It is now ten o'clock. At least I know where I am.

These first lines from Beverley Bryant's poem "From Inside Out" tell of the conflict family and friends have in dealing with PCS. If a loved one suffers such an injury, you can expect to undergo a series of reactions that are similar to the classic stages of grief, from denial to anger to depression to ultimate acceptance of the new reality. Of course, not everyone goes through the same reactions in the same order, or wrestles with each one for the same amount of time. Also, it is possible to experience two or more of these reactions simultaneously. As a general rule, however, friends and family members of a person with PCS can expect to experience something like the progression of emotional responses outlined below.

Denial

"To my three teenage sons, nothing changed after my accident except my unpredictability. They often complained about never knowing when I wouldn't be feeling well or what would cause me to lose my temper. I had my sons accompany me to my brain injury support group so they could meet other people who had problems like mine. Unfortunately, the impact of this meeting lasted for only a short time. I often wished that my children would read some of the material available for family members, but it seemed their denial and their desire to return to the old days were a stronger force.

After my original accident in 1990, I had two more concussions, each causing me months of recovery, and the reaction of my sons was still the same. They didn't want to discuss the symptoms of my brain injury; they just wanted me to be 'Mom.'"

—D.R.S.

Denial is the refusal to accept the reality of a problematic condition or event, and it is the biggest obstacle to coping with any injury. In the case of PCS, where the injury is invisible and the person looks, sounds, and functions (at least in some arenas) as he or she previously did, denial is almost a certainty.

Often, denial starts at the scene of the injury, because police or others in authority make a decision about an individual's need for medical care based upon his or her appearance. You may assume that the injury, if any, must be minor, since the person either was not taken to the hospital at all or was released after a superficial examination. If medical help is sought later, the person's complaints are often treated individually—as fatigue or headaches, say—and they may not be linked to the earlier head trauma. If symptoms such as uncharacteristic forgetfulness, poor concentration, irritability, or behavior changes occur, you may first suspect an emotional problem or become impatient when your loved one fails to "snap out of it." Often the injured person, unable to change, becomes depressed.

Realization

If the injured person's symptoms persist or intensify, you eventually come to realize that something is wrong and you must give up your denial. With this unwelcome awareness comes fear, worry, and a sense of vulnerability, for you have somehow lost the person you knew and depended upon, and you do not know what the future may bring. Financial issues become a concern, as do home issues such as household responsibilities and the care of children.

Helplessness

"My mother, who has had several strokes, was very understanding, because she had gone through many of the same experiences as I did. However, my extended family offered limited support because they did little to educate themselves about my problems. Sometimes I felt like I was the caregiver and had to enlighten everyone, and this was a burden I did not want. I wanted to feel free to just get better and get on with my life. My saving grace was psychotherapy, my Internet confidants, and my steadfast friends, who accepted me and my unpredictability without judgment."

—D.R.S.

IF YOU see someone you care about suffering and behaving in a strange and unpredictable manner, you may feel helpless. Not knowing where to turn or what to do creates an awkwardness that often leads friends and colleagues to stop calling or visiting. Extended family may behave in a similar manner. The immediate family, who cannot practice this kind of avoidance, may instead become withdrawn and extremely impatient.

Frustration

Frustration is an outgrowth of the feelings of helplessness that result from your inability to make things return to normal. There is no question that it can be extremely difficult to deal with a PCS sufferer's inability to acknowledge his or her deficits and reluctance to make needed lifestyle changes. Often, the injured individual sees his or her primary caregiver as bossy and domineering, and may respond with stubbornness or uncooperativeness, or by giving up household responsibilities. Almost any interaction with the person with PCS can quickly turn into a control issue, leading to anger and conflict in the home.

Anger

Frequently, both the individual with a concussion and his or her family feel anger that the injury has affected their lives. If the trauma was a result of carelessness or some other fault (real or perceived) on the part of the person with PCS, feelings of anger are intensified. The anger response strains many marriages, and often causes extended family to withdraw emotional support. Friendships that have withstood the stresses so far may fall apart at this point because the friend's anger may not permit him or her to deal with the injured person's unpredictability. As a family member or friend, you may feel angry that your loved one has changed dramatically, often permanently so.

Guilt

Anger at the injured loved one leads to feelings of guilt, as you regret your anger and short-temperedness with someone who badly needs your assistance. You scold yourself for not being more understanding, and feel guilty about not being completely supportive. The fact that you are clearly trying to help does not make you any less ashamed of the annoyance you feel when the person with PCS is being difficult.

Sadness

At some point, perhaps after much time spent going from frustration to anger to guilt and back again, you realize that life with your loved one simply may never be the same. You may get an empty feeling when you look at old photos or when you study the person as he or she is today. Reminiscing about the past and planning for the future may become occasions for feelings of sadness and resignation. There is a genuine loss to be dealt with.

Acceptance

Finally, you learn to accept your injured loved one for who he or she is now. You may not like what has happened to your life, but you accept that your friend or family member, though changed, still has wonderful qualities and many contributions to make to the relationship. You begin to care for and relate to the new person rather than bemoaning the loss of the old. Frustration and anger diminish, and loving interaction returns.

PRACTICAL SUGGESTIONS

"My then-husband and I went to marital counseling to help us cope with my PCS. I had learned to accept my limitations, lack of reliability, and unpredictability. I also discovered that it was okay to have someone look out for me. My husband discovered that my responses weren't always reliable, and that it wasn't productive to get angry when I did things that he felt were unwise or unsafe. For several years, he did try. However, he ultimately was unable to accept who I became and experienced caregiver fatigue. This resulted in our divorce."

—D.R.S.

Living with an individual who undergoes the personal changes associated with TBI is not easy. It is important to remember that feeling anger or frustration at times is normal, and that despite these feelings, you deserve a great deal of credit for the support and assistance you offer daily. The following are a number of tactics that can help make it easier to deal with a loved one who has had a concussion:

- Ask your loved one's neurologist about the medical reasons behind his or her behavioral and other problems. Simply understanding what is really going on may help reduce your frustration.
- Educate yourself about the nature of your friend's or family member's deficits. Refer to the various chapters of this book for hints on coping with specific problems.
- Realize that a person with PCS passes through several very different phases during recovery. Learn about each stage and try to devise fresh approaches to dealing with them.
- Ask the brain-injured person about how he or she feels, and accept these feelings as real.
- Talk openly about the loss of the "old" person and your frustration with the "new" person's unpredictability.
- Help the injured person set realistic goals and formulate strategies for achieving them. Track your loved one's progress with a success log, and give him or her full credit for everything he or she accomplishes.

- Get to know the new person, and appreciate him or her not in comparison to the old person, but as a valid and worthwhile individual.
- Accept your frustration as normal, but express angry feelings to someone other than the injured person. Find other people in similar situations through support groups and online groups.
- Consider counseling by a professional who specializes in post concussion issues to help you cope with your loved one's difficulties.
- Avoid letting your physical or emotional reserves become drained. Discover what activities refresh and rejuvenate you, and schedule time every week to pursue them. When possible, ask other family members or friends of the person with PCS to help out.
- Approach memory deficits by taking time to reeducate the person with PCS about his or her life. For example, look together at old photo albums and family movies and videos.
- Address the person with PCS by name before asking or telling him or her something important. Doing so increases the chance that your message will be received.
- Focus on the strengths and talents that your loved one still possesses.
- Help your friend or family member learn to live in the outside world again by taking walks together around the yard, neighborhood, and town.
- Find out about services that provide assistance to people with PCS in the home, workplace, and community. Your local rehabilitation center can advise you as to the types of help that are available.
- Consider personal, couples, or family counseling if coping with your loved one's PCS is causing emotional or marital problems.

Nursing homes, hospitals, and hospice facilities have respite care programs that last for five days and allow families time to recover from overwhelming circumstances. These programs, covered by Medicare, permit caregivers time to reduce their stress levels while ensuring that the recovering patient's medical needs are filled by professionals. Hospice care is required, and qualifications include stroke; TBI; cancer; dementia; heart, kidney, lung, or liver disease; multiple sclerosis; or Parkinson's disease. This option may not be for everyone. Please contact your local hospital or home hospice agency for assistance.

Finally, it is important to realize that you need not be solely in charge of your loved one's recovery. Many types of assistance and support are available to you and the person with PCS. If you are not sure what type of help you need or where to begin looking, call the Brain Injury Association for advice and referrals. Or, feel free to contact me for assistance via the information listed on page 367.

Caring for a friend or family member after a concussion is a huge undertaking, but you need never shoulder the job alone. The ordeal can be lessened by the realization that many post concussion symptoms lessen with time. As Jeff, whose story opens this chapter, says, "Dealing with a person with PCS takes patience . . . patience . . . patience."

TO OUR CAREGIVERS

As we struggle to understand ourselves,
Please understand us too.
As we struggle to learn to accept ourselves,
Accept us too, please do.
As we aspire to reach our goals
Please urge us in that direction.
If we fall short a step or more
Please help us achieve perfection.
Urge us on, but do not push.
Encourage, but do not shove.
We'll be doing our very best
And we will need your love.
The times we are not loveable,
We'll need you all the more!
We'll need you most at the times
When ourselves we do abhor.
And we will promise one thing
Though our progress may be slow;
We'll be doing our very best
As onward we do go.
Onward where? We have no way
Of knowing what the test.
But one thing you can know for sure,
We'll be doing our very best.

—RITA SMITHUYSEN

CHAPTER 31

OUTCOMES OF CONCUSSION/ MILD TRAUMATIC BRAIN INJURY

■

UNLIKE THE PREVIOUS CHAPTERS, THIS CHAPTER DOES NOT BEGIN WITH A real-life story that illustrates a specific problem. This is because each concussion experience is as unique as the affected individual, and one story alone cannot illustrate the range of outcomes. Since your recovery is unlikely to follow a straight and sure course, your doctor's ability to measure the residual effects of your injury and predict long-term results is limited. Years after suffering a concussion, also called *mild traumatic brain injury* (mTBI), some people are fully recovered, while others have learned to accept ongoing symptoms of *post concussion syndrome* (PCS). Still others may yet be healing, unable to guess at their eventual outcome.

FACTORS THAT INFLUENCE YOUR PROGNOSIS

The outcome of any individual concussion hinges on the many variables that have been discussed in earlier chapters—among them the site of the injury, the solidity of the person's support system, and the appropriateness of treatment. Your recovery will also be influenced by your pre-injury personality and by how determined you are. Age is another factor. Young children and older people, for example, appear to be better able to accept changes in personality and behavior than do young adults. Finances also figure in concussion outcome. Research has shown that navigating stressful insurance and legal processes related to an accident can hinder recovery. However, while the pace, time frame, and degree of recovery from a concussion may be uncertain, the healing process itself tends to follow a pattern.

The loss of predictability plays a role in recovery from a concussion. Prior to your injury, your life had a certain routine, based in part on your knowledge of how you thought, felt about, and reacted to things. You knew your strengths and weaknesses, what made you angry or sad, and how effective you were on the job. Also, you could plan and organize. Now, no one—including you—may have any idea how you will feel or act at any given time. This loss of predictability is a result of injury and dysregulation to your brain that may make you feel as if you are always adapting and adjusting your life. Even the experts cannot be certain whether the symptoms of PCS will affect you once a week or once in a lifetime— or, when fatigue, pain, and other maladies do occur, how intense or long-lasting they will be. Therefore, your ability to grieve the loss of who you were before is an extremely important factor in your outcome. Once you let go of the need for predictability and accept your present self, you can once again enjoy life—maybe not as before, but with a new outlook.

STAGES OF RECOVERY

There are several consistent stages in recovery from a concussion. During the first phase, your visible injuries heal enough to make you truly aware of the emotional and cognitive damage left by your concussion. Often, you notice these changes only when you feel well enough to resume your daily routine and are faced with evidence that you are not the same person as before. As part of this stage of evaluation, you may experience a jumble of feelings, including lack of awareness, denial, anger, depression, and grief. (See Chapters 23 and 27 for more about emotional reactions and grieving the loss of self.)

The second phase of recovery—often the most difficult—has to do with accepting that you may never be the same again. Coping with this realization is made harder each time you catch a glimpse of your "old self" and recognize that some of your former capabilities are out of reach. You live with uncertainty, you struggle to establish new ways of doing things, and you experience setbacks that make you wonder whether you will ever get better. It may be hard to allow others to assist you, but a support system that includes family, friends, and brain injury support groups is invaluable during the periods of vulnerability and sadness that characterize the second stage of recovery.

As you gradually accept the changes in yourself, you will enter the third phase of healing: regaining independence and a sense of control. You will get a feeling of accomplishment from driving, balancing your checkbook, or recalling a phone number without first writing it down. As you discover that your reactions to situations are quite different from before, you will also learn that there are things about your new personality that you like. You will regain your self-confidence through seemingly minor accomplishments, learn to accept your limitations, and begin to explore previously untapped potential. You will once again make progress, although on a different, perhaps bumpier, path than before.

Healing from a concussion is unlike recovering from an illness. You cannot say at the outset when you will begin to feel better, how you should pass the time, or how much care you would like from others. Instead, you wrestle with unfamiliarity and with friends and family who seem overprotective one minute and pushy the next. But you will achieve a positive outcome when you let go of the "old you," become confident about your new capabilities, and fine-tune the coping skills that allow you to return you to some form of independence.

CONCUSSION OUTCOMES

Throughout this book, you have become acquainted with the thoughts and stories of a number of real individuals as they struggled with the aftermath of their concussions and PCS. In this chapter, we will revisit some of these people as they are today, as well as meet several others who have experienced a concussion and PCS. Some of these stories are immensely encouraging, while others may inspire understanding and empathy. Taken together, they serve to illustrate the various and unpredictable courses of recovery from concussion. You may also recognize elements of your own recovery in these stories.

Beverley's Story

Beverley, the gymnastics judge and real estate broker whose story was told in Chapters 16 and 17, was in an automobile accident seven years ago and began experiencing *complex partial seizures* a month afterward. She also completely lost interest in physical intimacy with her husband. Since that time, she has experienced marked improvement. She looks well, her seizures are regulated by medication, and she has completely recovered from her sexual problems. She has written two books, *In Search of Wings* and *To Wherever Oceans Go*; she lectures throughout the United States; and she is active in her family's real estate firm and is a support counselor at Bayside Neurorehabilitation Services in Portland, Maine. Beverley is also the only TBI survivor who was director of a state head injury association. (As of this writing, the Maine Brain Injury Association is no longer in existence. Thus, Maine residents with TBI no longer have the assistance and resources this organization used to provide.)

Since the publication of *Coping with Mild Traumatic Brain Injury*, Beverley learned strategies that allowed her to return to community living. Although she had many deficits to overcome, the hardest was living as a new person in her old body. Everything about her changed, and who she had once been disappeared completely. Beverley notes that she was fortunate to have been blessed with an optimistic attitude and outlook, as well as a tremendous determination to succeed.

Beverley has successfully held a full-time job as a support counselor working in a brain injury day treatment center for six years. She has given keynote addresses and lectures in twenty-two states while using the very strategies she speaks about. She co-founded Brain Injury Voices (braininjuryvoices.org), a group of acquired brain injury survivors that meets monthly to help educate people, advocate for better services, and support those who need help in their journey. The field of brain injury needs survivors who are high functioning and can help the general public to better understand brain injury.

Kimberly's Story

Kimberly's concussion, the result of a car accident seven years ago, left her with headaches, dizziness, fatigue, confusion, memory problems, and other mental deficits, as described at the beginning of Chapter 19. Her memory problems improved dramatically after she was taken off several medications for depression. She still has many problems related to organizing, planning, and remembering, but she has devised alternative ways of doing things. For instance, she kept putting freshly made coffee into the garbage. Now she keeps a note on the coffeemaker that says "Drink it, don't toss it." To avoid the possibility of starting a fire while cooking, Kimberly removed the stove from her kitchen and installed a microwave oven.

She is still getting used to the unpredictable new person she has become, but she likes herself more each day. Kimberly attributes much of her positive outcome to the unfailing support of her companion and caregiver, Melanie. She also feels that taking care of her pets has forced needed certainty and meaning into her life.

Jack's Story

Jack, the retired law-enforcement officer whose story introduced Chapter 27, still grieves his loss of self from his accident six years ago. He feels he has not yet discovered who he is, because he never knows from moment to moment whether he is going to stutter, feel fatigued, or experience a headache or black mood. He compares his life to an amusement park ride that takes you into a dark tunnel where you never know what to expect.

Jack has undergone neuropsychological testing and psychotherapy. His participation in a local brain injury support group has helped him get out of the house and spend time among people who understand him. His clinical depression is being treated with medication, but litigation relating to his accident is pending, and this has caused ongoing stress because he is pressed to report on what he can and cannot do—abilities that vary greatly from day to day. Jack's recovery waxes and wanes, and he senses that he has a long road ahead of him.

Since the publication of my first book, Jack has been diagnosed with Sjögren's syndrome (an autoimmune disease), suffered a major heart attack, and endured three incidents of sepsis, retina surgery, treatment for melanomas, and massive dental issues. He also deals with excessively dry eyes. According to doctors, some of his many illnesses and symptoms might be attributable to his brain injury. Regardless, since his car accident, Jack has never returned to the strong, active life he led before. The accident was a true turning point in his life, and not for the better.

Jack, like many others with a concussion, lacked the support, resources, and medical and psychological guidance that are available to people in his circumstances. Jack and his wife were unaware of how to find solutions and assistance that would help them. Hopefully, this new book will provide the necessary information to help with his recovery and yours.

Carol's Story

Since the skiing accident that caused Carol's concussion five years ago (described in Chapter 10), she has succeeded both professionally and academically. She is currently a program research specialist at Hudson Valley Community College in New York and also teaches three courses there. Her husband, Ray, ultimately found he could not accept that he was living with a new person, and the couple separated. However, Carol's colleagues and her close friend Lauren have been extremely supportive throughout her recovery.

It is Carol's sense of self—of knowing who she is—that has suffered the most. Two years after her injury, she was diagnosed with major depression and placed on medication to help relieve the symptoms, but four months after that, she was nevertheless diagnosed as suicidal. Carol describes herself as having been killed on the mountainside that day five years ago. However, she says she has made many friends through BrainInjurychat.org and Neurotalk.org and is learning to grieve and go on living with her new, unpredictable self. She calls herself a "functioning dysfunctional."

Darlene's Story

Darlene, whose story is included in Chapter 14, continues to cook, cater meals for friends, and enter recipe contests using her original recipes. Interestingly, she recently won honorable mention for a recipe she concocted after losing her sense of smell. Today, Darlene's phantom-smell problem is much less troublesome than it was in the months following her concussion. It comes and goes, both without any obvious cause and also when triggered by things like a sinus infection or the presence of perfume. In general, Darlene avoids new foods and food products because her missing sense of taste negates their appeal. She worries that in a few years, she will forget what familiar foods taste like.

Darlene says that her husband has been a great help. She asks him whether the house—or she herself—has an odor, and about things like the freshness of foods. She date-labels perishable foods just to be sure. She makes a point of bathing, brushing her teeth, and laundering her clothing quite often so as not to risk body odors. For safety, she has a smoke detector and gas alarm in place in her home.

Coping with her sensory problem has taken time, partly because Darlene's doctors initially offered hope that her sense of smell might return, leaving her uncertain as to whether to view her condition as temporary or permanent. Now she has become resigned to both the loss of smell and taste and her problem with phantom smells.

Chad's Story

Chad, whose story opens Chapter 24, used to live at home with his mother and was trying on his own to put an end to his substance abuse. When this failed, he had to move out and is currently in assisted living in which part of his rent is paid by the Department of Housing and Urban Development and the rest through his Social Security check. He has made some strides in his recovery and no longer takes Suboxone. Unfortunately, with the current poor economy and his inability to find a job or resources, Chad continues to live with the symptoms of PCS on a daily basis. He still has hope that he will someday recover from his post concussion symptoms.

Carolyn's Story

The details of Carolyn's experience are discussed in Chapter 19. After Carolyn completed her consultation with me, we were able to find the appropriate treatment program for her in New York City. Today, Carolyn is once again performing onstage, delighted to have resumed her acting career.

Dawn's Story

Dawn, whose story is told in Chapters 19 and 20, has experienced improvement in her post concussion symptoms. Today, she is able to plan a grocery list and follow a recipe. She can focus on simple tasks and has learned to handle both interruptions and excess stimulation through a variety of coping skills. Dawn finds herself implementing these strategies on a daily basis, though she finds that doing so continues to require a good deal of effort and concentration.

Nancy's Story

With time, rest, and the understanding and support of her family, physician, and high school personnel, Nancy, from Chapter 22, was eventually able to resume playing basketball and other sports. She is keenly aware that she has had a concussion and that sustaining another in the future is likely to have greater consequences than the first. Nancy, along with her family, has learned the importance of eating a brain diet, getting restorative sleep, and inquiring about services that are available to people with PCS.

D.R.S. (My Own Story)

It took time to get used to the new me—a composite of the old and new. I continue to live with physical, emotional, and cognitive problems related to my brain injury, and for a long time, I was never sure when I woke up in the morning if I would be able to achieve my goals for the day.

For the first six years after my accident, each day challenged me to find new ways of learning to manage pain, compensate for lost skills, and cope with my emotions and ever-changing symptoms. I used to have an exceptional memory; then it became unpredictable. I could no longer do simple math problems in my head, my judgment was sometimes extremely poor, my mental endurance was compromised to the point that I could not work for more than an hour or two without resting, and I could no longer think and express myself in complicated analogies, but rather had to express myself more simply. Happily, my sexual dysfunction improved with time and the termination of various medications. There are still some times when I feel absolutely no desire, but this is now the exception rather than the rule.

My fatigue and attention problems affected me the most. For example, my daily activities did not interfere with my work on my first book, but I was unable to write new chapters in the presence of my children, a ringing phone, or even my cat entering my office. To prevent myself from losing my thoughts, I needed to be able to control my environment. My solution was to isolate myself in a local motel to do my writing.

In the years since *Coping with Mild Traumatic Brain Injury* was published, I have made significant progress with the use of a brain diet I developed, nutrition response therapy, and the Burdenko method, acupuncture, craniosacral therapy, therapeutic massage, homeopathics, biofeedback, neurofeedback, Bach Flower, energy psychology, spiritual training with a mentor, and psychotherapy. My ability to do math has returned, my atypical migraines are under control, and my balance, coordination, and mobility are restored. However, not until six years after my accident, when I discovered the benefits of neurofeedback, did my cognitive problems begin to improve markedly. After fifty sessions, I no longer feel fatigued, and my attention, organization skills, and judgment are more consistent. An added bonus was that this treatment eliminated my chronic pain. Now I feel pain only when there is an actual injury to my muscles.

Since my original accident, I've had two subsequent concussions, one from a second motor vehicle accident and the other due to a faulty chair. What was remarkable was my recovery from both of these incidents. In a recent visit to my neurologist, he was amazed at the progress I had made. He said, "Whatever you are doing, keep it up!"

In the years since my first concussion, each day has been a challenge to me. There is no question that my spirit and determination to recover are core factors in my progress, along with the love and support of family, close friends, and colleagues and the care and understanding I received from my local brain injury support group, friends in the community, and my brain-injured friends online. Since the publication of *Coping with Mild Traumatic Brain Injury*, some of the online chats have stopped, but there is now a vast variety of forums that provide both valuable information and welcome emotional support. My personal experience and awareness of what has worked for me led to a career shift. When I resumed working as a neuropsychologist and board-certified health psychologist, my focus became helping people like me. I employ my Five-Pronged Approach to recovery, first discussed in Chapter 6, considering every individual and organization from five distinct views: physical, psychological, emotional, spiritual, and energy. Often, these areas intertwine, yet each needs to be addressed during treatment. In my work, I look for a patient's core issue, and from this vantage point we begin their journey to overcome life's challenges and reach their potential. With this new book that you're reading, my goal is to help you find what is helpful and healthful for your recovery.

Recently, I was asked to serve as the expert on post traumatic stress disorder (PTSD) and TBI for the federal government's Defense Centers of Excellence. I turned down the opportunity, because I would have had to move and lose the support system that has helped me in my recovery. Instead, I agreed to become an independent consultant for them. This will allow me to help wounded warriors while still keeping my commitment to providing the consulting services for those of you who are looking for answers and treatment—what I term "Solutions and Resources."

Sometimes I still wish I could take a vacation from myself, but most of the time I am thankful that the new, composite me had the opportunity to meet the challenge of concussion and watch my children grow up.

YOUR OWN OUTCOME

No one can predict your eventual outcome. Your symptoms may be permanent, come and go unpredictably, or fade altogether. The one factor that can determine your outcome in the way that really counts is you—how you see and accept yourself.

Gail, whose story begins Chapters 7, 14, and 18, wrote the following in the *Headliner*, a newsletter of the Brain Injury Alliance of Oregon:

Our own inner peace will come when we have the strength of mind:

- to be satisfied with our own self,
- to be accepting of the way we are now,
- to be forgiving of ourselves,
- to be mindful of our own integrity, and
- to let go.

Normal? Been there.
Brain damaged? Done that.
Both together? Now there's a real challenge.

It is my hope that with the information in this book, together with your own acceptance of what you can and cannot do, you can meet this challenge.

PART 6

FUTURE INNOVATIONS

INTRODUCTION

∎

I
N OUR PREVIOUS BOOK, *COPING WITH MILD TRAUMATIC BRAIN INJURY*, WE DID not include the chapter that follows, because at that point there were very few innovations and programs for people with brain injury. At the time, the computer world was just coming into its own, and the Internet was called the World Wide Web, or "Web" for short. Many places in the world used the term *head injury* to refer to a brain injury, but now a day does not go by that you don't read of someone sustaining a concussion, also called *mild traumatic brain injury* (mTBI), from an accident, fall, sports collision, or blast injury.

Technology is changing the way we are diagnosed; the forms of treatment available; the development of automobiles, sports equipment, and military equipment; and one's ability to gain support from others with TBI. At the same time, previously used medications are being used in new ways, along with revolutionary medications that can be specific to a particular symptom.

Ancient methods that once were thought of as bogus or alternative are now part and parcel of many integrative rehabilitation programs for brain injury. Some that were once considered alternative, such as acupuncture, are now considered part of complementary medicine in many hospitals. Hyperbaric oxygen therapy (HBOT), once used solely for the military and for scuba divers, is covered by insurance in many states for the treatment of TBI.

When our first book was written, you had to be physically present to obtain most of the treatments that were available for post concussion symptoms, but with telemedicine and virtual treatments, it is possible (as I currently do) to work with people all over the world. With the use of credit cards, even the type of currency is no longer an issue. I can work with someone in Germany without worrying about how to convert euros to dollars. The credit card company does this, thus allowing such international consults and treatments to take place.

Along with advancements in technology, medicine, traditional methods, and worldwide access, concussion and *post concussion syndrome* (PCS) are now recognized as real injuries. As a result, there are new and innovative treatment programs being developed. Part 6 of this book deals with what is being proposed in the field of concussion, and what is being done in different aspects of recovery, rehabilitation, insurance coverage issues, and brain injury prevention. The future innovations, programs, and recognition of treatment and health care changes can hopefully allow us all to recover without regard to income level or where we live in the world, enabling us to return to achieving our greatest potential.

CHAPTER 32

ADVANCES IN THE PREVENTION, ASSESSMENT, AND TREATMENT OF CONCUSSION/ MILD TRAUMATIC BRAIN INJURY

■

WITH THE WORLDWIDE NEWS MEDIA DETAILING EVERYTHING FROM SPORTS injuries to war casualties, brain injury, and specifically concussion, has been brought to the forefront. This new awareness has brought advancements in technology and implementation for concussion prevention diagnosis, treatment, and support.

DEVELOPMENTS IN CONCUSSION PREVENTION

Worldwide, motor vehicle accidents are the major cause of concussion, also called *mild traumatic brain injury* (mTBI). Part of this is concussion caused by the very airbags made to prevent bodily injury. Newer, safer airbags are being developed and tested, along with extenders for gas and brake pedals for people who are of below-average height. Crash testing now includes side crashes along with head-on collisions.

The Centers for Disease Control and Prevention have a subdivision for the prevention and control of TBI. They suggest buckling children in the back seat of the car in safety seats and special harnesses based on size and weight. In recent years, great improvements have been made to these types of seats. Military jeeps and helmets are being tested for effectiveness against blast injury, and there is research suggesting that taking the medication NNZ-2566 prior to combat may help the brain during a blast. There is also a test to look at biomarkers for help in the diagnosis and treatment of blast injury.

Another major area linked to concussion is drug and alcohol abuse. Awareness programs such as Drug Abuse Resistance Education (DARE), Mothers Against Drunk Driving (MADD), and Students Against Destructive Decisions (SADD) are helping in this area.

Slips and falls are another primary cause of concussion. Helpful improvements and innovations include grip-soled footwear, nonslip pavement, the addition of handrails and nonslip surfaces in bathtubs and showers, and brighter lighting inside and outside homes. For children, there are window guards and shock-absorbing surfaces at playgrounds.

In the world of sports and recreational activities, there has been a huge shift in awareness of the potential for, and consequences of, head injuries among participants. Protective helmets and helmets with built-in impact detectors are being developed, along with mouth guards that absorb most of the force from a hit to the jaw. There is now protective headgear available for soccer, lacrosse, basketball, skiing, snowboarding, horseback riding, and skateboarding, as well as safer helmets for football, baseball, and ice hockey. The biggest development may be in bicycle helmets, with many states and provinces now making it mandatory to wear one. In track and field, where brain injury can occur in the pole vault and shot put, the padding and surfaces are being changed to better absorb impact, and regulations are being put in place to ensure greater safety. In football, new rules ban specific types of plays such as head butting and helmet-to-helmet hits. Cheerleading, formerly considered an extracurricular activity rather than a sport, is under review due to the number of concussions suffered, and guidelines are being developed to protect the participants.

Various organizations have stepped up the focus on brain injury prevention. For instance, Pilot International has developed "BrainMinders . . . Protecting Your Brain for Life," a signature project targeting TBI and brain disorders. The project encompasses a public service campaign to promote brain awareness, prevention education programs for both children and adults, workshop and speakers bureau materials, a partnership with Project Lifesaver, an injury tracking program, and support for brain-related programs. The award-winning BrainMinders programs feature safety tips for children presented by Pilot Clubs around the world. The BrainMinder Buddies program, a part of BrainMinders, weaves a "Play Safe, Play Smart" theme throughout its stories about helmet safety, playground safety, and seat belt safety.

Technology

Every day brings new, cutting-edge technology in the areas of diagnosing, treating, and preventing concussion. For example:

- Pulsed electromagnetic field therapy (PEMF) is being used to treat body and brain trauma. Through advancements in quantitative encephalography (qEEG), LORETA, and functional magnetic resonance imaging (fMRI), the assessment and treatment of such injuries has vastly improved. The advent of MRI technology such as susceptibility weighted imaging (SWI) and diffusion tensor imaging (DTI) now allows doctors to see small lesions that were once not apparent. For years prior to this technology, many concussion symptoms were dismissed as an attempt by a malingerer to get money from an insurance company.

- Today, there are bicycle helmets in development that will be able to detect brain injury in the wearer. Football helmets with the same capability already exist.

- A company called NeuroSky is developing headgear to help people with brain injury communicate just through thoughts. This project, with which I've been personally involved, entails the technology of brain-computer interface (BCI), through which the computer translates brain waves to brain wave recognition (similar to voice recognition) and speaks for the individual who is unable to communicate naturally. Another company, Emotiv, has developed a BCI wireless headset and software that allows you to compose emails through thoughts alone.

- Children's Memorial Hermann Hospital (UTHealth) and the Cord Blood Registry are enrolling individuals for the first safety study approved by the Food and Drug Administration to investigate the use of a child's own umbilical cord stem cells for treatment of TBI in children. In preliminary research, it has been found that stem cells have gone to the injured site and helped with healing.

- The U.S. Army's Telemedicine and Advanced Technology Research Center joined with the American Telemedicine Association to present a symposium called "Innovative New Technologies to Identify and Treat Traumatic Brain Injuries: Crossover Technologies and Approaches Between Military and Civilian Applications." Discussion centered on the increase in TBI and PTSD as a result of combat. The U.S. Army is interested in pursuing technological solutions for early detection and treatment of TBI to reduce its lasting impact on the war fighter.

- General Electric and the National Football League have established a joint initiative to better manage mTBIs. In their "Head Health Challenge

I: Methods for Diagnosis and Prognosis of Mild Traumatic Brain Injuries" they will award up to $10 million for improved technologies and methods that enable more accurate diagnoses and better prognoses for recovery following acute and/or repetitive injuries. I have been invited by NineSigma to participate in this initiative, which will also benefit soldiers and civilians who suffer head trauma.

As the technology used in the diagnosis, assessment, and treatment of brain injury continues to advance, physicians will be able to make more accurate predictions about an injured patient's prognosis. With compassionate counseling, families of TBI patients will therefore be able to reach life-changing decision points in their loved ones' medical management. While the technology needed to predict future quality of life is not currently available, it remains within an arm's reach. In the future, doctors will be able to better avoid uncertainty, thereby helping families immeasurably while reducing both highly controversial cases and related news media coverage.

Programs

The Traumatic Brain Injury (TBI) National Data and Statistical Center, funded since 1997 by the National Institute on Disability and Rehabilitation Research (NIDRR), has developed practice guidelines in important areas of medical care for people with TBI. The guidelines call for:

- Development of innovative approaches and procedures for rehabilitation immediately after injury
- Creation of new diagnostic procedures and assessment tools for complications that were previously difficult to measure objectively
- Identification of common long-term problems that occur after TBI and the reasons why they occur
- Development and validation of new assistive technologies for use by people with cognitive impairments, to help them live independently. This is the model for community-based rehabilitation, which has as its primary goal that individuals with TBI participate and integrate in their communities.

Many states, provinces, and countries worldwide have organizations and programs that offer information and support groups. One example is the

Massachusetts Rehabilitation Commission's (MRC's) Brain Injury and Statewide Specialized Community Services. The American Academy of Neurology (AAN) has developed new guidelines for concussion, including new recommendations covering an athlete's ability to return to play. In addition, many schools now have trained personnel who can gather baseline cognitive data, evaluate students after a concussion, and make appropriate recommendations.

The Military

A pilot program, Assisted Living for Veterans with Traumatic Brain Injury (AL-TBI) is being advocated by the Brain Injury Association and the Wounded Warrior Project. This program will ensure that war fighters can maximize their recovery after TBI, allowing access to a wide range of post-acute services and supports. The goal of the project is the improvement and maintenance of skills to allow brain-injured veterans to reside in noninstitutional settings.

Support Groups

Some of the support groups mentioned in *Coping with Mild Traumatic Brain Injury* are still in existence but are not actively used. After my initial concussion, Prodigy and its TBI chat rooms were where I met and networked with many fellow brain injury survivors. This is long gone, yet its purpose has been met by other social media support, such as Facebook and LinkedIn groups, blogs on concussion, and websites such as Neurotalk.org and brainline.org. With today's explosion of social media, people worldwide can connect, share, and support one another in a way never thought of prior to the computer age. No longer does someone have to feel alone, isolated, and without caring support. Skype and the various social media have provided individuals coping with post concussion symptoms the means to connect, be seen, and be understood.

Support Organizations and Websites

A number of organizations exist that provide information, assistance, programs, and/or support groups to assist people living with *post concussion syndrome* (PCS). A check of their websites can lead to helpful information and valuable connections. Here are some examples:

* www.avbi.org is the site of a nonprofit organization for veterans with a brain injury and their families.

- biacolorado.org offers support group meetings through the Brain Injury Alliance of Colorado.
- www.mass.gov/veterans/health-and-well-being/tbi/state-tbi-agencies/ offers information on support groups, programs, and rehabilitation services for military veterans with TBI in Massachusetts.
- bianys.org/bianys-support-groups.htm provides a list of support groups in New York state.

The Brain Injury Association once had chapters in all fifty states that provided educational programs and support groups. Since the publication of our first book, this number has been reduced. Maine's program, for instance, is no longer in existence, while in Massachusetts, the BIA remains very active in presenting programs and groups.

It is wonderful—and it is a great relief to those with PCS—that concussion is no longer being denied or dismissed. By the time you read this book, even more wonderful advancements in technology, cutting-edge programs, and support will be available than anyone could ever have conceived when our first book was written.

CONCLUSION

On with Living Again

■

"Life breaks everyone, but some people become stronger in the broken places."
—ERNEST HEMINGWAY

YOU LOOK IN THE MIRROR AND YOU APPEAR THE SAME, BUT YOU KNOW THAT A part of you has died. You struggle on a daily basis, wondering why you are no longer reliable, dependable, or predictable. Often, you feel that you are going crazy.

These thoughts and feelings are the same for every person with a concussion, also called *mild traumatic brain injury* (mTBI). The purpose of this book has been to help you understand and cope with the residual problems—*post concussion syndrome* (PCS)—from your brain trauma. You need to know that even if you don't walk, see, or process information the way you once did, you still are a worthwhile person who has much to offer yourself, your family, and society.

It is my hope that this book has provided you with the resources you need to continue your life with dignity and purpose. Use the information to educate yourself about your injury, its aftereffects, and the unpredictability of the healing process. Rely on its chapters to help you select the best treatments and professionals, and to teach the people in your everyday life to help you and listen to you. Ask for help when you are tired, in pain, or unable to do things for yourself. Allow yourself to be emotionally supported by your loved ones, and encourage them to accept you as you are now, rather than focusing on who you were before.

There will be days when your judgment is off, when your memory is unreliable, or when you cannot seem to get past your pain. So too will there be times when you are able to function very well. Don't forget that before your concussion, you had good days and bad days, too. Remember that conditions as varied as the barometric pressure, hormonal changes, foods, medications, and the stress of daily living can affect you. Be kind to yourself and use your energy wisely—but don't be afraid to live life. Mourn the loss of the "old you" and enjoy learning all the good things about the "new you." Take a few risks, find humor in everyday life, and reconnect with friends and family at your own pace and on your own level.

The message of the Serenity Prayer provides excellent advice to help you forge through adversity to a new quality of life: Accept the things you cannot change, change the things you can, and try to recognize the difference. Here's wishing you life, and living, again!

GLOSSARY

∎

THERE ARE MANY TECHNICAL TERMS ASSOCIATED WITH CONCUSSION, ALSO called *mild traumatic brain injury* (mTBI), and post concussion symptoms. Understanding these can help you to educate yourself about your problem and work with your physician and other practitioners toward recovery. Some of the most frequently encountered terms are defined below.

absence seizure. A generalized seizure in which consciousness is altered, but without convulsive symptoms. Formerly called *petit mal*.

acetylcholine. A brain chemical that controls activity in the brain area connected with attention, learning, and memory. Also active in controlling skeletal muscles and responses of the central nervous system.

acupuncturist. A practitioner of acupuncture, a type of treatment based on the principles of traditional Chinese medicine, in which extremely fine needles and herbal treatments are used to restore the proper flow of *qi*, the body's vital energy, to stimulate healing and relieve pain. An acupuncturist must be licensed to provide this service by the state in which he or she practices.

acute concussion. A concussion in which loss of consciousness (if any) was less than one minute, and symptoms resolve without complication within seven to ten days. No further intervention is required during the period of recovery.

adhesion. A band of fibrous material that forms an abnormal connection between the surface of one internal organ or structure and that of another. Adhesions usually form as a result of scarring (for example, after surgery).

agitographia. Rapid writing movements with the omission or distortion of letters, words, or parts of words.

agnosia. The loss of comprehension of sensory input, such as sounds or sights. Also, the inability to recognize a familiar object, even though all the physical senses are intact and functioning.

agnosia alexia. The inability to comprehend and understand written words.

agraphia. The inability to express thoughts in writing. This can be due to a brain lesion or to muscular coordination problems.

alexia. The inability to read or recognize written words.

alexia agraphia. The inability to read and write letters, words, numbers, or musical notes.

amino acids. Molecules containing nitrogen that combine to form proteins.

amnesia. The loss of memory. See also *anterograde amnesia*; *retrograde amnesia*.

analgesic. Any member of the group of drugs used to relieve pain.

aneurysm. A weak spot in the wall of a blood vessel that may balloon outward and, eventually, rupture. If an aneurysm in a blood vessel in the brain ruptures, brain hemorrhage results.

anomia. An inability to remember names of persons and/or objects.

anosmia. The loss of the sense of smell.

anoxia. The lack of oxygen. Anoxia in brain tissue causes brain injury.

anterior. Pertaining to the front part of a structure.

anterograde amnesia. The inability to remember a traumatic event, such as a brain injury, and events that occurred afterward. Also called post traumatic amnesia.

anticonvulsant. A medication used to prevent seizures by suppressing irregular electrical discharges in the brain.

antidepressant. A medication used to treat depression.

aphasia. A language impairment ranging from having difficulty remembering words to being completely unable to speak, read, or write. See also *conductive aphasia*; *expressive aphasia*; *receptive aphasia*.

apraxia. Difficulty starting, continuing, and stopping movements, even though there is no actual muscle weakness, paralysis, or sensory change or damage. Apraxia may affect speech or the movement of the arms and legs. Also called motor planning problems.

articulation. The ability to correctly pronounce the speech sounds in words.

ataxia. An inability to coordinate muscle movements and actions that is not due to apraxia (see above), to the extent that the ability to walk, talk, eat, work, and perform self-care tasks is compromised.

attention. The ability to focus on specific messages for a period of time while screening out irrelevant information.

audiologist. A professional who assesses hearing deficits through the interpretation of an audiogram, or hearing test.

aura. An early neurological symptom that may precede a migraine or a seizure. An aura may manifest itself as bodily sensations, sounds, smells, visual images, flashing lights, the sudden development of a blind spot, and/or a feeling of spaciness.

behavior. The total collection of overt actions and reactions exhibited by a person.

behavioral neurologist. A medical doctor who is a specialist in neurology and the treatment of organic personality disorder, also called organic personality syndrome.

benzodiazepine. A medication such as Valium that uses GABA receptors to help with relaxation and sleep.

beta-blocker. A drug, such as atenolol, used to reduce anxiety, headaches, and hypertension. Musicians, public speakers, and actors use beta-blockers to avoid performance anxiety and stage fright. Beta-blockers in sports are banned by the Olympic Committee.

biofeedback. A technique utilizing an external monitoring system to help an individual become conscious of usually unconscious body processes, such as the activities of the muscular, thermal, and electrical systems. This makes it possible to gain some measure of conscious control over these processes, and thereby learn to manage headaches, chronic pain, and other problems.

blast injury. A complex type of physical trauma resulting from direct or indirect exposure to an explosion. Blast injuries occur with the detonation of high-order explosives as well as the deflagration of low-order explosives.

brain stem. The rear lower part of the brain, just above the spinal cord. It contains structures that control breathing and heartbeat and serves as a relay station for all motion and sensation.

brain wave. An electrical impulse given off by rhythmic fluctuations of voltage within neurons in the brain. Measured by an electroencephalogram (EEG).

Broca's area. An area of the brain responsible for producing language.

Burdenko method. A system of water and land exercises based on a holistic approach to rehabilitation, conditioning, and training.

calcium-channel blocker. A drug used to relieve hypertension (high blood pressure). Calcium-channel blockers are also used to treat headaches.

central nervous system (CNS). The part of the nervous system made up of the brain and spinal cord.

cerebellum. The portion of the brain that is located below the cerebrum and is concerned with coordinating movements. Damage to this area may result in ataxia.

cerebral cortex. See *cerebrum*.

cerebrospinal fluid (CSF). A colorless solution of sodium chloride and other salts that circulates around the brain and spinal cord.

cerebrum. The largest and most advanced part of the brain. It consists of two hemispheres connected by a band of tissue. It is the area where most cognitive functions (thinking, understanding, and reasoning) take place. It is divided into four lobes: the frontal, temporal, parietal, and occipital. Also called the cortex or cerebral cortex.

chiropractor. A practitioner of chiropractic, a hands-on technique of manipulating the spine and/or joints to promote healing and relieve pain. A chiropractor must be licensed by the state in which he or she practices.

chronic traumatic encephalopathy (CTE). A progressive degenerative disease, diagnosed postmortem in individuals with a history of repeated concussions and other forms of head injury.

clinical social worker. A social worker who specializes in emotional and mental disorders. Many clinical social workers provide psychotherapy services.

CNS. See *central nervous system*.

cognition. The process of thinking, understanding, and reasoning.

cognitive flexibility. The ability to shift from one task to another.

coma. An unconscious state that lasts longer than 24 hours.

complex partial seizure. A seizure that involves only part of the brain—usually the frontal or temporal lobe—and causes an alteration of consciousness.

comprehension. The ability to understand things that are heard, seen, and/or touched.

computed tomography (CT) scan. A diagnostic test that uses X-rays and computer analysis to produce a picture of the brain.

concentration. The capacity to maintain undivided attention on a specific message or task.

concussion. An injury to the brain that causes momentary to one-hour loss of consiousness along with amnesia. Also called mild traumatic brain injury.

Concussion Resolution Index (CRI). An online assessment tool designed to track resolution of symptoms following a sports-related concussion, measuring reaction time, visual recognition, and speed of information processing. Also called HeadMinder.

conductive aphasia. A language problem characterized by halting speech with word-finding pauses and repetition of words.

contusion. An injury that results in localized bruising, swelling, and hemorrhaging from capillaries. A contusion in the brain can result in a concussion.

convulsion. An involuntary, spasmodic, usually full-body muscle contractions. At one time, the word *convulsion* was used interchangeably with *seizure*, but this is no longer the case.

cortical blindness. The severe loss of vision in both eyes caused by damage to the vision nerves in the brain's occipital lobes.

cortisol. A sterol hormone secreted by the adrenal glands, released in high levels during stress. Can negatively interfere with the functioning of the immune system. Also known as hydrocortisone.

Coup/contrecoup. Literally, "blow/counterblow." A type of brain injury in which impact on one place on the head causes the brain to bounce against the opposite side of the skull, thereby causing injury to both sides of the brain.

cranial electrotherapy stimulation (CES). A treatment that applies a small, pulsed electric current across a patient's head. It has been shown to have beneficial effects in conditions such as anxiety, depression, insomnia, and stress.

CSF. See *cerebrospinal fluid*.

CT scan. See *computed tomography scan*.

déjà vu. A sense that you have seen, done, or experienced something before, whether or not you actually have. In a person with a concussion, this can occur because of a total lack of awareness that he or she is recalling past information. Can also be seizure related.

diffuse axonal injury (DAI). Momentary alteration or loss of consciousness with no observable disruption of nerve impulses, resulting from a mild blow to the head.

diplopia. Double vision; the perception of two images from a single object.

disorientation. A disturbance in the recognition of people, places, and/or time and day; not knowing where you are or who you are.

dopamine. A neuromodulator, with either activating or inhibiting properties, that controls arousal levels in several parts of the brain and is essential for the control of sustained attention and attention to sensory input. It also is involved in control of the motor system.

dopamine agonist. A compound that activates dopamine receptors in the absence of dopamine.

dysarthria. A problem with the muscle movements needed to form, or articulate, words. Dysarthria affects the pronunciation of spoken sounds.

dyscalculia. A partial inability to perform mathematical functions.

dysfluency. Stuttering; the repetition or drawing out of initial word sounds.

dysgraphia. A partial inability to perform the motor movements required for writing.

dyslexia. A partial inability to read words, characterized by the misperception of letters and letter sequences, misidentification of words, and/or an inability to distinguish text from its background.

dysnomia. A difficulty finding and retrieving words.

dysosmia. An altered sense of smell.

dysregulation of the brain. When the brain is out of balance (regulation) due to neurological, structural, hormonal, vascular, or chemical changes.

dyssymbolia. A partial loss of the ability to use or understand symbols, such as those used in mathematics, chemistry, or music.

EEG. See *electroencephalogram*.

electroencephalogram (EEG). A diagnostic test that records electrical activity in the brain.

emotional lability. Intense fluctuations of emotion that appear to be exaggerated or inappropriate responses to situations or thoughts, or that occur without any reason.

epilepsy. A disorder characterized by recurring seizures.

executive functions. The highest functions of the brain, which help a person plan, organize, remember facts, start and finish a task, control emotions, self-monitor, and problem-solve.

expressive aphasia. A problem with expressive language, such as difficulty in articulation, fluency, and written communication. The most common type is Broca's aphasia.

factitious disorder. The intentional falsification of illness by pretending or by inflicting injury on oneself, even though one does not stand to gain anything by doing so.

fascia. A fibrous connective tissue between muscles or organs that permits adjacent muscles to glide smoothly over each other.

Fatigue Impact Scale (FIS). A clinical measure to guide intervention and the treatment of fatigue as well as to assess change over time. It consists of forty questions that rate the extent to which fatigue causes problems in one's life.

Fatigue Severity Scale (FSS). A method of measuring the impact of fatigue. It is a short questionnaire that rates the level of fatigue on a scale from 1 to 7.

feverfew. An herb used to reduce fever and treat headaches, migraines, arthritis, and digestive problems.

floaters. Tiny bits of solid matter that develop in the vitreous fluid, the gel-like substance that fills most of the space within the back half of the eyeball, between the lens and the retina, causing one to see tiny floating spots.

frontal lobe. The area of the brain located at the front, closest to the forehead. It is responsible for emotions, behaviors, social and motor skills, abstract thinking, reasoning, planning, judgment, memory, and speech.

gamma-aminobutyric acid (GABA). An inhibitory neurotransmitter used to induce sedation.

Glasgow Coma Scale. A neurological scale used to reliably and objectively record the conscious state of a person after a head injury. Assessment consists of three tests (eye, verbal, and motor responses); the lowest GCS (sum) is 3, or deep coma/death, and the highest is 15, or fully awake.

grief therapy. A form of therapy that uses clinical tools to treat a severe or complicated traumatic reaction to death or a major life change when normal coping mechanisms are shut down.

gustatory. Pertaining to the sense of taste.

health maintenance organization (HMO). A health insurance plan where a person receives most or all of his or her care from a network provider. Plan subscribers are required to pick a primary care physician to coordinate their care.

heart rate variability (HRV). The variation in the time interval between heartbeats. HRV is a noninvasive measure of nervous system activity and heart health.

hematoma. An accumulation of blood outside of a blood vessel. This can occur anywhere in the body and is the cause of brain swelling that can occur after a concussion.

hemiparesis. The weakness of one side or part of the body due to injury to motor areas of the brain.

hemiplegia. The paralysis of one side of the body.

hemorrhage. An abnormal discharge of blood.

herbalist. A practitioner who prescribes various types of herbal remedies to stimulate healing and harmony within the body.

hippocampus. The brain area that is important in the creation of new memories and the transition of short-term to long-term memory. It is centrally located next to the temporal lobe near the base of the brain.

homeopath. A practitioner who treats illness by prescribing homeopathic remedies, which consist of highly diluted plant, animal, and mineral substances. Remedies are prescribed based on a detailed, multifaceted evaluation of symptoms.

hormones. Chemical messengers in the brain produced by glands or organs that cause a variety of metabolic functions in near or far organs or cells by sending specific signals that produce specific responses.

hypersomnia. A disorder characterized by excessive sleepiness, extended sleep time in a twenty-four-hour cycle, and the inability to achieve the feeling of refreshment that usually comes from sleep.

hyposmia. A partial loss of the sense of smell.

hypothalamus. The part of the brain that influences sex drive, sleep, long-term memory, and the expression of emotion.

ictal event. A medical term for a seizure of any type.

initiation. In behavioral terms, the ability to carry out tasks you have set for yourself.

interictal behavior syndrome. A feeling of disorientation, confusion, spaciness, and fatigue following a seizure. This behavior, sometimes called "postictal," is usually temporary and disappears after a period of rest.

lesion. A visible localized abnormality of the tissues of the body; any damage to the nervous system.

libido. The sex drive.

limbic system. A group of interconnected deep-brain structures that helps the hypothalamus prioritize incoming information and also plays a part in controlling memory and emotion.

lobe. Any of the four sections of the cerebral cortex, the largest part of the human brain. The frontal lobe is associated with reasoning, planning, emotions, problem-solving, and speech; the parietal lobe is associated with movement, orientation, and the perception of stimuli; the occipital lobe is associated with visual processing; and the temporal lobe is associated with the perception of auditory stimuli, memory, and speech.

long-term memory. A system for permanently storing, managing, and retrieving information for later use.

magnetic resonance imaging (MRI). An imaging test that uses a magnetic field and a computer to produce an image of the brain or other internal structures; it produces a clearer picture than X-rays or a computed tomography (CT) scan.

malingering. The intentional falsification of illness by pretending or inflicting injury on oneself in order to gain financial compensation or to avoid work, military duty, or criminal prosecution.

memory. A complex process of storing and retrieving information for later use. Types of memory include sensory, or information that lasts for a second; short-term (or working, or buffer), or information that lasts up to one minute; and long-term (or remote, or secondary), or information that lasts longer than thirty seconds.

Ménière's syndrome. A condition characterized by one-sided low-frequency hearing loss with a sensation of fullness in the same ear; ringing or buzzing noises in the ear; and severe, even violent, attacks of vertigo.

meninges. Any one of three membranes—the dura mater, pia mater, and the arachnoid—that encase the brain and spinal cord.

migraine. A neurological disorder caused by blood-vessel or electrical-impulse changes in the brain and characterized by intense headache, often affecting only one side of the head, that may be preceded by an aura and/or accompanied by nausea, vomiting, and/or sensitivity to light and noise. In some cases, symptoms can be almost identical to those of a seizure. A migraine preceded by an aura is termed a classic migraine or migraine with aura; a migraine not preceded by an aura is called a common migraine or migraine without aura.

mixed mood state. A condition in which symptoms of mania and depression occur together; for instance, feeling like a failure while at the same time having a flight of ideas.

MRI. See *magnetic resonance imaging*.

muscle tone. The tightness in muscles when they are at rest.

myelin. The electrical insulation around the axon of a neuron that allows impulses to transmit quickly and efficiently along the nerve cell.

nerve conduction velocity (NCV) study. A test to see how fast electrical signals move through a nerve.

neuroconnectivity hub. Any of the clusters of neurons that together form functional systems (much like the digestive or respiratory system) that cooperatively interact to form perceptions, memories, emotions, movements, executive functions, and various psychiatric and psychological dysfunctions.

neurodiagnostic testing. A body of tests that analyze and monitor nervous system function, to promote the effective treatment of neurological diseases and conditions. The most common and most frequently performed test is the electroencephalogram (EEG), in which the electrical activity arising from the brain is recorded and interpreted.

neurologist. A medical doctor who specializes in the nervous system and its disorders.

neuromodulator. A substance released by a neuron that transfers information to other neurons, influencing (or modulating) the overall activity level of the brain. An example in this category is serotonin.

neuroplasticity. The ability of neural pathways to change due to changes in behavior, environment, and neural processes, as well as changes resulting in bodily injury. Previously, the brain was thought to be a physiologically static organ, but the study of neuroplasticity now explores how, and in which ways, the brain changes throughout life.

neuropsychological testing. Specifically designed tasks used to measure a psychological function known to be linked to a particular brain structure or pathway. Tests are used for research into brain function and in a clinical setting for the diagnosis of deficits.

neuropsychologist. A psychologist with special training in the relationship between behavior and the brain. Neuropsychologists assess problems with brain function and coordinate the rehabilitation of brain-behavior relationships.

neurotransmitter. Chemicals such as acetylcholine and GABA whose movement across the small gaps (synapses) between neurons allows for the communication of information between neurons.

norepinephrine. A hormone produced by the brain and the adrenal glands that is active during the startle response. It is critical to attentiveness, emotions, sleep, dreaming, and learning. Also known as noradrenaline.

nystagmus. An involuntary horizontal, vertical, or rotary movement of the eyeball.

occipital lobe. The posterior, or back, part of the brain. This area is involved in perceiving and understanding visual information.

occupational therapist. A specialist in upper-extremity rehabilitation. Occupational therapy improves the fine motor, social, and daily living skills of people challenged by a brain or bodily injury, and teaches people how to contribute to their own recovery and avoid reinjury.

olfactory. Pertaining to the sense of smell.

ophthalmologist. A medical doctor who specializes in the diagnosis and medical and surgical treatment of eye disorders.

optometrist. A practitioner who evaluates vision, prescribes corrective lenses, and provides testing for certain eye disorders. An optometrist must be licensed by the state in which he or she practices.

organic personality disorder. A condition in which a person begins to exhibit antisocial or harmful behaviors that he or she is not usually known for exhibiting. Sometimes called "organic personality syndrome," the new behaviors center around the damaged areas of the brain.

orientation. The awareness of self in relation to person, place, and time, in past or present environments.

orthopedist. A medical doctor who specializes in the musculoskeletal system and its disorders.

otolaryngologist. A medical doctor with expertise in the field of ear and hearing disorders; an ear, nose, and throat (ENT) specialist.

parasomnias. Disruptive sleep disorders that include bed-wetting, sleepwalking, nightmares/night terrors, and sleep apnea.

parasympathetic system. The part of the autonomic nervous system responsible for conserving the body's resources and energy during inactive times—for example, by lowering the heart rate.

parietal lobe. The upper middle section of the brain. This area is responsible for sensory and spatial awareness, giving feedback from and understanding of eye, hand, and arm movements during complex operations such as reading, writing, and numerical calculations.

peripheral nerves. Nerves that lie outside the brain and spinal cord.

perseveration. The uncontrolled repetition or continuation of a word, thought, or activity after the topic or task requirements have changed. This affects a person's ability to shift from topics or tasks and thus interferes with learning and social interactions.

phonophobia. An abnormal sensitivity to noise, often experienced during a migraine attack.

photophobia. An abnormal sensitivity to light, often experienced during a migraine attack.

physiatrist. A medical doctor who specializes in physical medicine and rehabilitation. (Pronounced *fizz-EYE-a-trist*.)

physical therapist. A therapist trained in muscle rehabilitation. Physical therapists use a variety of techniques, including massage, water therapy, hot packs, ice massage, ultrasound, and therapeutic exercises to reduce pain and help patients improve or regain physical functioning.

polarity therapist. A practitioner who uses Therapeutic Touch (TT) and relaxation techniques to promote bodily harmony and healing.

pons. A prominence in the brain stem located between the medulla oblongata and the midbrain.

post concussion syndrome (PCS). The label applied when concussion symptoms do not resolve within a week or two of disrupted brain function. Also known as post concussion disorder.

posterior. Pertaining to the back part of a structure.

post traumatic amnesia. See *anterograde amnesia*.

post traumatic headache (PTH). A type of headache that results from a brain injury, sometimes persisting for a year or longer after the trauma.

post traumatic stress disorder (PTSD). A type of anxiety disorder that can occur after a person has seen or experienced a traumatic event that involved the threat of injury or death.

preferred provider organization (PPO). A health plan that has contracts with a network of providers from which a person can choose. It is not required to have a primary care physician.

primary health care provider. A family physician, general practitioner, homeopathic physician, or other practitioner who sees to a person's routine health care needs and provides referrals to specialists for the evaluation of certain medical problems.

prognosis. A forecast as to the likely outcome of an illness or injury.

psychiatric nurse. A nurse with a master's degree in psychiatric mental health nursing who can prescribe and administer medication with special certification. He or she has expertise in medical issues and the diagnosis, treatment, and prevention of emotional and mental disorders.

psychiatrist. A medical doctor licensed to prescribe medication who has expertise in the diagnosis, treatment, and prevention of emotional, behavioral, and mental disorders.

psychologist. A doctor of psychology who is licensed to assess, diagnose, and treat emotional and mental disorders and who oversees the management of attitude and behavioral problems. Psychologists do not prescribe medication. Many psychologists hold board certification in specialty areas of psychology, such as behavioral medicine.

psychopharmacologist. A medical doctor who is a specialist in psychiatry and has expertise in the use and interactions of medication to treat neurological, psychological, and behavioral problems.

receptive aphasia. Problems with reading, interpreting, and comprehending spoken language. Called Wernicke's aphasia when caused by damage to Wernicke's area of the brain, this problem affects the ability to understand the meaning of spoken and written words.

rehabilitation. A program or process designed to reduce deficits following injury or illness, and to assist a person in attaining his or her optimal level of mental and physical functioning. Rehabilitation may involve working on an outpatient basis with one or more specialists. Pain management techniques may also be involved.

retrograde amnesia. The inability to recall events prior to a traumatic event. The "missing" memories may cover a specific span of time or certain information.

second impact syndrome (SIS). A condition in which the brain swells rapidly and catastrophically after a person suffers a second concussion before symptoms from an earlier one have subsided. This dangerous second blow may occur days, weeks, or minutes after an initial concussion, and even the mildest grade of concussion can lead to this syndrome.

seizure. A sudden temporary, unusual discharge of electrical impulses within one area of the brain that may quickly spread to other areas, causing uncontrolled stimulation of nerves and muscles. Seizures usually last only a few minutes and can cause abnormal or arrested movement, alteration of consciousness, disorders of sensation or perception, and behavior disturbances. Also called an ictal event.

selective serotonin reuptake inhibitor. A medication used in the treatment of depression and anxiety disorders.

sensory impairment. A problem with one or more of the senses caused by the brain's inability to react to stimuli and pass on the impulse. Most commonly refers to sight and hearing, but can include issues relating to smell, touch, taste, and spatial awareness.

sequelae. The consequences that follow an illness or injury.

serotonin. A brain neuromodulator essential for regulating mood. It relays messages between brain cells.

shearing. A type of brain lesion often seen as a result of an abrupt deceleration in movement that causes the brain to continue moving within the skull, tearing brain cells.

short-term memory. A system for temporarily storing and managing information required to carry out tasks such as learning, reasoning, and comprehension.

sleep/wake cycle disturbance. A disorder in which the body cannot adjust to a normal light/dark cycle and insists the day is longer than twenty-four hours, making it impossible to sleep at normal times.

somatoform disorder. The presence of one or more physical complaints for which a physical explanation cannot be found.

sound agnosia. The inability to understand environmental sounds, such as the barking of a dog, without an accompanying disturbance in the ability to understand speech.

spasticity. A condition of spasms or other uncontrollable contractions of the skeletal muscles.

speech/language pathologist or therapist. A practitioner who specializes in the evaluation of speech and language deficits and who devises individualized therapy programs consisting of tasks and exercises to improve concentration, articulation, and listening and comprehension skills.

Sports Concussion Assessment Tool (SCAT 2). A standardized method of evaluating people after a sports concussion. It is also called the Sideline Concussion Assessment.

stereognosis. The inability to recognize objects by the sense of touch.

sympathetic nervous system. The portion of the autonomic nervous system responsible for preparing the body to respond to challenges that call for survival.

synapse. The gap between two neurons through which electrical or chemical signals are passed.

syndrome. Not a disease, but a collection of signs or symptoms that together form a condition that has a known outcome or that requires special treatment.

temporal lobe. A part of the brain located beneath the frontal and parietal lobes that plays a part in remembering information, noticing things, understanding music, categorizing objects, the ability to smell and taste, and sexual and aggressive behavior. At the back of the left temporal lobe is Wernicke's area, which is responsible for hearing and interpreting language.

tension headache. A two-sided headache caused by muscle tension that feels like squeezing or the pressure of a tight band around your head. It may be accompanied by facial or back pain, particularly in persons who have had a whiplash injury.

thalamus. A part of the brain that acts as a nerve-impulse relay station for information coming into the brain, passing it to the cerebrum to be prioritized and transmitted throughout the body.

tinnitus. A condition characterized by persistent roaring, buzzing, or ringing in the ears.

tonic-clonic seizure. A type of seizure most commonly associated with epilepsy. In the tonic phase, a person will quickly lose consciousness. In the clonic phase, the muscles will contract and relax rapidly, causing convulsions.

tracking. The ability to maintain visual focus on a moving object.

tremor. A rhythmic, purposeless, quivering movement resulting from the involuntary contraction and relaxation of opposing groups of muscles.

vagus nerve. One of two cranial nerves that extend from the brain to the abdomen and that help regulate heartbeat, control muscle movement, keep a person breathing, and transmit chemicals through the body.

verbal apraxia. Impaired control of the sequencing of muscles used in speech; specifically, the tongue, lips, jaw muscles, and vocal cords. These muscles are not weak but their control is defective, causing speech to be labored and characterized by sound reversals, additions, and word approximations.

vertigo. A type of dizziness where there is a feeling of motion even when standing still and lying down.

vestibular system. The sensory system that contributes to balance and the sense of spatial orientation. Injury to the vestibular system can induce vertigo and/or instability, often accompanied by nausea.

vestibular testing. Consists of a number of tests to determine whether a problem exists with the vestibular system. These tests can help isolate dizziness symptoms and lead to treatment recommendations.

visual agnosia. The partial or complete inability to understand things that are seen, even though the sense of sight is functioning normally.

Visual Analog Scale for Fatigue (VAS-F). An instrument of measurement used to determine the amount of continual fatigue, from none to severe.

visual cortex. The part of the brain responsible for processing visual information. It is located in the back of the brain (occipital lobe).

visual field impairment. An inability to see something in a specific area of the visual field. Often, either the left or right half of the field of vision is involved.

Wernicke's area. An area of the brain associated with processing and understanding language.

CONSULT DIANE ROBERTS STOLER, ED.D.
(DR. DIANE®)

■

IF YOU NEED ADDITIONAL INFORMATION AND ASSISTANCE CONCERNING YOUR concussion or post concussion symptoms, Dr. Diane® can help. Please visit www.drdiane.com for up-to-date resources and further information.

I regained my life, and so can you! I can provide you with an individualized, integrative recovery program tailored to your specific needs. I also work with individuals and organizations worldwide to help them find Solutions & Resources^{SM} to overcome life's challenges and reach their goals.

Whether you wish to obtain a personalized treatment program or need someone to speak on your behalf to your doctor, lawyer, or school, Dr. Diane® and her team of experts are there to give you Help and Hope. There is a way!^{SM}

Start your road to recovery, and call for a consult today! Contact:

Diane Roberts Stoler, Ed.D.
P.O. Box 148
Georgetown, MA 01833
Telephone: (800) 500-9971
E-mail: book@drdiane.com
Website: www.drdiane.com

INDEX

◾